W0106114

D. W. Behrenbeck, E. Sowton,
G. Fontaine and U. J. Winter (Eds.)

Cardiac Pacemakers

Diagnostic Options · Dual Chamber Pacing
Rate Responsive Pacing · Antitachycardia Pacing

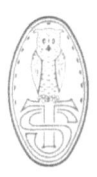
Springer-Verlag Berlin Heidelberg GmbH
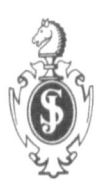

CIP-Kurztitelaufnahme der Deutschen Bibliothek

Cardiac pacemakers: diagnostic options; dual chamber pacing; rate responsive pacing; antitachycardia pacing / D. W. Behrenbeck . . . (eds.). – Darmstadt: Steinkopff; New York: Springer, 1985.

ISBN 978-3-662-06212-8   ISBN 978-3-662-06210-4 (eBook)
DOI 10.1007/978-3-662-06210-4

NE: Behrenbeck, Dieter [Mitverf.]

This work is subject to copyright. All rights are reserved, whether the whole or part of the material is concerned, specifically those of translation, reprinting, re-use of illustrations, broadcasting, reproduction by photocopying machine or similar means, and storage in data banks.
Under § 54 of the German Copyright Law, where copies are made for other than private use, a fee is payable to the publisher, the amount of the fee to be determined by agreement with the publisher.

Copyright © 1985 by Springer-Verlag Berlin Heidelberg
Originally published by Dr. Dietrich Steinkopff Verlag, GmbH & Co. KG, Darmstadt in 1985.
Softcover reprint of the hardcover 1st edition 1985

Medical Editorial: Juliane K. Weller – Copy Editing: Cynthia Feast – Production: Heinz J. Schäfer

The use of registered names, trademarks, etc. in this publication does not imply, even in the absence of a specific statement, that such names are exempt from the relevant protective laws and regulations and therefore free for general use.

Prefaces

The original concept of pacing as a treatment for heart block has expanded so dramatically that there is a continual need for meetings at which information can be exchanged and results compared. This book is the result of such a Symposium. It covers a wide variety of present day techniques and the actual numbers of patients involved in these presentations was far less important than the concepts which their treatment represented. Within this monograph can be found reference to all the growth areas in pacing, and several presentations with different methods of managing similar problems. There are extensive references to software pacemakers, antitachycardia pacing and implantable defibrillators and clinical results are available for comparison from major centres. A particular feature of this Symposium was the co-operation between manufacturers and research workers in producing presentations dealing in depth with particular apparatus. One result is that many papers provide practical hints and tips not often included in papers, as well as giving more development details than usual.

The monograph will clearly be an important reference point to detail the state of the art, and document the application of the technologies in Europe.

The Editors

Cardiac pacing is now 25 years old.

The only parameter unchanged from its early days is the electrical spike, the basis of this therapy.

However, artificial cardiac pacing design has completely changed over the past 25 years. The physician's theories, together with the engineer's ability, have lead to increasingly reliable electronic wonders, with improved adjustment and efficiency within the therapy (rate responsiveness and tachycardias), while featuring memory capacities which make new prospects possible.

This book, gathering together the great names of cardiac pacing and electrophysiology, gives an accurate overview of the situation in 1985, for which the authors should be sincerely thanked.

Jacques Mugica, M.D.

Head of the Cardiac Pacing Department
Val D'Or, Saint Cloud, France

Contents

II Physiologic and Rate Responsive Pacing

1. Rate Responsive Pacing

2. DDD Pacing

3. Hemodynamics

III Antiectopic and Antitachycardia Pacing

1. Pathogenesis and Ventricular Tachycardias

2. Pre-Implantation Examinations

3. New Stimulation Techniques

4. Tachycardia Recognition

5. Holter Functions in Antitachycardia Pacemakers

6. Antitachycardia Pacemaker

7. Antiectopic and Tachycardia Preventing Pacing

8. Problems with Antitachycardia Pacemakers

9. Antiarrhythmic Surgery

The "Philosophy" of the Diagnostic Pacemaker

P. Attuel, A. Ripart, and J. Mugica

Summary: When a syncope occurs in patients, even with sinus rhythm or with IV block, controversial and debatable studies have led cardiologists to progressively enlarge their indication. In fact in the beginning, pacemaker implantation based only on certitude came to include arguments of mere probability. To increase diagnosis and prognosis accuracy, a diagnostic function was introduced in 1978 with a capacity to record the onset of cardiac pause or bradycardia thanks to a specific and pre-programmed built-in memory.

By 1980 the diagnostic function evolved into the notion of an implantable Holter, not only to distinguish bradycardia from tachycardia syncopes but to easily establish the relationship between the clinical event and the occurrence of arrhythmias. Moreover the permanence and reliability of sensing allowed us to realise a quantitative evaluation at least as accurate as that made by external Holter monitoring.

Incorporated monitoring systems of many parameters will improve the diagnostic pacemaker (PM) to the level of a software PM with more and more automatic therapeutic applications. Thus various logic functions provided by selected data processing open an extremely wide range of cardiac PM applications, not only in the diagnosis and treatment of arrhythmias but also and increasingly in the physiological domain.

With regard to cardiac syncope occurring in patients with sinus rhythm or with IV block, most indications for cardiac pacemakers depend on both extensive clinical and pharmacological studies.

During the last decade and up to the present day etiological studies have often been based on debatable and controversial parameters. In fact, endocavitory and ambulatory ECG investigations have very often led to presumptive arguments.

For instance, a prolongation of the IV interval demonstrated by a His bundle recording of a pharmacological test with Ajmaline may be considered by some to be pathological and by others to be at the limit of normality. To increase diagnostic and prognostic accuracy, in 1978 we developed a diagnostic pacemaker capable of recording one or more pauses in excess of a selected cycle length.

This pacemaker was triggered by a specific and adjustable hysteresis thanks to a built in memory. The recording of a pacing pulse delivered by this pacemaker enabled us to affirm that a pause at least as long as the escape interval had occurred.

The diagnostic function was based on a programming code where the escape interval was initiated at twice the normal pulse period.

Very quickly, this kind of diagnostic function, despite some technical limits such as a difficulty in distinguishing pauses from the demand defect, came to include patients with a pacemaker in whom syncope continued to occur. It was the multitude and diversity of causes of syncope or dizziness which naturally led us to request an implantable Holter monitoring device from engineers, capable of continuous and reliable recording of endocardial activation and data processing permitting a quantitative evaluation of cardiac arrhythmias enabling an analysis of arrhythmias comparable to that of the external Holter (Tables 1 and 2). With such a device we could detect paroxysmal arrhythmias, picked up by the diagnostic function, and more generally the spontaneous occurrence of this type of arrhythmia or of other types such as sinus defect after implantation.

Table 1. Holter function of an implantable pacemaker (1980).

● Continuous and reliable recording of endocardial activation
● Quantitative evaluation of cardiac arrhythmias

Table 2. Capabilities of a diagnostic pacemaker.

Technical principles	Processing
● Adjustable hysteresis	● Quantitative evaluation
● Memory of pause duration and occurrence	● Histogram trends
● Resetting possible	● Arrhythmia classification
● Easy reading by magnet	

Despite the impossibility of long-term ECG recording due to limited memory capacity, the storage of compressed data, basically the R-R interval, permits data processing or arrhythmia detection and classification. An AV sequential pacemaker permits all classifications of supraventricular or ventricular arrhythmias, or more simply the possibility of an R-R histogram (Fig. 1).

This kind of histogram allowed us to detect and distinguish the occurrence of paroxysmal tachycardia, premature beats or bradycardia from normal sinus rhythms. This type of result also permits the analysis of drug efficiency.

These different possibilities of data storage on the one hand and data processing on the other led to a decision-making function of the pacemaker. And so, in this way, the most recent software pacemaker has enabled the evolution from diagnosis to therapy.

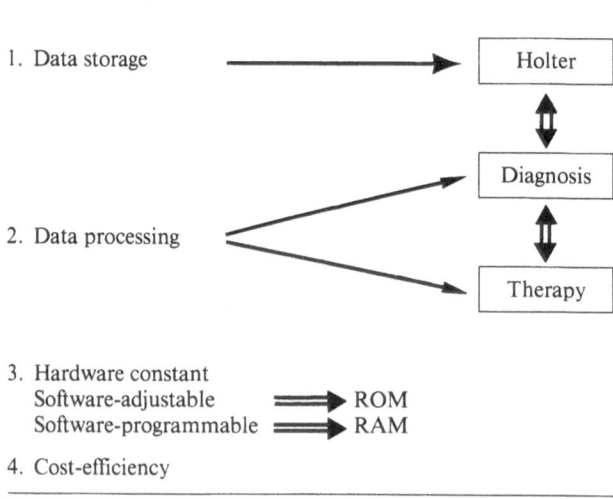

Fig. 1. Microcomputer capabilities.

The most sophisticated of these recent pacemakers is without doubt the automatic implantable defibrillator developed by Mirowski, a therapeutic pacemaker which can be used in patients with severe arrhythmias resistant to treatment.

For the future, attractive prospects await us through the development of multiple and correlated sites of encocardial sensing and different kinds of associated physiological sensors.

Authors' address:
P. Attuel, M.D.
Centre Chirurgical Val d'Or
Dpt. de Stimulation Cardique
16, rue Pasteur
F-92211 Saint-Cloud Cedex, France

Comparison of Different Pacemakers with Holter Functions

A. W. Nathan*

Summary: The advent of small memory chips with very low power consumption, coupled with advances in radiofrequency telemetry, has enabled implantable cardiac pacemakers to become diagnostic as well as therapeutic devices.

Different types of devices are available. The simplest type merely indicates whether or not a bradycardia or tachycardia has occurred or has been treated. This may be indicated by the amplitude of a marker pulse, by the number of pulses on magnet application or on the magnet rate of the pacemaker. Some pacemakers are capable of counting paced and sensed beats over a given time period instead of, or as well as, indicating bradycardia or tachycardia. The most complex Holter functions currently available in an implantable device, in addition to the above features, allow the construction of a histogram of spontaneous heart rates, as well as being able to count premature beats or to give information about sensed tachycardias. Typical "random access memory" store is 256 bytes (8 bit), although such pacemakers require up to 2 kbytes of "read only memory" to control the pacing and diagnostic functions. An external microprocessor based device is then required to interpret, structure and present all the information that is telemetered out.

Increasing electronic sophistication will permit increased data storage and more versatile data processing, and although devices capable of storing short durations of electrographic waveforms will shortly become available, the future lies in improved "front-end" processing enabling the efficient storage of preprocessed data.

There is no reason why an implantable device without pacing functions should not be used for arrhythmia monitoring in certain selected patients, perhaps using subcutaneous electrodes. Finally, implantable ambulatory monitors could be used for other physiological variables, for example, systemic or pulmonary artery pressure, or concentrations of oxygen, glucose or other biological substances, depending on the sensor used.

Introduction

There are many advantages to be gained from the use of totally implantable devices for long-term ambulatory monitoring. Currently the only implantable devices with diagnostic functions are cardiac pacemakers. Initially pacemakers had no sensing function at all, and were ventricular asynchronous fixed rate systems ("VOO"). Then atrial synchronous ("VAT") and ventricular demand units (VVI) were made available, and these paced according to sensed signals. The advent of large-scale integrated circuits with extemely low power consumption, coupled with the advances that have been made in radiofrequency telemetry, have enabled the construction of pacemakers with diagnostic features. Although real-time electrographic telemetry is now commonplace, the memory capability of CMOS (complementary metal oxide semiconductor) circuits is not sufficient, at present, to store the waveforms themselves. Current devices rely on front-end processing to enable the efficient storage of data.

---

* Supported by the British Heart Foundation.

Currently available devices

This is not an exhaustive list of devices but does illustrate examples of available technology.

1. Devices which can indicate bradycardia or tachycardia

Two devices have been designed expressly to indicate whether or not a significant bradycardia has occurred. The Siemens P38 system (1) indicates the occurrence of a bradycardia if there have been three consecutive intervals in excess of 2000 ms. The pacemaker is fully programmable and is based on the Siemens 668 device. When programmed to a rate of 30 ppm the bradycardia indicating feature is activated. It will then pace on a demand basis at 30 bpm (2000 ms interval) but if three consecutive pulses are given will revert to the conventional demand mode at 70 ppm. Stimulation due to perceived interference is not indicated. On follow-up, if the pacemaker is pacing at 70 ppm, then bradycardia has been indicated. However, in the type of patient in whom this device would normally be implanted (that is, one with possible intermittent bradycardia) normal sinus rhythm will usually present at follow-up. In this case, a magnet is applied and if bradycardia has been logged the rate will be 120 ppm and if not, it will be 100 ppm.

The Telectronics bradycardia counting pacemaker will count the number of pauses in excess of 2600 ms. It will then pace at 50 ppm with a 2600 ms hysteresis. This device can actually count the number of pauses of 2600 ms or more and indicates this by its response to magnet application. If no episodes of bradycardia have been sensed, 128 pulses are generated, but for each episode sensed one pulse less is emitted. This pacemaker is non-programmable.

Both of these devices were designed for implantation into patients with suspected but perhaps unproven bradycardias or those thought to be at risk of developing significant bradyarrhythmias and who might require prophylactic pacing. They are therefore principally research tools and both are relatively crude.

The Intermedics Cybertach 60 is a pacemaker with a memory "flag" to indicate whether or not a tachycardia event has been detected. When used with a special telemetry monitor it can transmit, using high energy inductive coupling, a waveform to an ECG recorder. When the flag is set the waveform is tall, and when no event has occurred or the memory is cleared by programming it is short. The pacemaker may be interrogated over the telephone. The number of episodes cannot be determined using this marker flag.

2. Devices with paced and sensed beat counters

Advanced radiofrequency telemetry allows more data to be obtained from pacemakers than is available from the relatively simple devices described in the previous section. The CPI Command Ultra I is capable of counting paced beats and total paced/sensed events, but not bradycardia or tachycardia events.

The Telectronics Optima MPT and Siemens Dialog series pacemakers can telemeter similar paced beat data (with up to a maximum of 2^{24} counts, approximating to 6 months of data in the average patient) but will also count the number of tachycardia interventions. They can also function in a mode similar to the Siemens P38 but with an alpha-numeric hard copy print-out from the telemetry link and programmer. In future models, the total number of perceived events will also be recorded. The Siemens Dialog 718 is a single chamber device but the 704 is a dual chamber pacemaker capable of storing either atrial or ventricular events.

3. A device capable of rate and interval analysis

The most sophisticated diagnostic pacemaker currently available is the Vitatron Quin-tech DPG ("diagnostic pulse generator"). This is a microprocessor based device con-trolled and programmed with an external microcomputer. The pacemaker contains a mi-croprocessor, 2 kbytes of read only memory (ROM), 256 bytes of random access memory (RAM), a programmable pacer controller, functional hardware and a communications link. The external device used for programming and telemetry is a Hewlett-Packard HP85 microcomputer together with a special radiofrequency programmer head.

This pacemaker not only has more versatility than most other single chamber pace-makers in terms of its ranges of programmable features, but also utilizes the RAM to store data. There are counters capable of recording the total number of inhibitions, the total number of stimulations and the number of sensed beats to pace. The number of epi-sodes of tachycardia may be counted as well as their total duration. A unique feature is the rate histogram. Eight classes of heart rate may be set with a 250 bpm maximum. The limits of the rate range depend on the programmed pacing and hysteresis rates as well as the programmed refractory periods. The rate counters register the values of all beats within the various classes and store them for later telemetry. Data retrieval and display is both numeric and graphical. The histogram may be set in continuous operation which will allow data to be acquired and stored over at least a six month period or may be set to alternating operation to give access to both recent and more distant data. Finally, there is a programmable premature beat counter which may be set to count beats that are either 12.5% or 25% shorter than the previous pacing or inhibition interval.

The rate counter/histogram has been useful in the detection of either bradycardia or ta-chycardia and has been particularly useful in the management of patients with atrial fi-brillation, when it has been helpful in determining the response to digoxin and other AV nodal blocking agents. The premature beat counter is not useful in patients with atrial fi-brillation as it will be triggered by the variation in rates, but in patients with relatively stable sinus rhythm it may be of use for counting ectopic beats and to determine the re-sponse of such beats to medical therapy. Unfortunately, supraventricular and ventricular ectopics cannot, at present, be distinguished.

The future

Larger (e.g. 1 kbyte) CMOS static RAMs are now becoming available to the necessary standards required for implantable devices. These memories will allow the capability of devices like the Vitatron Quintech DPG to be extended, with distinction of the different types of ectopic beats being possible by morphological analysis, and dual chamber opera-tion becoming realistic.

However, the storage of actual electrographic waveforms is not possible as up to 140 million bits of memory store are necessary for a single day's recording, assuming 100 Hz band width, two samples/cycle, 8 bits of resolution/sample (2). Magnetic bubble memories at one time seemed to present a possible answer, but their capacity (e.g. 256 kbytes) would not solve the storage problem and their power consumption is high. Biotechnology may eventually produce tiny memory components capable of mega- or even giga-byte storage, but these are at present little more than figments of the imagination. In the foreseeable future, CMOS technology will continue to be used, and larger memories will allow very limited amounts of electrographic waveform to be stored when significant events are detected. These waveforms will be used together with the front-end processed data.

Conventional Holter recorders, modified to record, over a 24 hour period, the electrograms telemetered from current generation pacemakers (e.g. Pacesetter AFP), are being developed (3) and this will become an area of considerable interest in the near future.

Other devices

Implantable diagnostic devices of many types may emerge in the future. A system to analyse the electrocardiogram using subcutaneously implanted chest electrodes is a possibility for patients suffering from frequent arrhythmias although this type of device would lack therapeutic power, in comparison with a pacemaker, unless coupled with a drug infusion pump. The electro-encephalogram could also be monitored, as could systemic arterial pressure and pulmonary artery pressure, providing that suitable transducers become available. Pulmonary artery pressure monitoring would be particularly pertinent in patients with left ventricular failure or pulmonary hypertension and preliminary studies have already shown the feasibility of monitoring pulmonary artery pressures over periods of up to 96 hours (4). Finally, chemicals such as oxygen or glucose could be measured in the bloodstream and the latter would almost certainly be part of the implantable "artifical pancreas".

References

1. Edhag KO, Elmqvist H, Vallin HO (1983) An implantable pulse generator indicating asystole or extreme bradycardia. PACE 6: 166
2. Bhatt S, Schober RC (1982) Holter monitoring using implanted pacemakers. In: Barold SS, Mugica J (eds) The Third Decade of Cardiac Pacing: Advances in Technology and Clinical Applications. Futura, New York, p 333
3. Amundson D, Renger L, Mann B, Sholder J (1983) Long-term intracardiac Holter monitoring in man. PACE 6: A-105
4. Nathan AW, Perry SG, Cochrane T, Banim SO, Spurrell RAJ, Camm AJ (1983) Ambulatory monitoring of pulmonary artery pressure. A preliminary clinical evaluation. Br Heart J 49: 33

Author's address:
Dr. A. W. Nathan
Department of Cardiology
St Bartholomew's Hospital
West Smithfield
London EC1A 7BE
England

Clinical Evaluation of a Diagnostic Pulse Generator (DPG) with Special Analysis Functions in Pacemaker Patient Follow-up

U. J. Winter, D. W. Behrenbeck, Th. Brill, M. Höher, and H. H. Hilger

Summary: Recent progress in computer technology has enabled the design of software-guided pacemakers. Earlier devices offered only 1 or 2 diagnostic functions, such as pacing threshold measurement and telemetry of the intracardiac electrogram. Software pacemakers like the DPG 1 (Vitatron) have a whole variety of analysis functions.

The aim of the study was to investigate the clinical reliability of the DPG 1's analysis functions for pacemaker adjustment and follow-up. Twenty-three patients (3 female, 20 male) with symptomatic bradyarrhythmias were treated with the DPG 1 and a Helifix lead (AAI, n = 4; VVI, n = 19). A HP 85 personal computer was used for the 300 pacemaker telemetries. The telemetry procedure lasted 20 ± 5 minutes, for trained users also. The DPG 1-HP 85 system offers the following analysis functions: telemetry of the programmed parameters, R- and P-wave amplitude, pacing threshold, lead impedance and battery/output status.

The repeatedly performed threshold measurements revealed an accuracy of ± 0.05% and a variability of ≧ 50% at very low threshold values. Due to the simplicity, reliability and the strength-duration curve, threshold-guided pacing was possible in each patient. Examination of the lead impedance revealed an accuracy of ± 10% and a variability of ± 10%. The telemetry of the R-wave amplitude had an accuracy of ± 0.5 mV and a variability of ± 1.0 mV.

The telemetry functions were of great help for the adjustment of the pacemaker and the treatment of pacemaker dysfunctions. To apply the pacemakers and program functions correctly special training is necessary. Diagnostic pacemakers like the DPG 1 are considered to be an intermediate stage of development towards autodiagnostic pacemakers.

Introduction

In recent years pacemaker technology and clinical pacemaker therapy have made considerable progress. Transvenous stimulation, demand pacing and a reduction of the pacemaker size due to the incorporation of large integrated electrical circuits have thus become possible, for example (Table 1). CMOS technology opened up the possibility to design software-based pacemakers of acceptable size and handling with the capability of bi-directional telemetry (i.e. percutaneous interrogation and programming of the pacemaker even after the implantation). A new generation of software-based, single chamber pacemakers have improved diagnostic (interrogation) options, such as analysis and Holter functions. The components of these pacemakers are shown in Fig. 1 (1). The main functions of the VVI and AAI pacemakers are directed by the functional hardware which cannot be changed by percutaneous programming. The memory capacity of the diagnostic pacemaker is conducted by a microprocessor (μP) which has a ROM (a non-programmable read only memory) and a RAM (a programmable readable addressable memory). Percutaneous programming of these pacemakers can be realized by a programmer (= computer) and a programmer head which has to be positioned on the skin upon the implanted pacemaker (Fig. 1).

Table 1. Improvements of pacemaker technology and clinical pacemaker therapy.

Implantation technique	Pacemaker	Electrode
Epicardial implantation (1961)	Demand pacing (sensing circuit) Lithium batteries	Energy density Sensing Active fixation
Transvenous implantation (1965)	Integrated circuits and microprocessors – bidirectional telemetry – diagnostic and adaptive pacing (threshold, sensitivity) Dual chamber pacing Antitachycardia and antiectopic pacing Rate responsive pacing	Non-traumatic fixation

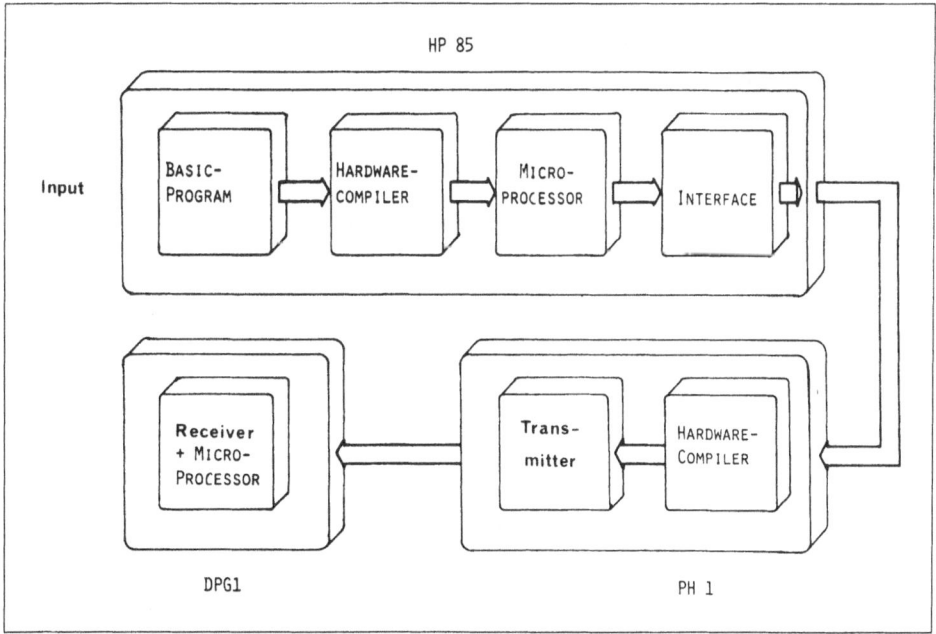

Fig. 1. Flow chart of data from the HP 85 terminal to the Vitatron DPG 1 pacemaker.

Objective

The aim of the study was to investigate the clinical value and limitations of the analysis functions of a new single chamber, software-controlled pacemaker in clinical follow-up of pacemaker patients.

Patients

Twenty-three patients were treated with a DPG 1 pacemaker (Vitatron) and a Helifix lead (Vitatron): age, 56 ± 15 years; 3 female, 20 male patients; implantation of 19 VVI and 4 AAI pacemakers. In all patients sinus bradycardia or bradyarrhythmias combined with complex cardiac diseases were indications for a VVI pacemaker with analysis functions (see Table 2).

The patients were followed up for 19 ± 4 months after the implantation.

Table 2. Patients – DPG 1 study.

N = 23	
VVI: N = 19	AAI: N = 4
	Permanent: N = 3

Age: 56.3 ± 15.3 years	
Sex: ♀ = 3, ♂ = 18	

Underlying diseases:	
Sinus bradycardia	N = 5
CHD + VES	N = 510
Atrial fibrillation	N = 3
SV Tach.	N = 4
WPW-syndrome	N = 1
HOCM	N = 1
Follow-up period (until 12/31/84)	
18.6 ± 3.6 months	

Methods

Interrogation and programming

The data processing flow chart from the HP 85 to the pacemaker is shown in Fig. 1. The different, so-called screens (menu technique) which can be seen on the display of the programmer during the interrogation process are shown in Fig. 2. The *status listing* represents the programmed parameters of the pacemakers including stimulation mode, pacing rate, impulse duration, output voltage, sensitivity, hysteresis and technical refractory period of the pacemaker. The hemodynamic side effects of cardiac stimulation are influenced by the stimulation mode and rate, as well as by hysteresis. The sensing behaviour of the pacemaker is determined by the sensitivity and the technical refractory period of the pulse generator. The amount of energy consumption depends on the stimulation mode, the pacing rate, the stimulation parameters such as impulse duration and amplitude, the hysteresis and the pacing threshold. The present energy reserves and power con-

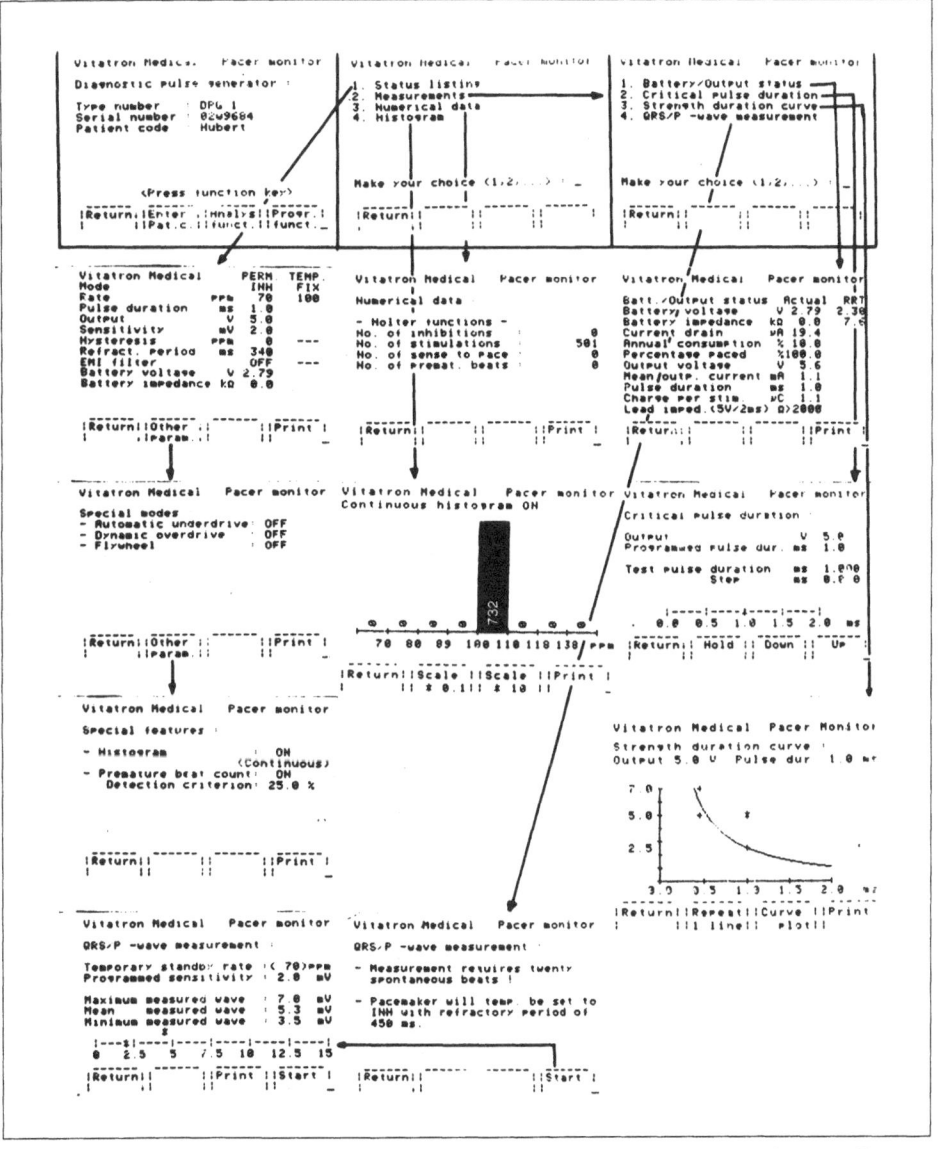

Fig. 2. Different screens of the HP 85 performing bidirectional telemetry with the Vitatron DPG 1.

sumption can be controlled in interrogating the so-called *battery and output status*. The components of the power consumption in the DPG 1 are also shown in Fig. 2. For the differential diagnosis of pacemaker dysfunctions the telemetry of the status listing (phantom programming?), the battery and output status, the lead impedance (sudden increase?), the numerical data (increase of number of stimulations?), the pacing threshold (sudden thereshold increase?) and the R-wave amplitude (R-wave decrease) may be helpful.

Measurement principles in the DPG 1

Measurement of the battery impedance

The measurement of the battery impedance R_{Batt} is calculated by dividing the battery voltage U_{Batt} actually measured in vivo (during conditions equal to the I_{Batt} measurement) by the I_{Batt} value measured in vitro, which is stored in the pacemaker.

Calculation of the annual (power) consumption

The annual power consumption (AC) of the pacemaker is calculated by the division of the product: current drain of the microprocessor plus (pacing rate multiplied by the charge per stimulus) multiplied by 8, 760 (365 day multiplied by 24 hours) by 1.7 Ah (true value: 2.5 Ah), which is the capacity of the lithium iodide power source.

Measurement of the pacing threshold

In the DPG 1 pacing threshold determination is performed in programming 3 different output voltages (2.5; 5.0; 7.5 volts) and decreasing the impulse width stepwise automatically from 2.0 to 0.025 ms (see Fig. 3). In this way both mean and high threshold curves

Fig. 3. Comparison of the measuring range of the Siemens-Elema vario principle and the Vitatron DPG 1 threshold measuring system.

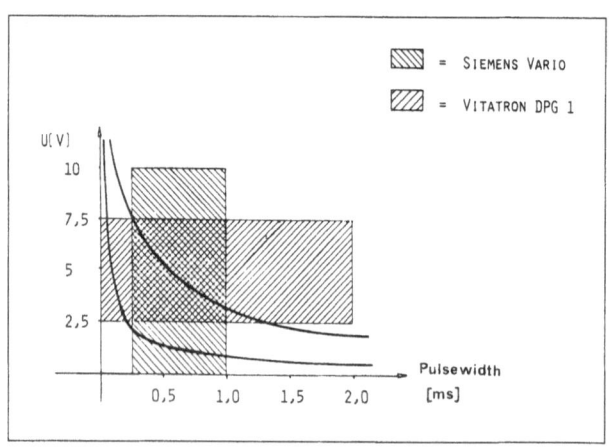

are covered. In contrast, the Siemens vario principle (Fig. 3) works by programming the impulse widths from 0.25 to 1.0 ms and in decreasing the output voltage automatically (stepwise) from 10.0 to 0.0 volts. The graphic design following the semi-automatic determination of the pacing threshold is shown in Fig. 4. The accuracy is described by the manufacturer as $\pm$ 12.5 mV at 2.5 V, $\pm$ 2.5 mV at 5.0 V and $\pm$ 37.5 mV at 7.5 V.

Measurement of the lead impedance

The components of the measured lead impedance are demonstrated in Fig. 5. This parameter includes the impedance between the electrode tip and the endocardial surface (R_E),

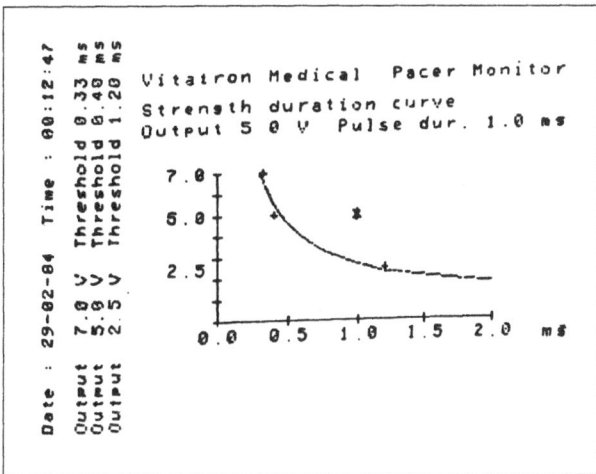

Fig. 4. Graphic design (strength-duration curve) after semi-automatic determination of the pacing threshold by the HP 85. (Vitatron DPG 1)

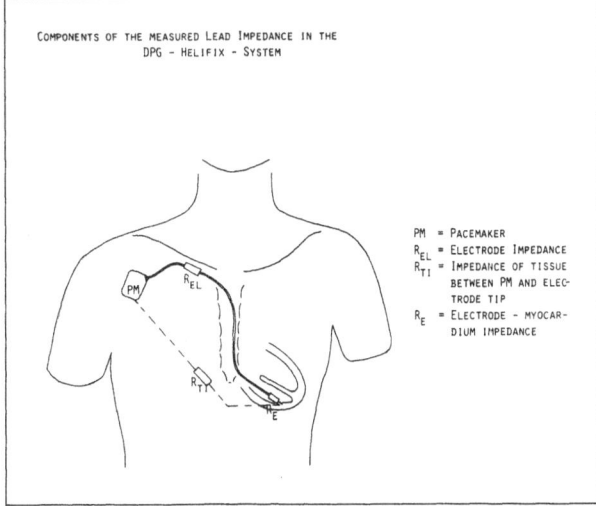

Fig. 5. Components which influence the measured value of the lead impedance.

13

the impedance between the implanted pacemaker and the electrode tip (R_{Ti}) and the electrode impedance itself. The lead impedance is determined by a voltage measurement device using a nearly rectangular impulse of a certain duration (see Fig. 6). The measurement steps are shown in Table 3. They have different values since the measuring steps are expressed as a constant percentage (e.g. 10%) of differing underlying numbers (10% of 300: 30; 10% of 500: 50).

The manufacturer declared an accuracy of about 10% between 400 and 1200 ohms (Table 3). Our own in vitro measurements revealed an accuracy of 5% between 450 and 900 ohms and of 10% below 450 ohms and between 900 and 2000 ohms.

Fig. 6. Measuring principle of the lead impendance determination (DPG 1). 'V' is measured by a voltmeter. Using a special algorithm (lower part of the figure) 'R' can be calculated from the known and measured parameters.

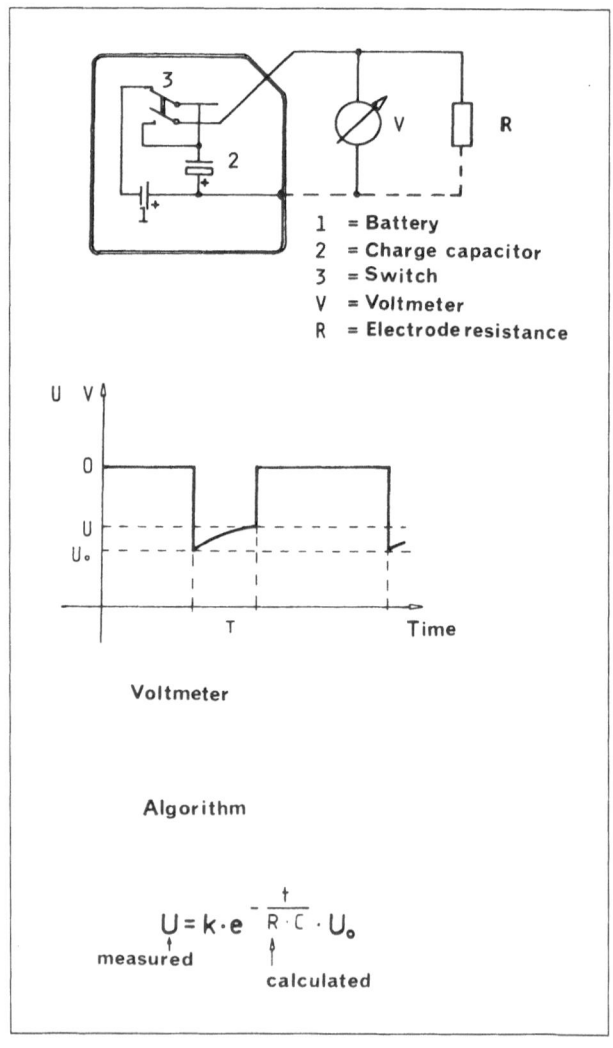

1 = Battery
2 = Charge capacitor
3 = Switch
V = Voltmeter
R = Electrode resistance

$$U = k \cdot e^{-\frac{t}{R \cdot C}} \cdot U_o$$

measured   calculated

Table 3. Measuring steps of the lead impedance (DPG 1) $[\Omega]$.

250	440	730	1200
250	460	770	1280
270	490	810	1360
290	520	850	1460
320	550	900	1570
340	380	950	1700
360	620	1010	1860
390	650	1070	2000
410	690	1130	

Precision of the DPG's measuring system (manufacturer's data)

Lead impedance*	
400–1200 Ω	10%
400 und 1200 Ω	20%

* measured at 5.0 V / 2.0 ms

R or P-wave measurement

The principle of measuring the endocardial signal amplitude is representative of the sensing circuit of the demand pacemaker (2). After automatic reduction (in a stepwise fashion) of the sensitivity threshold to a value where the sensing of the endocardial signals becomes possible (at a stimulation rate below the spontaneous rhythm) the minimal, maximal and mean signal amplitudes can be determined.

Site of stimulation and measurement

The Helifix electrode was positioned in the right ventricular apex or the appendix of the right atrium, guided by the threshold measurement during the implantation procedure. The helical configuration of the electrode tip leads to non-traumatic fixation at the endocardial trabeculac.

Results

Clinical reliability of the programmer and the programming procedure

The HP 85 computer was used for repeated (n = 300) programming procedures and for analysing measurements. Even after a training period each measurement lasted 20 ± 5 minutes. This was mainly caused by the loading procedures and changing from the analysis program to the programming procedure. In 4/300 interrogations data transmission could not be realized. It was always necessary to keep a distance of a least 1.0 m between the programmer head and other electrical devices. During the repeated controls the programmer head had to be exchanged after six months due to mechanical defects.

15

Clinical reliability of the different analysis functions

Status listing:

The status listing shows current programming. Phantom programming, which may be due to misprogramming, dysprogramming or iatrogenic phantom programming, was observed only twice during a follow-up period of 19 ± 4 months.

Battery and output status:

It is difficult to validate the battery status in implanted pacemakers by external means. During the repeated controls, the data were reproducible and realistic. Whether or not the battery and output status can predict the end of life of a pacemaker more precisely than the conventional magnet test will only be clarified in a few years' time when a sufficient number of pacemakers have been implanted for a period of 4 to 5 years. Whereas in the battery and output status a decrease of the battery voltage and an increase of the battery impedance indicate that the end of life is close, a significant (≥ 10%) drop of the magnet rate during the magnet test is the EOL criterion. The parameter 'annual consumption' gives a reliable prediction of the EOL if only a few programming procedures changing the stimulation characteristics are performed during the follow-up period.

Measurement of the pacing threshold

Methodological considerations:

The output voltage was measured in 8 patients at 0.1 to 2.0 ms impulse width (Fig. 7). It was found to be 5.6 V at 0.1 ms, slowly falling to 4.95 V at 2.0 ms. The measurement of the pacing threshold was difficult or impossible during the following circumstances:
1. bipolar stimulation (pacemaker spike difficult to identify);

Fig. 7. Dependence of the value of the output voltage on the given impulse width, measured in 8 patients with VVI pacemakers. (Vitatron DPG 1)

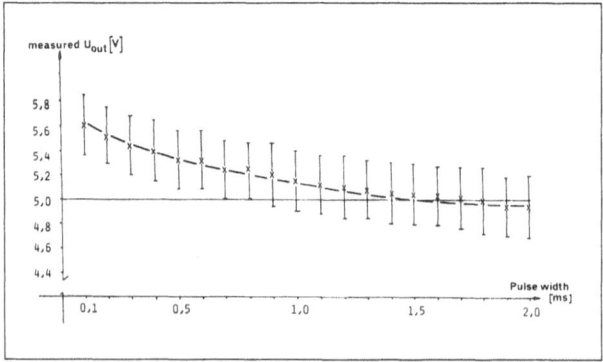

2. atrial stimulation (differentiation between stimulation artefact and pacing response difficult);

3. intermittently occurring exit block.

In all determinations the automatic reduction of the impulse width lasted longer than the amount of time for which the button of the keyboard was switched down. The pacing threshold was not significantly dependent on the stimulation rate (80, 100 and 125 ppm) at 2.5 volts in 13 VVI pacemakers (see Fig. 8). The day-to-day variations of the measured pacing threshold in 25 determinations during the chronic implantation period were significant (> 50%), but at very low threshold values (Fig. 10). A remarkable influence of electrolyte concentration or drugs on the pacing threshold curves could not be detected.

Follow-up

VVI pacemakers:

The typical threshold increase until the 4th or 5th day after implantation is shown in Fig. 9. The differences in the threshold curves at the 3 given output voltages were seen in all

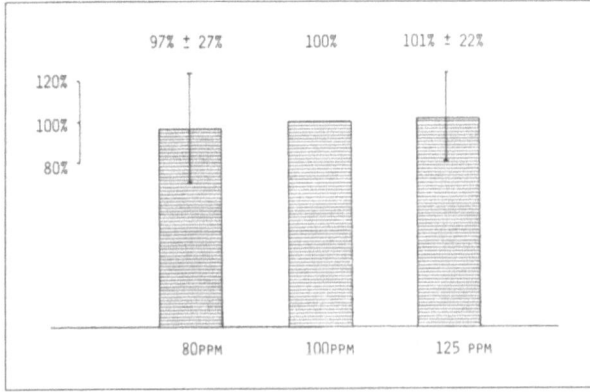

Fig. 8. Pacing threshold measured in 13 patients with VVI pacemakers at 2.5 V using varying pacing rates ($\bar{x}$ ± S.D.) (Vitatron DPG 1)

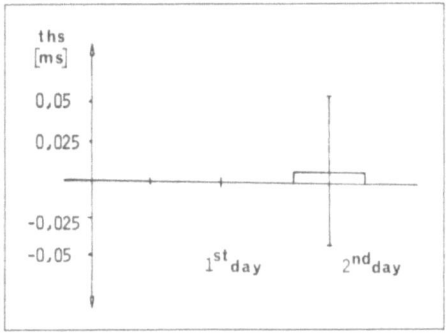

Fig. 9. Day-to-day variations of the pacing threshold in 25 VVI pacemakers ($\bar{x}$ ± S.D.). (Vitatron DPG 1)

17

patients, with the most prominent changes at 2.5 volts. In the VVI pacemakers type I was seen in 3 patients, type II in 8 and type III in 4 patients. In AAI pacemakers 1 patient showed type II behavior, 2 patients type II and none type III. A high threshold curve was observed in 1 male patient with a VVI pacemaker. Figure 10 illustrates the large standard deviations (> 300%) if the data are put together from 13 patients with different underly-

Fig. 10. Threshold course at 2.5 V in 10 patients with VVI pacemakers ($\bar{x} \pm$ S.D.). (Vitatron DPG 1)

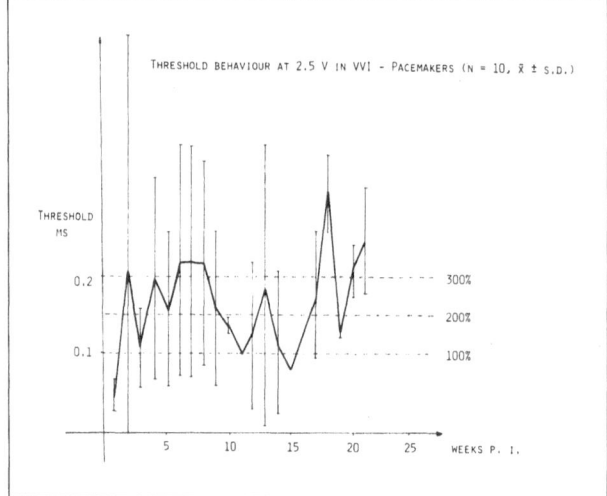

Fig. 11. Course of the pacing threshold after a new pacemaker implantation (upper part; right part of the lower figure) and a battery exchange (middle figure; left part of the lower figure). (Vitatron DPG 1)

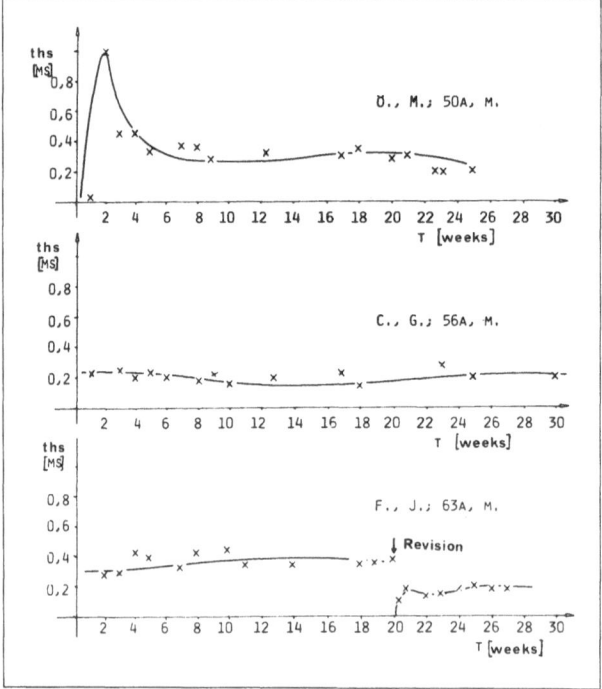

18

ing diseases etc. During a follow-up period of 20 weeks a biphasic or undulatory curve was found, revealing culminating points in the 7th week (+ 320%) and in the 18th week (+ 400%). In a 61 year old patient who was treated with amiodarone (dose: 300 mg p.o. because of recurrent ventricular tachycardias due to WPW-syndrome) and by cortisone (dose: 20 mg because of severe bronchial asthma) a very similar course of threshold development was observed. The difference between the acute and chronic threshold course is demonstrated in Fig. 11.

AAI pacemakers:

A threshold increase until the 5th day post implantation, quite comparable to VVI pacemakers (see Fig. 10), is shown in Fig. 12. As in VVI pacemakers the threshold behaviour at the 3 given voltages differs, with the most prominent effects to be seen at 2.5 volts (Fig. 13). As already demonstrated with VVI pacemakers interindividual comparisons of the threshold behaviour can be neglected due to the large standard deviations.

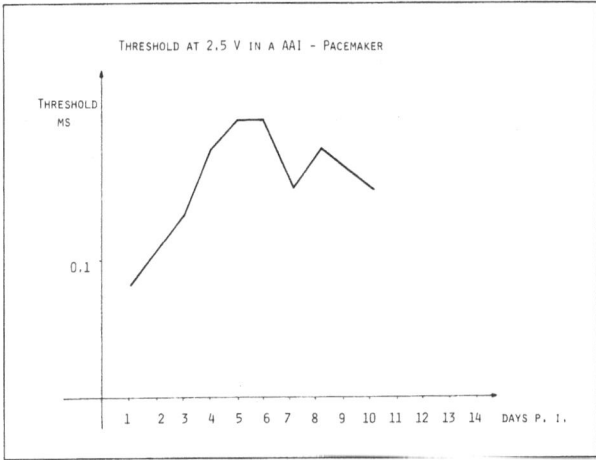

Fig. 12. Threshold course in an AAI pacemaker a few days after implantation. (Vitatron DPG 1)

Measurement of the lead impedance

Methodological considerations:

Determination of the lead impedance was always possible. In vitro measurements revealed an accuracy of 5% between 450 and 900 ohms. Also the in vivo, i. e. minute-to-minute and hour-to-hour variability, was in the range of 5% (see Fig. 14). The day-to-day variations in lead impedance were not significant (see Fig. 15), as demonstrated during 30 measurements.

19

VVI pacemaker follow-up:

In 2 patients with battery exchange and a Helifix lead the initially measured, chronic value (> 40 months after implantation) of the lead impedance was 650 Ω, whereas in 2 patients (> 40 months after implantation) with a ball-tip electrode the chronic lead impedance was 850 or 900 Ω.

Fig. 13. Threshold behaviour at 3 given voltages in an AAI pacemaker during the first 20 weeks. (Vitatron DPG 1)

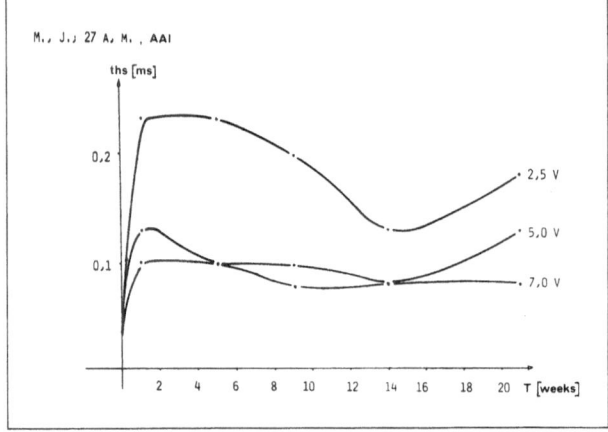

Fig. 14. Minute-to-minute and hour-to-hour variability of the lead impedance. The variations are in the range of 1 measuring step. (Vitatron DPG 1)

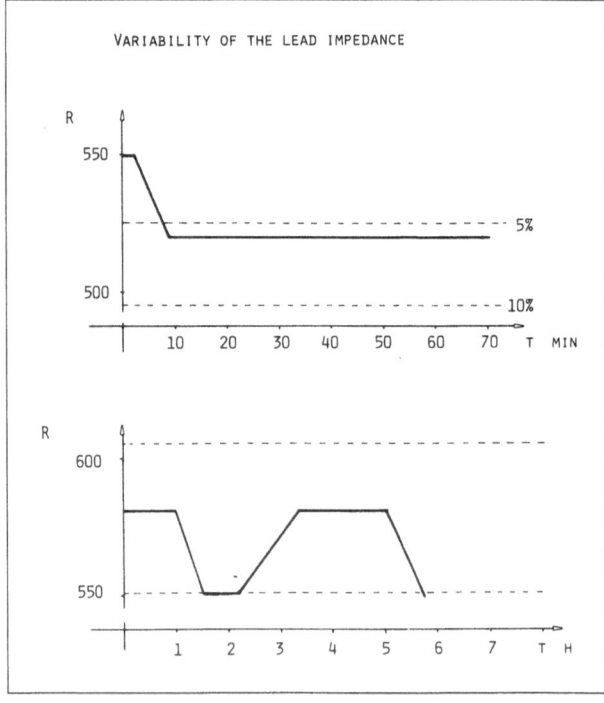

In 10 patients with VVI pacemakers the lead impedance was followed up for 21 weeks after the implantation.
During a period of 2 weeks after the implantation oscillatory-like behavior of the lead impedance was observed in 3 VVI and 1 AAI (Fig. 16) pacemakers.
A decrease of lead impedance in the range of 1 measurement step was observed in 1 VVI patient. The lead impedance remained constant in 2 patients (VVI). An increase of lead

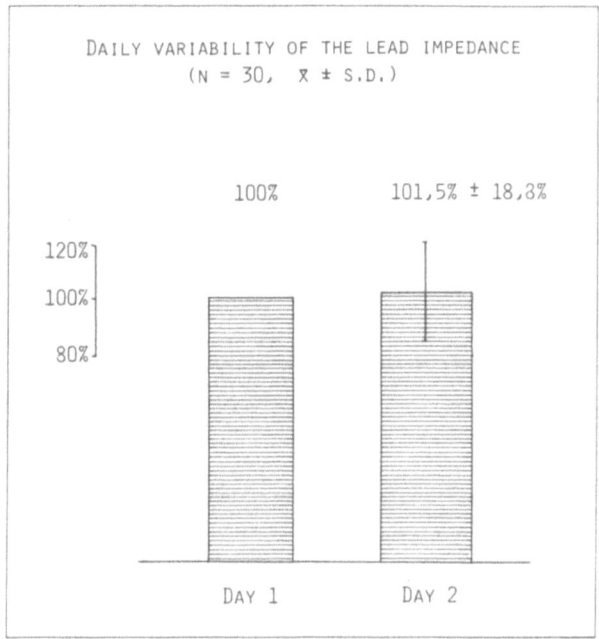

DAILY VARIABILITY OF THE LEAD IMPEDANCE
$(N = 30, \quad \bar{x} \pm S.D.)$

Fig. 15. Day-to-day variability of the lead impedance, measured in 30 VVI pacemakers ($\bar{x} \pm$ S.D.) (Vitatron DPG 1)

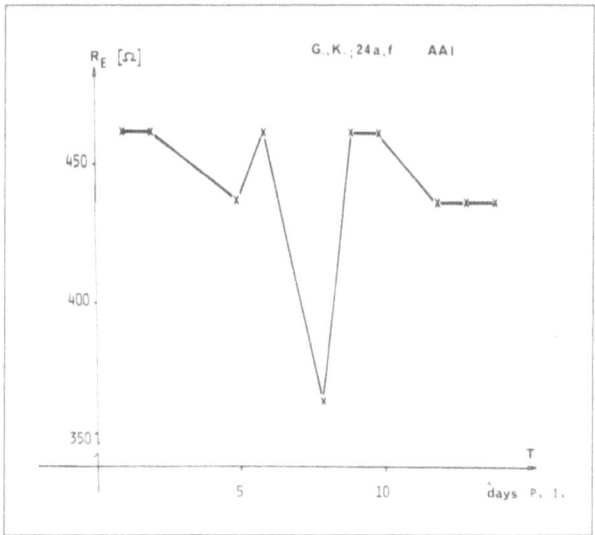

Fig. 16. Remarkable variation ("oscillation") of the lead impedance in an AAI pacemaker during the first 14 days after implantation. (Vitatron DPG 1)

21

impedance in the range of 1 measurement step was detected in 17 patients (15 VVI, 2 AAI), and of 2 measurement steps in 1 patient. The values showed biphasic or undulatory behaviour with culminating points in the 7th (+ 7%) and 14th week (+ 10%) post implantation. The standard deviations were large, showing again that the graphic display of repeatedly measured parameters is more suitable for intraindividual comparisons than interindividual ones.

AAI pacemaker follow-up:

The lead impedance was followed in 2 patients with AAI pacemakers for 20 weeks following implantation. The values showed a slight, insignificant increase (Fig. 17)

Fig. 17. Variability ("oscillation") of the lead impedance in 2 patients with an AAI pacemaker for 20 weeks after implantation. (Vitatron DPG 1)

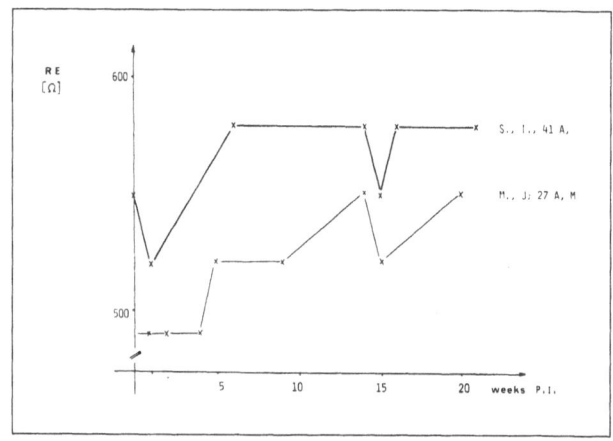

Measurement of the R-wave and P-wave amplitude

This will be discussed in our next paper in this volume (p. 33).

Clinical value of the analysis functions for the regular pacemaker control

Pacemaker telemetry itself lasted 20 ± 5 minutes, its interpretation another 5 to 10 minutes. Due to the complexity of the pacemaker programmer system the telemetry had to be performed by a physician. After each of the 300 measurements we had detailed knowledge of the pacemaker and the myocardium-pacemaker interaction which could not be achieved by the conventional pacemaker control. In the future the procedure should be simplified and shortened.

Clinical value of the analysis functions for pacemaker adjustment ("fine tuning")

Pacing threshold-guided pacing:

Energy conservation can be achieved by reducing the output voltage by 50% (e.g. from 5.0 to 2.5 V) or by halving the impulse width (e.g. from 1.0 to 0.5 ms). The power reduction achieved is increased by reducing the output voltage. In most cases the halving of both the output and impulse duration leads to a very slight safety margin.

The charge per stimulus can be taken as a parameter of the pacemaker's longevity, dependent upon voltage and impulse duration. A charge of 5 V / 1 ms was regarded as 100%. If the impulse duration is prolonged or the voltage increased the charge per stimulus will also increase. Shortening of the duration will reduce charge consumption and output voltage. If the output voltage is halved the effect is greater than by using duration shortening by a factor of 2. Due to the reliable pacing threshold estimation method, threshold-guided pacing with an optimum of power conservation could be achieved in all 23 patients. They could all be programmed to 2.5 volts or 0.5 ms. The parameter "annual consumption" indicated misleading values if the pacemaker output or impulse duration was repeatedly programmed.

Discussion

Programming procedure

Recently developed programs for single or double chamber pacemakers are no longer based on conventional personal computers, have reduced and simplified software-menus and are easily programmed by using touch screens or light pencils. Programming has thus become quicker and easier.

Battery and output status

Apart from the lead impedance (see above) hardly any clinically interesting information is displayed here. A drop in magnet rate of $\geq 10\%$ indicates an exhausted battery. This rate drop is caused by a circuit which will prolong the magnet rate interval as the battery voltage decreases below a certain level, pacemaker aging, prolonged sensing interval, and a lower magnet rate. After all, a differential diagnosis of these factors can be realized without the parameters of the battery and output status. These parameters are nevertheless scientifically interesting and should be optional, but not combined with a crucial measurement as is the case with the lead impedance.

Pacing threshold measurement

Measurement method:

The Vario system allows accurate investigation of the voltage pacing threshold and a construction of a strength-duration curve in conjunction with the programmability of the impulse duration (3).

The DPG 1 system has two major advantages over the Vario principle:

1. The construction of the strength-duration curve is easier and performed quicker due to the incorporated graphic program in the HP 85's software;
2. the DPG's measuring area covers particularly high threshold curves (see Fig. 3).

Our own data show that the method is extremely accurate. The measured output was only equal when compared with the programmed output at 1.5 ms impulse duration (Fig. 7). Since these values also show this slight deviation during the pacing threshold measurement procedure this can be neglected clinically. The variability can reach $\leqq 50\%$, but at very low threshold values.

Clinical follow-up:

As already described for the Vario system the DPG is suitable for the detection of individual, atypical threshold courses. In reviewing the literature (3, 4), three major types of threshold behavior after the implantation can be described:

1. type I or classic type, found in most patients: early threshold peak in the first two (5, 6) to four weeks;
2. type II, found only in a small proportion of pacemaker patients: slow threshold rise reaching the peak value in the second or third month (or even later) followed by a gradual decrease or stabilisation;
3. type III, found in 20% of patients, with a progressive increase of the threshold (7, 8). In our patient population we could also find these 3 types with the DPG 1 system. An interindividual comparison has to be neglected since the mixture of the 3 different curve types and the differing underlying diseases cause an undulatory or biphasic course and large standard deviations. The latter oberservation was also made by El-Gamal and van Gelder (9) for the Helifix electrode in the atrium, by Scoblionko and Rolett (10), Ramdohr and v. Leitner (11) and by Schulten et al. (12). Compared with the reported data in the literature there was no significant difference between the Helifix electrode and other lead types with respect to the threshold course.

Explanation of the threshold course:

The initial increase of the pacing threshold (type I) was found to occur with and without the lead. Thus, this rise was understood to reflect the local foreign body reaction (13, 14). The slow threshold rise over a more prolonged period (type II) was interpreted as the consequence of current flow during cardiac stimulation (15). The course of the threshold curve is highly influenced by the following factors (S. 10):

1. the site of stimulation;
2. the degree of morphological changes around the implanted electrode (early edematous and late fibrotic lesions);
3. the constitution of the surrounding myocardium:

24

a) the oxygen supply,
b) the extracellular/intracellular electrolyte content,
c) the local hormone or drug effects;
4. the type of electrode configuration, surface and metal; ·
5. the kind of stimulation (unipolar/bipolar; anodal/cathodal; impulse width; output voltage);
6. the constitution of the autonomous nervous system. The pacing threshold increases during sleep (vagotonia) and during treatment with procainamide, diphenylhydantoine, sparteinsulfate, lidocaine and β-receptor blockers. The stimulation threshold decreases during exercise, sharp movement into the upright position, and therapy with sympathomimetic drugs. The undulatory or biphasic course which could not be detected during the individual follow-up is explained by the fact that the addition of 3 types of threshold behavior (types I to III) is characterized by an increase phase and a following undulatory period (Fig. 18).

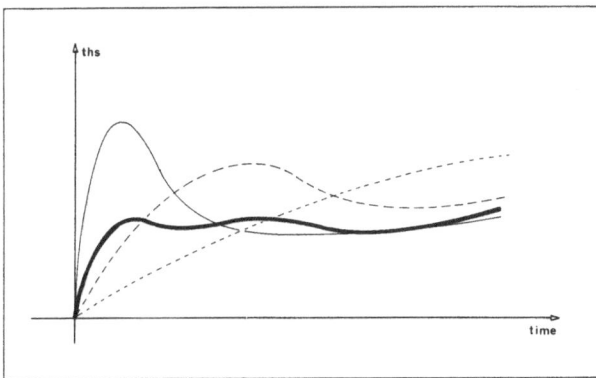

Fig. 18. The addition of the 3 different types of threshold behaviour reveals an undulatory course.

Lead impedance measurement

Measurement method:

Accuracy in the range of 450 to 900 Ω was high (5%) and variability was low (5%). There are only a very few reports in the literature dealing with the accuracy etc. of lead impedance measuring systems in implanted pacemakers.

Clinical follow-up:

The slow increase of the lead impedance which we found in the atrium and ventricle was also described for porous tip electrodes in dogs by Gebhardt-Seehausen et al. (16). A slow decrease in the electrode resistances and lead impedances in VVI pacemakers with Osypka VY 61 screw-in electrodes was reported by Höltmann (17).

25

Explanation of the lead impedance courses:

The values of the lead impedance are dependent on the following factors:
1. the constitution of the myocardium: the site of stimulation and the degree of tissue alteration (dependent on the duration of the postimplantation period);
2. the electrode configuration, surface and metal;
3. the kind of stimulation: impulse width and output voltage.

Since the site of stimulation, the electrode configuration, surface and metal, as well as the stimulation parameters remained constant until the chronic phase the curves demonstrated above may reflect the time course of tissue alteration ("maturation") close to the electrode.

Our findings are that the DPG's lead impedance measuring system is very accurate. The measurement is reliable and easy to perform. Looking at the literature only a few articles state influencing parameters such as electrode type, site of stimulation, etc. We could not find any dependence of lead impedance upon electrolytes. The stability of this parameter is good if the measurement is repeated after 24 hours. It does not seem to have a circadian rhythm which exceeds the precision of the measuring system. After all, it can be said that the lead impedance is a stable parameter which changes slowly after a stabilization period of 1 to 2 weeks. The lead impedance curve has a convex, slightly biphasic course. These findings correspond with those of Gebhardt-Seehausen et al. (16), who performed a similar study using Osypka VY 61 electrodes. There is no significant rise in lead impedance after 20 weeks. But if one looks at stabilized Helifix electrodes which have been implanted for over 40 months, a difference of approximately 200 Ω can be seen. Comparing Helifix with ball tip electrodes after a similar period of implantation it can be observed that the latter have an impedance about 280 Ω higher. Corresponding to the literature it can be said that the lead impedance increases with implantation time (slow reaction of the myocardium to the electrode).

Endocardial signal amplitude measurement

This will be discussed in our next paper in this volume (p. 33).

Pacemaker control, adjustment, differential diagnosis and therapy
of complications or dysfunctions

As demonstrated above the analysis functions of the DPG 1 greatly improved regular pacemaker control, threshold-guided pacing and the diagnosis as well as therapy of pacemaker complications or dysfunctions. Major disadvantages are the following:
1. the excessive duration of the telemetry procedure due to the complex software program;
2. its inability to transmit the intracardiac electrogram;
3. its inability to store patient data from repeated controls for further graphic evaluation (trend analysis).

Proposed improvements

Monitor program of the HP 85

The bidirectional telemetry could be accelerated by using:
1. a more condensed menu-technique and touch screen or light pencils;
2. erasable programmable read only memory (EPROM);
3. a programming language as low as possible.

Futhermore it should be possible to store patient data in the HP 85 in order to perform a trend analysis of the investigated parameters with the help of a special graphic program. This proposal was also made by G. Fontaine at the International Congress on Cardiology in Marilleva in 1984.

Pacemaker functions

As mentioned before the capability to transmit the intracardiac electrogram should be incorporated to achieve improved sensitivity adjustment. With regard to the threshold measuring system, the step down mode should be improved. Additionally marker signals should be integrated in order to signalize sensing and pacing.

References

1. Winter UT, Behrenbeck DW, Brill Th, Höher M, Hombach V, Hilger HH (1985) Value and limitations of the Holter functions of a single chamber diagnostic pacemaker (this volume)
2. Winter UJ, Höher M, Behrenbeck DW, Liertz KP, Missler T, Hilger HH (1985) Determination of the endocardial signal amplitude in single chamber demand pacemakers: comparison of two measurement methods (this volume)
3. Barold SS, Ong LS, Falkoff MD, Heinle RA (1982) Programmable pacemakers: clinical indications, complications and future directions. In: Barold SS, Mugica J (eds) The third decade of cardiac pacing. Futura Publishing Co, New York, pp 27–76
4. Starke ID (1978) Long-term follow-up of cardiac pacing threshold using a noninvasive method of measurement. Br Heart J 40: 530–533
5. Furman S, Hurzeler Ph, Mehra R (1977) Cardiac pacing and pacemakers IV: threshold of cardiac stimulation. Am Heart J 94/1: 115–124
6. Furman S, Escher D, Fischer J (1979) Seven year experience with programmable pulse generators In: Meere C (ed) Cardiac Pacing: Proceedings of the VIth World Symposium on Cardiac Pacing, Montreal, Ch 19-1
7. Luceri RM, Furman S, Wurzeler P, Escher DJW (1979) Threshold behavior of electrodes in long-term ventricular pacing. Am J Cardiol 40: 184
8. Rossi P, Palma G, Marino B, De Bellis F, Solina A, Vercelotti F (1979) Long-term follow-up myocardial pacing threshold measurement with an external radiofrequency transmitter in patients with an implanted pacemaker and an independent radio receiver (Radiocor).
9. El-Gamal M, Van Gelder B (1979) Preliminary experience with the Helifix electrode for transvenous atrial implantation. 2: 444–454
10. Scoblionko DP, Rolett EL (1981) Short-term threshold behavior of human ventricular pacing electrodes: non-invasive monitoring with a multiprogrammable pacing system. PACE 4: 634
11. Ramdohr B, Leitner E-R (1973) Zur Methodik der Reizschwellenbestimmung nach Herzschrittmacherimplantation. Acta Med 21 Nr 2: 35–37

12. Schulten HK, Grosser KD, Steinbrück G (1972) Langzeitmessungen von Reizschwellen bei endokardialen Schrittmachersonden. Z Kardiol 62/7: 617–624
13. Westerholm C-J (1971) Threshold studies in transvenous cardiac pacemaker treatment. Scand J Thorac Cardiovasc Surg 5 (Suppl 8): 53
14. Contini C, Papi L, Pesola A et al (1973) Tissue reaction to intracavitary electrodes: effect on duration and efficiency of unipolar pacing in patients with AV-block. J Cardiovasc Surg 14: 280–282
15. Marchand P, Jaros GG, Obel IWP (1969) Long pulse stimuli for cardiac pacing. Ann New York Acad Sci 167: 706–721
16. Gebhardt-Seehausen U, Recker S, Müllges W, Keusen H, Hollweg G (1982) Evaluations with a new porous tip electrode: ingrow- and electrophysiological behavior. Proceedings of the World Congress on Medical Physics and Biomedical Engineering, Hamburg. 1982, No 12, 18
17. Höltmann B (1984) Zur Problematik der Elektrodenimpedanz: Telemetrische Messung und Impulsformanalyse bei Schraubelektroden. Herzschrittmacher 4, Nr 3: 191–194

Authors' address:
U. J. Winter, M.D.
Medizinische Universitätsklinik III, Kardiologie
Josef-Stelzmann-Straße 9
5000 Köln 41
West Germany

Clinical Importance of the Analysis Functions of a Multiprogrammable Pacemaker

M. J. L. de Jongste and D. Nagelkerke

Summary: The recent introduction of microprocessor based pacemakers with full bidirectional telemetry has greatly improved the flexibility of multiprogrammable pacing systems. In addition to "standard" programmable options, these pacemakers offer the possibility of measuring such parameters as battery status and lead impedance, of making strength duration curves, and of recording intracardiac ECG and Holter monitoring data. All of these functions can be useful in the analysis of pacemaker and/or lead related problems (insulation defects, electrode dislocation and sensing errors), in the development of new electrodes and in the evaluation of drug therapy. The possibility of storing data in the pacemaker can also be of importance in cases where patients are admitted in an emergency. This would become a significant advantage if some form of standardisation could be achieved with respect to the various programming devices.

The increased amount of time needed for follow-up, the lack of compatibility between and the complexity of the different pacemaker systems are disadvantages that can be solved by making these systems autoprogrammable.

In this article we will discuss these various aspects in relation to the Vitatron DPG 1 pacemaker.

Introduction

The incorporation of integrated circuits and full bidirectional telemetry in implantable pulse generators has greatly increased the possibilities of storing data and of analysing the various pacemaker functions.

A very sophisticated and highly flexible software VVI pacemaker, the Diagnostic Pulse Generator (DPG), contains such an integrated circuit, which is used as a hardware Central Processing Unit connected to the necessary peripheral circuits.

Flexibility in such a system is necessary because of the continuing changes in electrophysiological, haemodynamic and metabolic states of the patient. In addition, it also has scientific as well as clinical implications. For example, by having the possibility of reprogramming the pacemaker a second invasive procedure might be prevented.

1. Measurements in the analysis function program

The DPG has special features that can be programmed by using an HP 85 personal computer in combination with an interface and special software. After selecting the option "Measurements" in the analysis program a choice can be made from:
1. Battery and output status (including lead impedance).
2. Critical pulse duration,
3. Strength duration curve, and
4. QRS/P-wave measurement

Fig. 1. Battery and output status

```
Vitatron Medical    Pacer monitor

Batt./Output status   Actual   RRT
Battery voltage       V  2.80   2.30
Battery impedance     kΩ  0 0    8.2
Current drain         µA  23 6
Annual consumption    %  12 2
Percentage paced      %  99 9
Output voltage        V   5 4
Mean outp. current    mA  7 0
Pulse duration        ms  0.5
Charge per stim.      µC  3 5
Lead imped.(5V/2ms)   Ω  900

|Return| |          | |        | |Print |
```

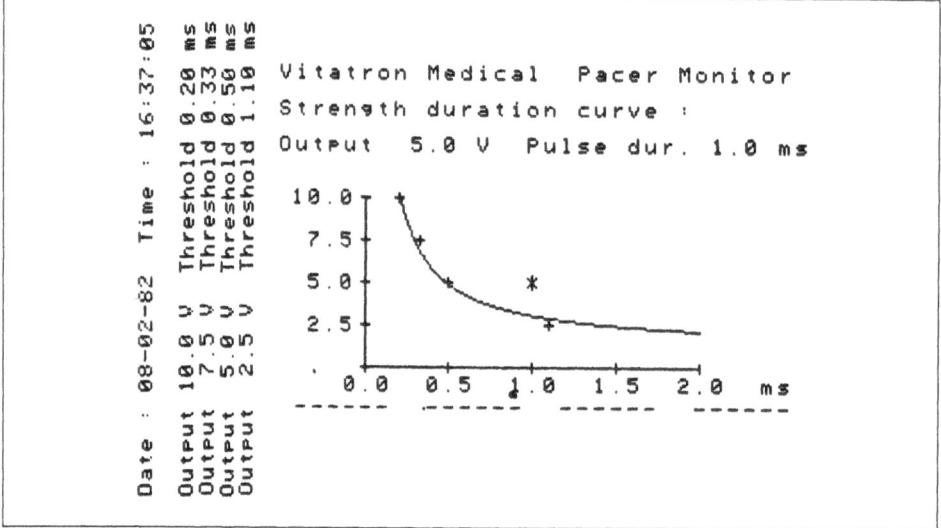

Fig. 2. Strength/duration curve

The battery and output status and lead impedance measurements are important for the prediction of pacemaker lifetime and for the analysis of lead related problems such as mechanical defects and insulation problems.

In combination with the strength duration curve (Fig. 2) it is also possible to program the pacemaker parameters to economic values and so conserve energy.

Measurement of intracardiac signal strength

Evaluation of the intracardiac ECG recording is convenient and can be useful in the analysis of problems related to interference and sensing.

In addition, the intracardiac ECG is useful for scientific purposes such as the development of new electrodes, for the evaluation of the influence of medication on the intracardiac signal, for rate responsive pacing (QT principle) and for the detection of macro and micro dislocation.

Holter monitoring

Holter monitoring and event counters (premature beat counters, sense to pace counters, inhibition and stimulation counters) in the pacemaker can be used for the evaluation of the influence of medication in stabilising heart rhythm (1).
Especially in patients with atrial fibrillation, frequent premature beats, or when the pacemaker is operating in the flywheel mode, the combination of histogram and premature beat counters can be useful.
In combination with the pace, sense and sense to pace counters, the Holter option can be used in patients with the pacemaker syndrome to program the pacemaker to a lower rate, with or without hysteresis. In addition the histogram (Fig. 3) can be useful in the detection of sensing problems or exit blocks, because the largest R-R interval has to be the lowest pacemaker rate.
By using the DPG as an external device bradycardias can be detected.

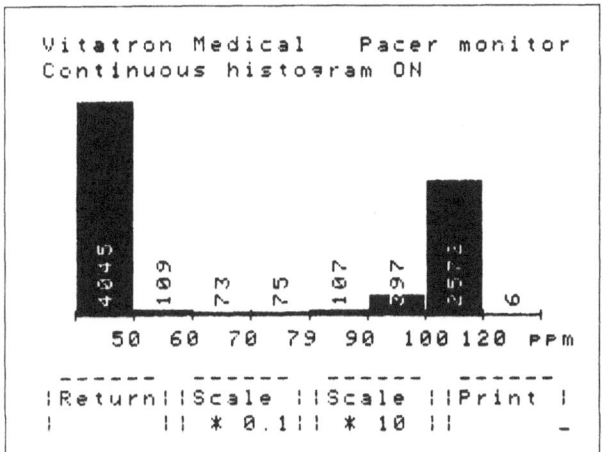

Fig. 3. Continuous histogram

2. Future perspectives

In addition to the size, shape, cost, settings and programming convenience there are some options that can be incorporated in the near future. The storage of data relating to personal (name, address etc.), technical (pacemaker settings) and medical information (drugs, diseases etc.) in the pacemaker will save time, especially in cases where patients are admitted in an emergency. In order to make this a real advantage, however, standardisation of programming devices is essential. In rate responsive pacemakers or arrhythmia treating devices it is sometimes necessary to have marker pulses to control and interpret these more complex systems.

31

3. Discussion

Although multiprogrammable pacemakers are now accepted as the primary choice of therapy, the value of the multiprogrammability is still under investigation. In a presentation during the 1st World Symposium on Cardiac Pacing, it was stated that the rate and output were the most useful parameters (2). Furthermore, pulse width and sensitivity programmability can save 9% of the patients from a second invasive procedure (3). In addition to the above mentioned advantage the clinical importance of the analysis functions is mainly in the field of research, with special regard to the intracardiac signal analysis (4). Research and development of new software pacemakers with full bidirectional facilities will undoubtedly make such systems even more flexible.

Although auto-programmability should be the ultimate purpose, this state of the art has some disadvantages, such as the increased amount of time needed for follow-up and the complexity of the system. As mentioned before the lack of compatibility between the different systems is a major problem that must be solved by the pacemaker manufacturers. In conclusion multiprogrammability still has disadvantages, but as Didinot stated "It is a feasible, practical, safe and convenient device" (5).

References

1. Attuel P, Ripart A, Mugica J (1984) Progress in Holter monitoring: towards an implantable system. Author abstract in: Herzschrittmacher 1
2. Djordjevic M, Milosevic U, Velimirovic D (1983) Programmable pacemakers to selected patients or to all patients. PACE Vol 6, No 3, part II: 376
3. O'Keefe JH Jr, Hayes DL, Holmes DR Jr, Vlietstra RE (1983) Clinical use of multiparameter programmability in the early and late follow-up period. PACE Vol 6, No 3, part II: 377
4. Thalen HJTh, Wittkampf FHM, Rickards AF, Norman J, Nagelkerke D (1982) Evoked response sensing (ERS) as automatic control of the pacemaker output. In: Feruglio GA (ed) Cardiac Pacing. Proceedings and Mini Courses of the Second European Symposium on Cardiac Pacing. Piccin Medical Books, Padova, pp 1229–1234
5. Dodinot B, Kubler L, Buffet J, Meunier JF (1983) Clinical investigation of a multiprogrammer. In: Steinbach K et al (eds) Cardiac Pacing. Proceedings of the VIIth World Symposium on Cardiac Pacing. Steinkopff Verlag, Darmstadt, p 29

Authors' address:
M. J. L. de Jongste, M.D.
Cardiology Department
University Hospital
Oostersingel 54
9713 EZ Groningen
The Netherlands

Determination of the Endocardial Signal Amplitude in Single Chamber Demand Pacemakers: Comparison of two Measurement Methods

U. J. Winter, M. Höher, D. W. Behrenbeck, K. P. Liertz, J. Missler, and H. H. Hilger

Summary: The causes of a failure to sense in demand pacemakers may be located in the myocardium, in the electrode or in the pacemaker itself. Alterations of the sensing behaviour often occur in patients with acute myocardial infarction close to the electrode, bundle branch blocks, slowing of the impulse propagation due to drug effects or premature contractions. Some pacemakers offer the possibility of transmitting the intracardiac electrogram, which is used for the sensing circuit of the pulse generator.
The aim of the study was to compare the clinical reliability of the transmission of the intracardiac electrogram (Medtronic Spektrax SXT) with the simple telemetry of the endocardial signal amplitude (Vitatron DPG 1). Thirty-three patients with symptomatic bradyarrhythmias were treated with the Spektrax SXT (VVI), 19 patients with the DPG 1 (VVI). During the postimplantation period the clinical reliability of both methods was investigated by repeated controls. The telemetry of the intracardiac electrogram (Spektrax SXT) and the determination of the different parameters (amplitude of the intrinsic deflection and ST elevation; slew rate; dV/dt max. etc.) was time consuming. The estimation of the different parameters of the intracardiac electrogram has to be performed under equal conditions, since respiratory excursions, changes in the body posture, filters etc. may highly influence the electrogram. With screw-in electrodes the ST elevation returned to nearly normal values about 90 minutes after the implantation. A significant reduction of the signal amplitude changes during respiratory excursions showed the finished connective tissue growth around the electrode tip and thus a stabilized lead position.
The determination of the R-wave amplitudes (DPG 1) was quite easy and did not take too much time. But 33% of the 300 measurements were not credible, since the mean, minimum and maximum R-wave values were equal. In 8/19 patients the measurement range was too small in the early postimplantation period. The variability was $\pm$ 1.0 mV. This can lead to problems of interpretation only in very small signal amplitudes.

Introduction

Sensitivity-guided pacing is one of the "neglected" topics in modern cardiac pacing, according to Barold et al. (1). Some of the single chamber devices, e.g. Siemens-Elema Dialog series and Medtronic Spektrax SXT, offer the capability of percutaneous transmission of the intracardiac electrogram to an ECG recorder. But due to different reasons this method could not succeed in clinical follow-up of pacemaker patients. One of the major reasons might have been the time consuming recording technique. Recently a software-based single chamber pacemaker (DPG 1) was built with simplified, computerized determination of the endocardial signal amplitude.

Objective

The aim of the study was to determine which of two different measurement principles, either the transmission of the intracardiac electrogram (ICEG), e.g. realized by the Spektrax SXT (Medtronic) or the measurement of the endocardial signal amplitude, performed by the software-guided DPG 1 (Vitatron), is more reliable for the adjustment of the pacemaker sensitivity to the intrinsic signal amplitude. Therefore in patients with bradyarrhythmias either the Spektrax SXT or the DPG 1 were implanted in combination with a Helifix (Vitatron) or DY- (Biotronic) electrode, both having an electrode surface area of 12 mm² (medium size).

Transmission of the intracardiac electrogram (ICEG): Spektrax SXT

Patients:

In 8 patients with bradyarrhythmias (3 female, 5 male; age: 59 ± 20 years) a new implantation of the Spektrax SXT (as VVI pacemaker) and a Helifix electrode was performed. An additional 25 patients with bradyarrhythmias (5 female, 20 male; age: 55 ± 10 years) were treated with a Spektrax SXT (VVI pacemaker) on the occasion of a battery exchange. In this patient population the following underlying diseases were observed: CHD (n = 11); hypersensitive carotid sinus (n = 7); AV or bundle branch block (n = 5); cardiomyopathy (n = 2); LGL-syndrome (n = 1). Furthermore, the Spektrax SXT was implanted as VVI pacemaker in 5 patients (φ = 3, δ = 2) with bradyarrhythmias connected to a DY-electrode (Biotronik). The underlying diseases were: mitral valve disease (n = 1); sinus node syndrome (n = 2); AV block II to III ° (n = 2).

Methods:

The Spektrax SXT 8423 (unipolar) has an input impedance of 10 to 20 K Ω. The pacemaker telemetry can be performed by the programmer Censys TM 9701 A. The transmitted electrogram and the lead I were recorded with a Siemens-Elema Mingograph at 1000 mm/sec paper speed. After new implantations recordings were performed 30, 60, 120, 150 and 180 minutes as well as 1, 2, 5 and 10 days after the implantation. In the chronic group the controls were realized 15 ± 13 months after the battery exchange. Beside other parameters, the R-wave amplitude was measured twice from the ECG recordings, taking finally the mean value of both.

Results

Methodological considerations:

In monophasic negative chamber signals of the acute stage (Fig. 1a, Type I), the R-wave is very small in comparison to a very large, deep negative S-wave. Monophasic positive endo-cardial signals of the acute phase have a small S-wave and a predominant R-wave. In endocardial signals with several positive and negative deflections the determination of the R-wave amplitude is difficult (Fig. 1, Type IV). Furthermore the original R-wave amplitudes were influenced by the kind of underlying disease, e.g. being lower in CHD patients and higher in younger patients with nearly normal myocardium (Fig. 2). In

34

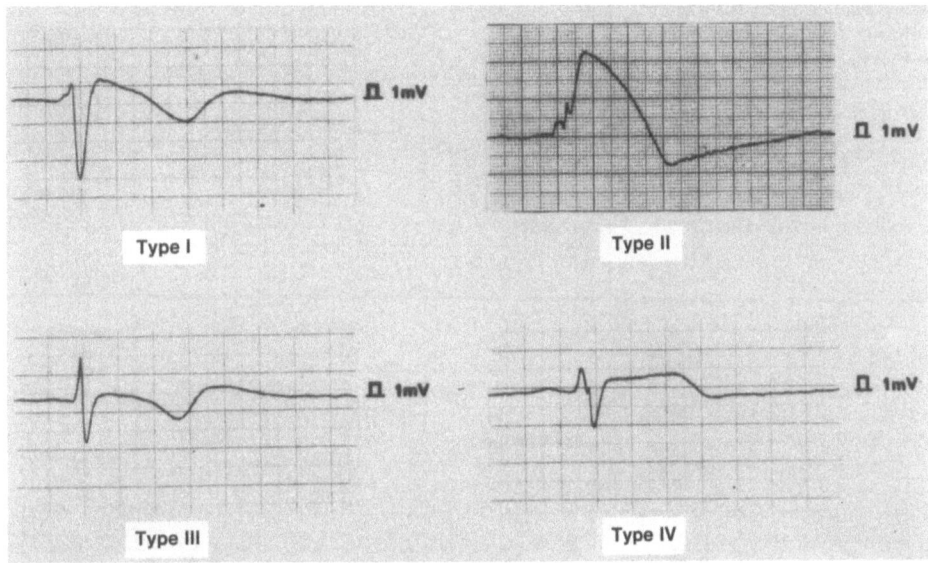

Fig. 1. Different endocardial signal morphologies: Type I: Monophasic negative; Type II: monophasic positive with monophasic ST-elevation (acute stage); Type III: biphasic; Type IV: biphasic with splitting. (Medtronic Spektrax SXT)

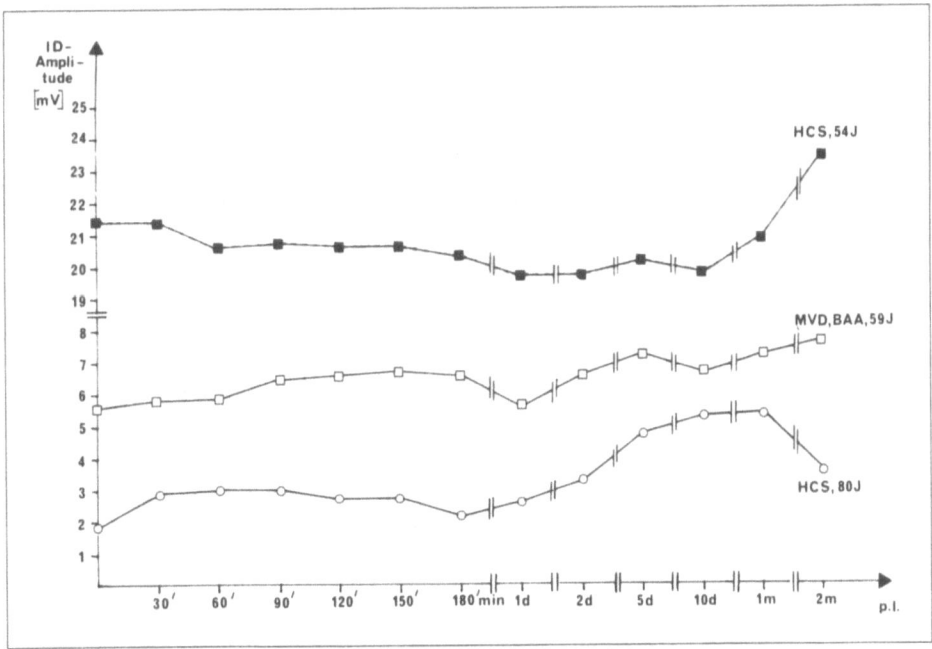

Fig. 2. Dependence of the amplitude of the intrinsic deflection (ID) on the underlying disease and age. (Medtronic Spektrax SXT)

Fig. 3. Reduction of the signal amplitude (intrinsic deflection/ ID) by the 50 Hz filter of the ECG recorder. (Medtronic Spektrax SXT)

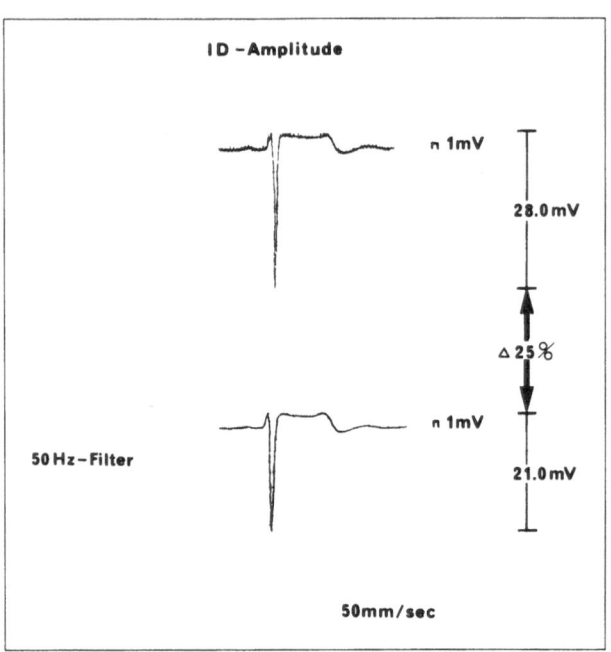

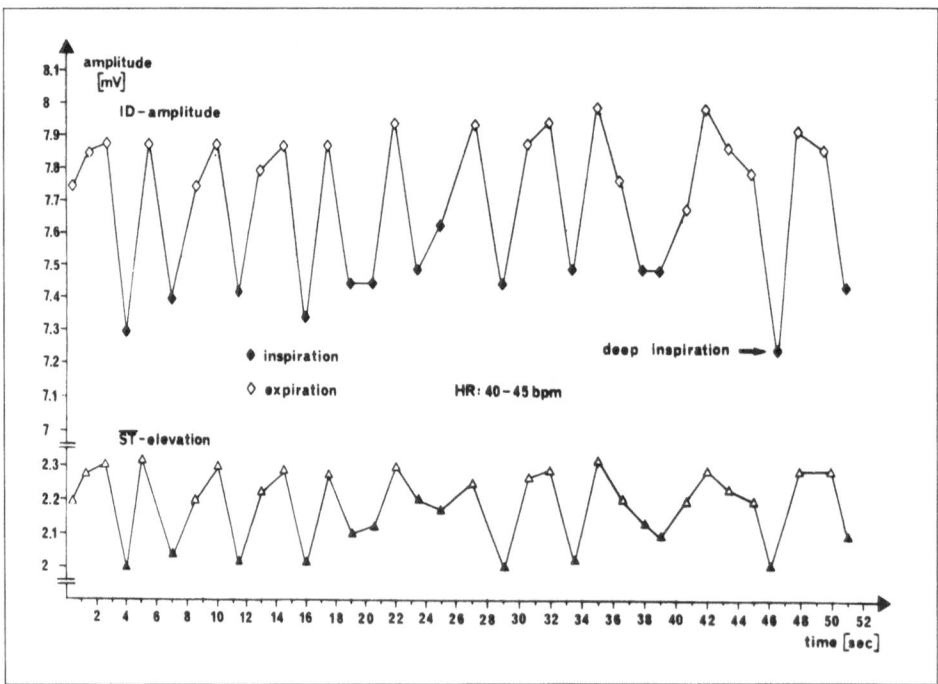

Fig. 4. Variations of the amplitude of the intrinsic deflection (ID) and the ST-elevation during respiration. (Medtronic Spektrax SXT)

noisy recordings of the ICEG, the Mingograph's 50 Hz filter leads to a reduction of the R-wave amplitude of up to 25% (Fig. 3). Furman et al. (2, 3), described respiratory induced variations of the R-wave amplitude in the range of ± 5.3%. We found similar variations (± 4.8%; Fig. 4).

Follow-up:

In the early post-implantation period an undulatory course was detected in all patients (see Fig. 5). Four out of five patients (DY electrode) showed a peak value of the R-wave amplitude in the fourth week (Fig. 5). In the interindividual comparison, an undulatory course and larger standard deviations were observed.

Discussion:

Barold et al. (4) described a reduction of the R-wave amplitude of about 15% from the acute (5 to 15 mV) to the chronic stage. Wirtzfeld et al. (5) observed no significant difference between the acute (8.1 ± 3.8 mV, SEM) and chronic stage (battery change: 9.8 ± 4.1 mV). Furman et al. (3) measured 12.4 ± 5.5 mV in the acute and 10.5 ± 4.8 mV in the chronic phase. In our own patient population we saw a slow increase of the R-wave amplitude until the fourth week (peak value), followed by a slow decrease. The different data reported in the literature may be explained by the following reasons:

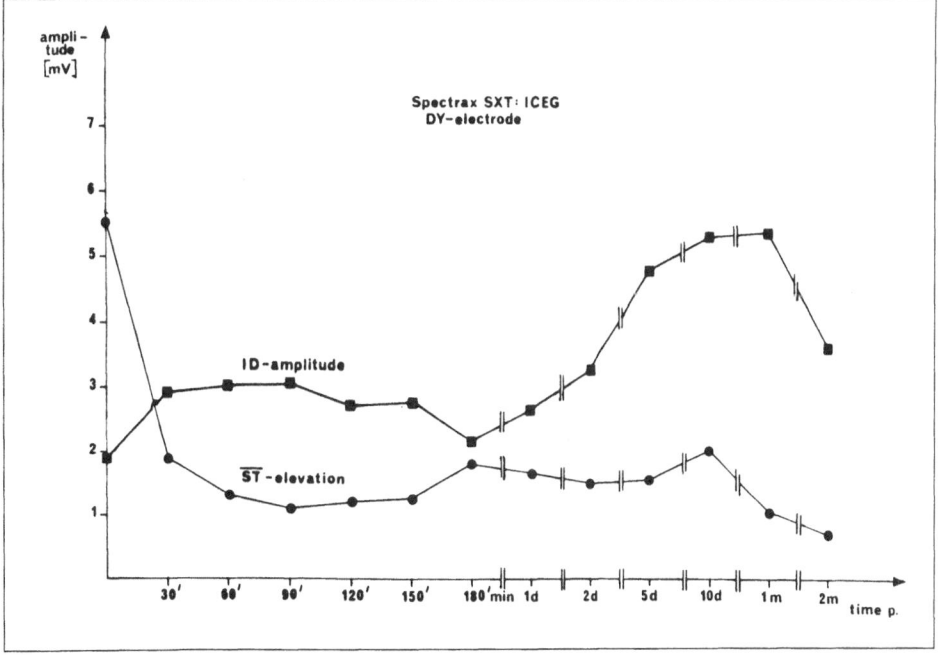

Fig. 5. Undulatory course of the amplitude of the intrinsic deflection (ID) in the early post-implantation period, as demonstrated in one representative patient. (Medtronic Spektrax SXT)

1. different electrode types (traumatic-non-traumatic, surface area : medium or large);
2. different times of measurement of the parameter;
3. different filter settings.

Similar curves of the R-wave amplitude were found in our institution by different measurement systems (Spektrax SXT; DPG 1) and different electrodes (Helifix: DY). The undulatory course was seen in the early postimplantation (e.g. 10 days) and during a longer follow-up period (e.g. 20 weeks).

Measurement of the endocardial R-wave amplitude: DPG 1

Patients:

Nineteen patients were treated with a DPG 1 pacemaker (Vitatron) and a Helifix lead (Vitatron): age 56 ± 15 years, 1 female, 18 male patients; 19 VVI. In 13 patients with coronary heart disease and complex arrhythmias, drug-induced bradycardia was the main indication for a VVI pacemaker with analysis functions. Furthermore, the DPG 1 was implanted in 3 patients with atrial fibrillation and drug-induced bradyarrhythmias as VVI pacemaker. Additionally, 1 patient with CHD and carotid sinus syndrome, 1 patient with WPW syndrome and amiodarone-induced bradycardia and 1 patient with hypertrophic, obstructive cardiomyopathy were treated with the DPG 1 as VVI pacemaker. The follow-up period was 19 ± 4 months.

R-wave amplitude measurement: methods:

The principle of measuring the endocardial signal amplitude, being representative of the sensing circuit of the demand pacemaker, is shown in Fig. 6. After having automatically reduced (in a stepwise fashion) the sensitivity threshold to a value where the sensing of the endocardial signals becomes possible (at a stimulation rate below the spontaneous rhythm) the minimal, maximal and mean signal amplitude can be determined (Fig. 6).

Results of the R-wave amplitude measurements

Methodological considerations:

The minimal R-wave amplitude is most important for the sensitivity adjustment. In about 33% of the 300 measurements the values of the R-wave amplitudes were not credible. In 3/23 patients the lower limit of the measurement range (1.5 mV) was not sufficient, in 5/23 patients the upper limit of 15.0 mV was too low (Fig. 7). The repeated measurements of the R-wave amplitude during 30 minutes revealed variations of about ± 1 mV (see Fig. 8). Shortly after the implantation where high R-wave amplitudes ($\geqslant 10$ mV) were found, variations of ± 1 mV are very slight. During the chronic phase, where R-wave amplitudes of about 3 to 4 mV are observed, variations of ± 1 mV become more significant (see lower part of Fig. 8). In the latter case a capability for the estimation of the slew rate would be helpful for the sensitivity adjustment. Variations of the R-wave

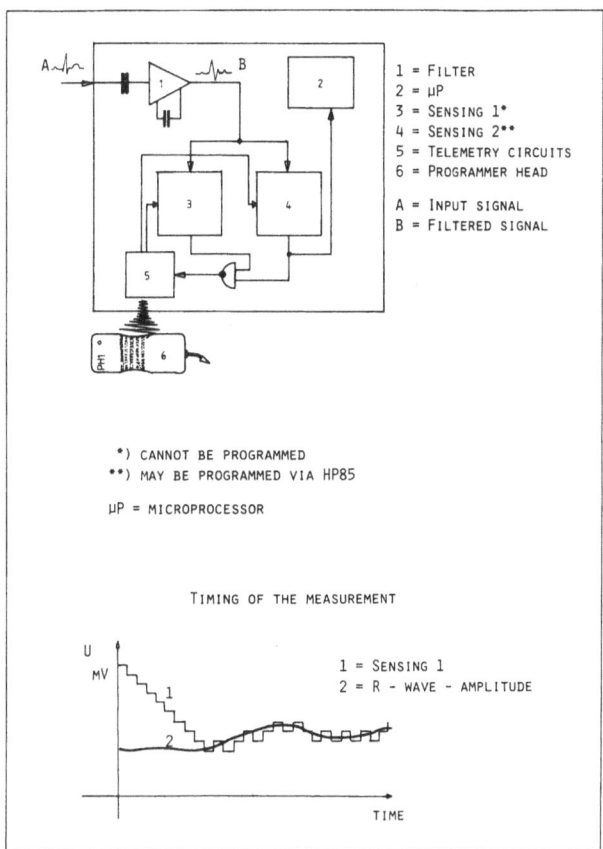

1 = FILTER
2 = μP
3 = SENSING 1*
4 = SENSING 2**
5 = TELEMETRY CIRCUITS
6 = PROGRAMMER HEAD

A = INPUT SIGNAL
B = FILTERED SIGNAL

*) CANNOT BE PROGRAMMED
**) MAY BE PROGRAMMED VIA HP85

μP = MICROPROCESSOR

TIMING OF THE MEASUREMENT

1 = SENSING 1
2 = R - WAVE - AMPLITUDE

Fig. 6. Measuring principle of the R-wave amplitude in the Vitatron DPG 1. The signal amplitude is determined in automatically reducing the sensitivity to a value where sensing becomes possible.

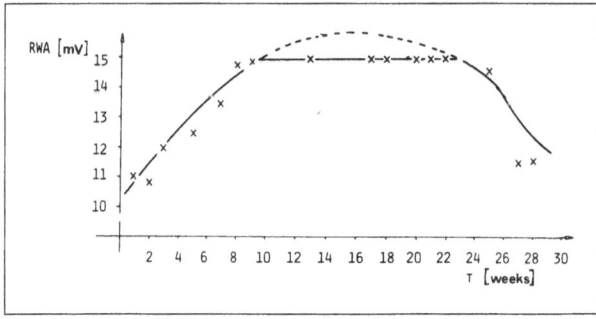

Fig. 7. Course of the R-wave amplitude, exceeding the upper measurement limit of 15.0 mV (RWA: R-wave amplitude). (Vitatron DPG 1)

amplitude, measured after 3.5 ± 3 minutes and again after 24 hours, are not significant (Fig. 9). Furthermore, the variations of the R-wave amplitude, determined during normal respiration, deep inspiration, deep expiration, during Valsalva-maneuver, in the left and right lying position, were not significant (Fig. 10).

39

Fig. 8. Variations of the measurement of R-wave amplitude 30 minutes and 6 and 52 months after implantation. In the chronic phase the R-wave amplitude is much lower. (Vitatron DPG 1)

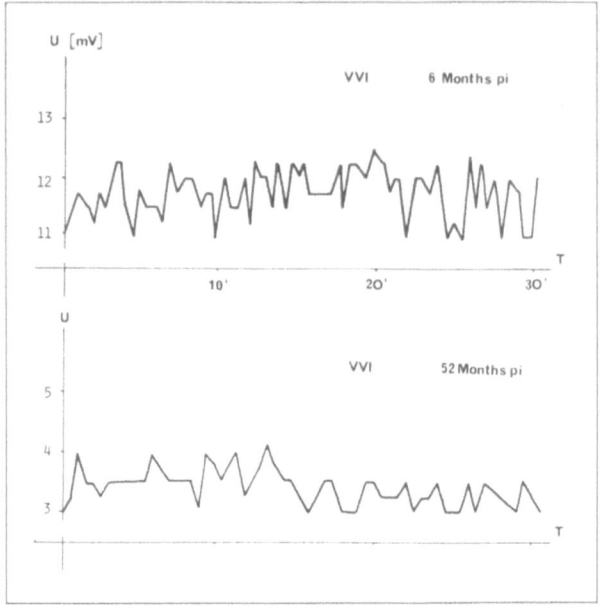

Fig. 9. Minute-to-minute and day-to-day variations of the measured R-wave amplitude in the chronic phase. (Vitatron DPG 1)

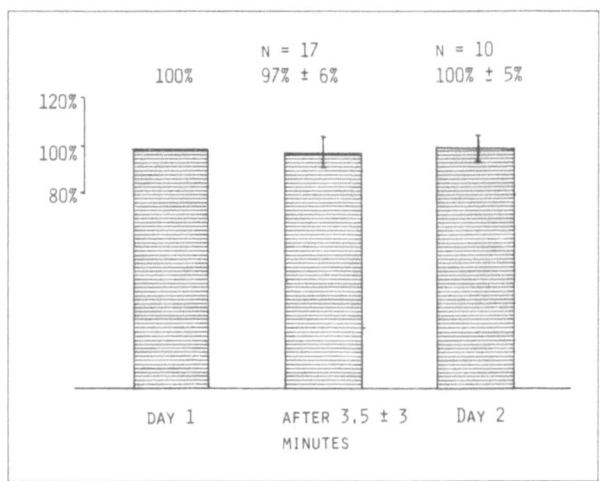

Follow-up: VVI pacemakers:

The R-wave amplitude typically decreases after implantation (Fig. 11, lower part) from 13 mV to about 7 mV in the 2nd week. After that, the amplitude increases up to 12 mV (7th week) and then decreases again. This kind of biphasic or undulatory course can also be seen in the chronic phase (Fig. 11, upper part) after a battery exchange in the same patient and in Fig. 12. In the interindividual comparison of 10 patients with VVI pacemakers a biphasic or undulatory course is demonstrated again, with culminating points in the 10th (+45%) and 17th (+30%) weeks. The standard deviations are large, showing that the graphic display is more suitable for intraindividual comparison.

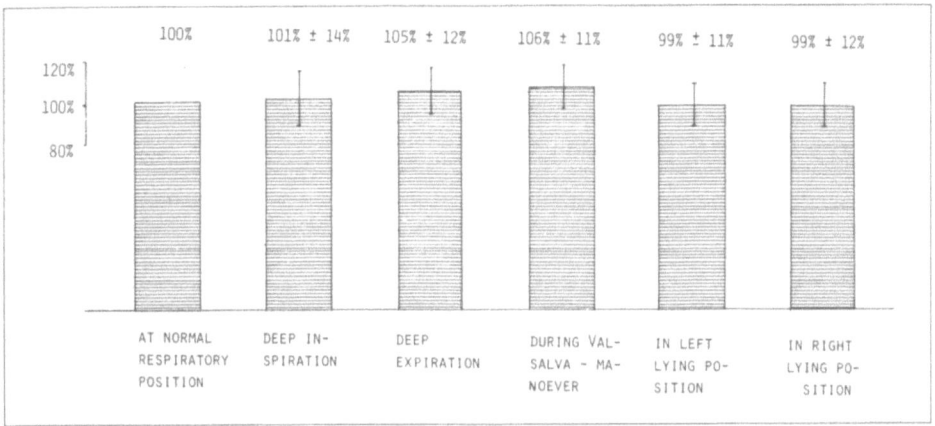

Fig. 10. Variability of the measured R-wave amplitude during respiration and different body positions. (Vitatron DPG 1)

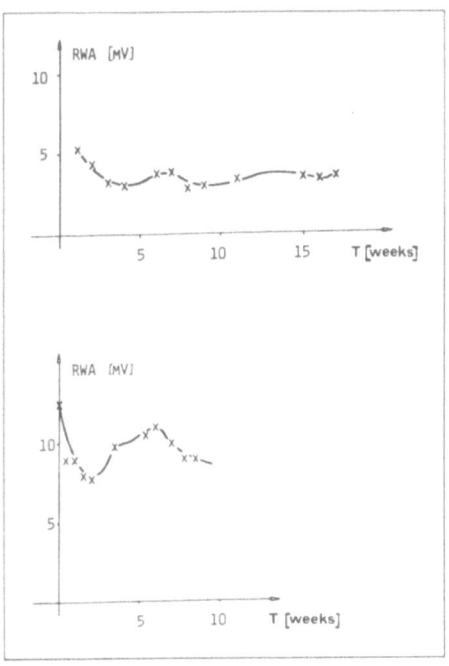

Fig. 11. Differing R-wave amplitudes in the same patient after battery exchange (chronic phase) and in a new implantation due to pacemaker pocket infection. (Vitatron DPG 1)

Discussion

Measurement method:

In about 33% of the 300 measurements, incredible R-wave values were printed out. The variations of the R-wave amplitude, determined minute-to-minute, day-to-day and at different respiratory or body positions, were not significant (about 12%). During the acute

41

Fig. 12. Undulatory course of the R-wave amplitude in 3 different patients at 3 different amplitude levels (RWA: R-wave amplitude). (Vitatron DPG 1)

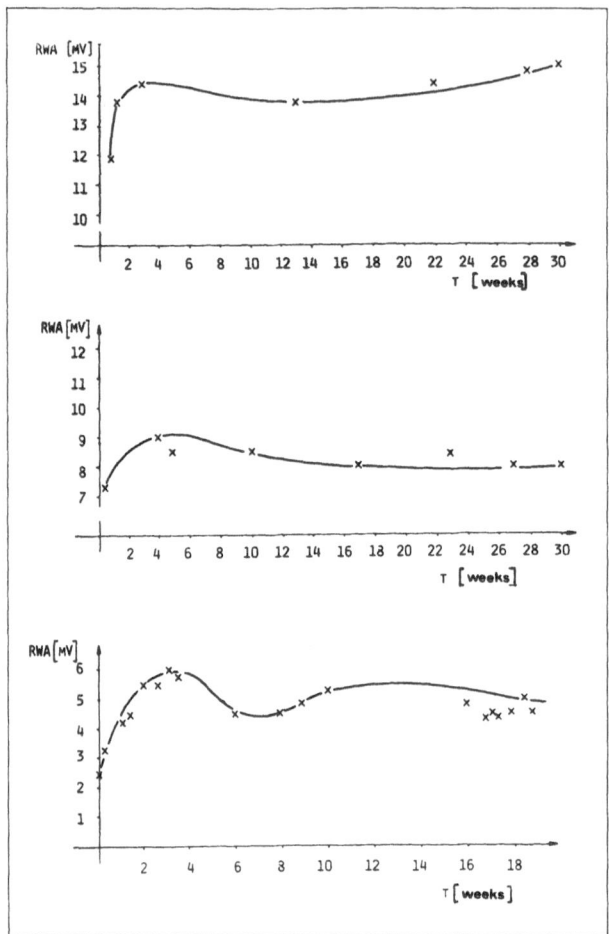

and chronic phase the variability of the R-wave amplitude was about 1.0 mV, being 10% and thus not significant in the acute period, but 33% and significant in the chronic stage. In the latter cases, the additional capability of a slew rate estimation would have been helpful.

Follow-up:

During a follow-up period of 20 weeks a biphasic or undulatory course of the R-wave amplitude was observed. The method of the signal amplitude determination seems to be more suitable for intraindividual comparison.

The biphasic course of the measured R-wave was confirmed by Stokes and Stephenson (6), who implanted Medtronic ring tip electrodes 6971 in dogs. They also found large standard deviations in looking at the interindividual comparison. According to our own experience the R-wave measurement system of the DPG 1 is not as sufficient as expected

42

for the follow-up of electrophysiological and morphological changes close to the electrode and for sensitivity adjustment.

Discussion

As reported before both measurement techniques have advantages and disadvantages. The DPG system is quickly and easily handled, but cannot be applied successfully in all cases. The Spektrax system is a time-consuming technique with recordings that have to be evaluated manually. The parameters have to be interpreted with caution since respiration and filters sometimes influence the signal amplitude significantly. But nevertheless this method has the advantage of enabling the physician to evaluate an ECG morphology, to measure parameters like slew rate, QRS width, intrinsic deflection, ST elevation etc. Thus, the information derived from the intracardiac electrogram is more complete. Especially with acute or chronic low signal amplitudes the slew rate gives additional help for the sensitivity adjustment. Low acute R-wave amplitudes may be due to:
1. reduced mass of the impulse generating myocardium (e.g. acute myocardial infarction);
2. early lead displacement; poor electrode position;
3. bundle branch block;
4. aberrant conduction pathways;
5. reduced contraction force;
6. cardio-active drugs.
Low chronic R-wave amplitudes are observed in the following cases:
1. reduced myocardial mass;
2. late lead displacement;
3. reduced contractility;
4. development of a fibrotic capsule around the electrode tip; active fixation electrodes; no fixation electrodes.
Thus, the decrease of the R-wave amplitude in the early post-implantation period may reflect the local tissue changes with temporarily reduced mass of impulse generating myocardium. This interpretation may be underlined by the observation that the ST elevation decreases in the first 90 minutes significantly (Winter et al., unpublished data). The late decrease of the R-wave amplitude may demonstrate the development of the fibrotic capsule around the scar.

Conclusions: sensitivity-guided pacing

During demand pacing the correct identification of the endocardial signals is an important prerequisite for the correct inhibition of the pacemaker. The estimation of the R-wave amplitude by the DPG 1 is not a complicated method, but was not so helpful for the sensitivity adjustment. The reasons for this are:
1. incredible R-values in 33% of 300 measurements;
2. in 8/23 (35%) patients insufficient measurement range;
3. variations of up to 33% in the chronic phase with low R-wave values;
4. impossibility of determining additionally the slew rate at low R-wave values.

The transmitted ICEG (Spektrax) in contrast delivered much more information for the "fine tuning" of the sensitivity. In future single chamber pacemakers the intracardially recorded electrogram should be transmitted to the monitor of the programmer in order to facilitate and shorten the total procedure. This is already realized in the dual chamber pacemaker AFP (Pacesetter). Furthermore, an automatic measurement device should be incorporated for the fast determination of the slew rate.

References

1. Barold SS, Ong LS, Falkoff MD, Heinle RA (1982) Programmable pacemakers: clinical indications, complications and future directions. In: Barold SS, Mugica J (eds) The third decade of cardiac pacing. Futura Publishing Co, New York, pp 27–76
2. Furman S, Wurzeler P, De Caprio V (1977) Cardiac pacing and pacemakers III. Sensing the cardiac electrogram. Am Heart J 93: 794–801
3. Furman S, Wurzeler P, De Caprio V (1977) The ventricular endocardial electrogram and pacemaker sensing. J Thorac Cardiovasc Surg 73: 258–266
4. Barold SS, Gaidula JJ (1971) Evaluation of normal and abnormal sensing functions of demand pacemakers. Am J Cardiol 28: 201–210
5. Wirtzfeld A, Himmler Ch, Lampadius M, Präuer H (1979) Analysen intraventrikulärer Elektrogramme für die Schrittmachersteuerung. Verh Dtsch Ges Kreislaufforschg 42: 251–254
6. Stokes K, Stephenson NL (1982) The implantable cardiac pacing lead – just a simple wire? In: Barold SS, Mugica J (eds) The third decade of cardiac pacing. Futura Publishing Co., New York, pp 365–416

Authors' address:
U. J. Winter, M.D.
Medizinische Universitäts Klinik III, Kardiologie
Joseph-Stelzmann-Straße 9
5000 Köln 41
West Germany

Progress in Holter Monitoring Towards an Implantable System

P. Attuel, A. Ripart, and J. Mugica

Summary: During the last decade, Holter recording has demonstrated good results in the diagnosis of paroxystic arrhythmias, improved knowledge of their induction mechanisms, and evaluation of therapeutic efficiency. Use of micro computers has allowed quantitative or semi quantitative evaluation of arrhythmias. Permanent recording of the endocardial signal leads to the determination of a rhythmic profile of implanted patients. New technical problems are seen. Unlike the external Holter, these difficulties are not related to the detection of electrocardiographic signals but are due to limited memory capacity. This constraint leads to statistical treatment of compressed or synthetic data, with edition of sequential classification of arrhythmias, frequency histograms, or numbered data. These possibilities make it as interesting as the external Holter.

Introduction

Long-term ambulatory electrocardiographic monitoring, Holter recording, has proven to be extremely valuable in detecting and treating cardiac arrhythmias. An implantable Holter device is justifiable because it can supply the electrocardiogram information obtained thanks to a continuous monitoring capacity with a higher quality due to an internal lead placement.

Technical limitations

There are three basic levels in external Holter monitoring.
- 24 h recording in an ambulatory patient analysis at 60 or 120 times the real time.
- The pre-processing unit can currently only take into account the R wave allowing the determination of the R-R interval, QRS duration and QRS polarity.
- A computerized quantitated evaluation classifies arrhythmias into different kinds of trends.

In an implantation Holter, we do not have a permanent storage medium, like for instance a magnetic tape, but a random access memory limited in its storage capacity. The daily output of a Holter needs about 16 Mbytes of memory per day. This capacity is not yet available, and will not be applied to pacemaker technology for several years.

For this reason, the implantable Holter realises real time pre-processing, usually taking endocardial ventricular activation into account with:
- an equal or a better detection of the QRS signal,
- a more difficult analysis of the duration,
- but on the other hand, better data analysis of polarity because of the possibility of cartography thanks to multiple leads.

Concerning the latter, the data processing is nevertheless comparable to the external Holter system to the extent that a microprocessor is as efficient as a large computer. Quantitative evaluation, histogram trend and arrhythmia classification are possible because of the storage of compressed data.

45

Clinical interest

All types of computerized data are thus theoretically available, which in practice permits us to expect the same results as in the external Holter device.

The first type of data is paroxysmal arrhythmia detection. Overall, the implantable Holter permits an appreciation of the relationship between the clinical evolution after pacemaker implantation and the occurrence of arrhythmias, and, furthermore, the study of triggering and mechanisms of arrhythmias (vagal tachyarrhythmia).

This type of tachycardia depends on bradycardia occurring generally at night or at rest. The analysis of such a case of interdependence could automatically command an overdrive of atrial stimulation which permits the prevention of tachyarrhythmias.

Of course, drug efficiency may not only be determined from a comparison of statistical data before and after treatment but also from histogram trends of the duration of effect of an i.v. drug in slowing down the rhythm of tachycardia without reduction.

However, a fundamental problem remains concerning the possibility of a long-term ECG recording. We have already stated that about a 16 Mbyte memory is necessary. For this reason, the implantable Holters available today are blind but generally if it is a question of statistical computerized evaluation, the event is already known and if this is not the case, simple answers to the onset of rapid tachycardias or abnormal bradycardias are of paramount importance in determining etiological investigations.

Authors' address:
P. Attuel, M.D.
Centre Chirurgical Val d'Or
Dpt. de Stimulation Cardique
16, rue Pasteur
F-92211 Saint-Cloud Cedex, France

Memory Technology and Implantable Holter Systems

A. Ripart and P. Jacobson

Summary: Progress made in the field of semiconductor integration has enabled the introduction of a Holter function into pacemakers. Various methods are used for the storage and selection of data. The memories must comply with the specific pacemaker characteristics: low current drain, high capacity, low voltage, high reliability. CMOS (complementary metal-oxide semiconductor) technology is now used with several circuit configurations. The CMOS circuit memories are directly linked to the silicium lithography and piling methods, which are regularly and rapidly improving. For a given circuit memory, the few seconds of ECG storage available with the technology of 1980 will be increased to several hours by 1990.

The introduction of microcomputers in implantable cardiac pacemakers has allowed the analysis and storage of various data concerning:
– the *patient file,* such as date, place and reasons for implanting a pacemaker, model and serial numbers of leads and pulse generator used, programmed pacing parameters, associated therapy,
– *pacemaker functions,* such as voltage values or current thresholds, lead impedance, R wave or P wave amplitude measured during follow-up,
– *electrophysiological* synthetic information, such as bradycardia detection, ratio sense to pace, number of premature beats, of detected PMTs etc. (1–3). And, with the advent of rate responsive pacemakers:
– *hemodynamic function* characterized by the value of various physiological parameters such as respiration rate and central venous temperature, which can be recorded by means of reliable implantable sensors.
With the added storage of sampled electrograms, the memorization of all this information leads to a wider concept of the "Implantable Holter Function" [4].
The aim of this paper is to outline the technical progress made in this field during recent years and the goals of the near future.
How much data does one need to record?
A moderate quality single channel ECG can be represented by taking 100 samples per second and storing 4 bit words (2^4 bits = 16 possible values) representing the amplitude at the points where the measurements are taken. A simple calculation shows that the complete recording of 24 h ECG needs a storage capacity of approximately 35 million bits (5).
How can one compress so much data?
The ECG consists of more or less rapid deflexions and mainly of isopotential portions. Real time analysis could be performed by a microcomputer driven pacemaker in order to keep only useful information (6). The isoelectric line which is the most common event can be described with only a few words of memory, and the characterization of P and T waves does not need as many samples as an intrinsic deflexion of the R wave.
With such rather complex techniques which increase pacemaker consumption, one can reduce the data to be stored in a proportion of 5 to 10.

47

Another interesting method is the storage of time intervals between combinations of atrial or ventricular events, as for example: P-P intervals, R-R intervals, P-R intervals, etc. To improve the reduction of space required in the memory, only particular sequences will be stored. As for a classical "Holter" recording, a particular sequence will be stored only if additional criteria, such as number of premature beats or cycle length are met.

A simple way to use the available memory is to generate histograms. One example of this representation method is a histogram of R-R intervals taken from a standard VVI or AAI pacemaker (Fig. 1). Some years ago, at Cardiostim 80, we showed that if we use a *1 k × 4 bits* memory, which at the time was the state of the art, and if we divide the possible values the interval could take into channels 100 ms wide regularly spaced from 300 to 1200 ms, one can demonstrate that the capacity of a channel would not be overloaded even for a constant heart rate during 6 days of cardiac activity, with histograms generated every 6 hours. With one histogram per week, the memory could store between 5 and 6 months of cardiac activity [5].

In conclusion, the size of the information to store in a single channel 24 hour ECG recording may be estimated between a few bits to $> 10^7$ bits according to the degree of analysis required.

Which are the most important criteria for selecting an implantable memory?

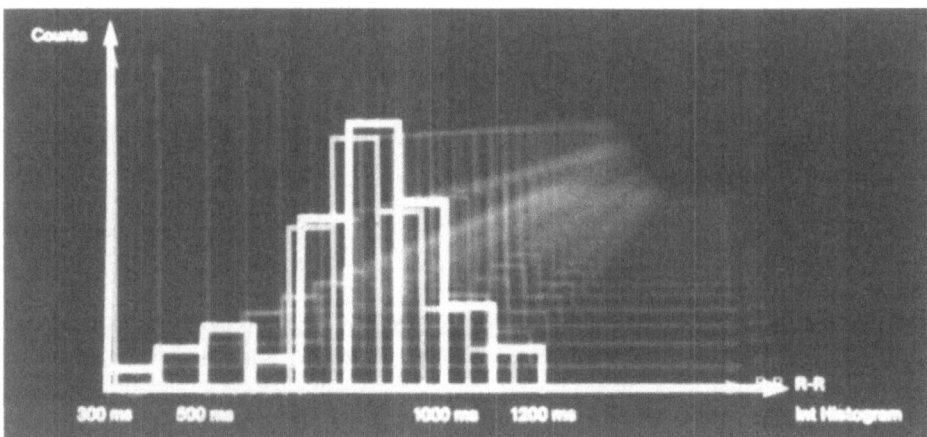

Fig. 1: The generation of histograms is another way to use the memory available. If we divide the possible values of the R-R interval into channels 100 ms wide, regularly spaced, with one histogram recorded per week, a 1 k × 4 bits memory included in a VVI pacemaker can store up to 5 months of activity. (Reproduced from Ripart and Jacobson (5) The Third Decade in Cardiac Pacing, with permission from Futura Publishing).

1. Quiescent current

This must be sufficiently low to avoid:
– lifetime shortening of the device first designed as an implantable cardiac pacemaker, and
– titanium case oversize, so that an adequate longevity is kept by increasing the capacity of the cell and then of its volume.

48

For a modern pacemaker, the current consumption needed for a Holter function should not exceed 3–5 μA, according to the complexity of the design (telemetry speed, anti-tachycardia function etc.).

The current drawn by the device when it is neither being read nor written must be very low, since if only synthetic information is stored, an implantable Holter will spend 99% of its time in this mode.

2. Capacity

The greatest possible storage capacity must be available, with low current and voltage operations. The size should be sufficient to store significant ECG segments and long-term synthetic information.

3. Reliability

As with any implantable component, the memory must feature maximum reliability.

4. Low voltage

The memory should operate directly with currently available lithium iodine cells, that is, at a voltage supply between 1.8 and 2.8 V. The requirement for high capacity led some years ago to the belief that the magnetic bubble memory could be used. Magnetic bubble memories store information in mobile magnetic fields created within an orthoferrite slab, a component which allows for magnetization much more easily in one direction than at right angles to that preferred direction [7]. In fact the large size of the chip, the awkward read/write mechanism, and the progress made in CMOS (complementary metal-oxide semiconductor) technology have decreased the interest in this component and bubble memories have now been abandoned by most manufacturers.

The requirement for minimum quiescent current makes CMOS technology the preferred choice for an implantable memory. Figure 2 shows a basic CMOS memory cell. Two

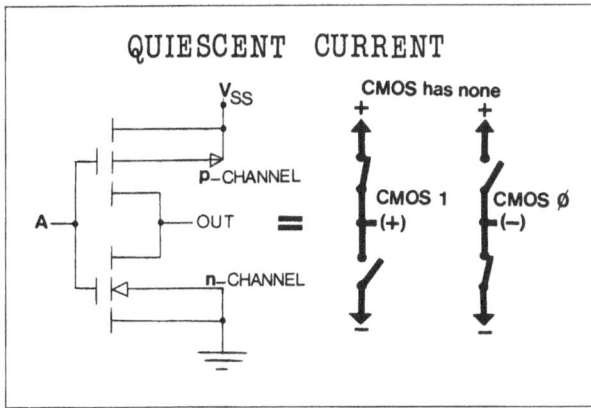

Fig. 2: Design and function of a CMOS switch. When the N channel is opened, the P channel is closed, so no quiescent current is requested in the steady state.

complementary switches are connected in series across the power supply. When the top switch (P channel) is closed the bottom switch (N channel) is open. The memory value is "1" as the output is at V_{ss}. In the opposite case (at right), the value of the memory cell is "O" as the output is at the ground. The value of the output follows the value of the voltage A. $V_{out} = \overline{A}$.

In either case, no current leaks from the supply during storage. Only a small current leaks when the device changes state, due to the fact that both switches close simultaneously for an instant, and also because of parasitic capacities, particularly on the transistor gates.

One common way to store information is to use this parasitic effect and to utilize the CMOS gate input capacitance as a memory cell. Another MOS transistor is then used to transfer the information from the data line to the capacitor (Fig. 3). The main advantage of such a structure commonly used in dynamic RAM (random access memory) cells is the low number of transistors used, 3 for a standard cell, which allows a high level of integration. The main disadvantage is the necessity of periodic memory refreshing as, because of the small value of the capacity, leakage currents tend to discharge the capacitor. Refreshing the memory increases current consumption and dynamic CMOS RAM cells are mostly used if the memory size is reduced, for example, a memory for programmed pacing parameters of a VVI or DDD pacemaker.

Fig. 3. Dynamic CMOS RAM cell: the input capacitor C of a CMOS gate is used as a memory. Another MOS transistor is used to transfer the information from the data line and charge or discharge the capacitor.

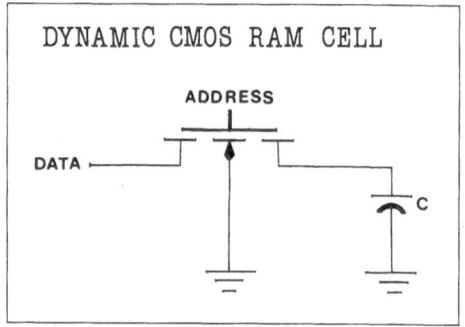

Fig. 4. Static CMOS RAM cell: C is the data line, R is the read/write command. No static current is needed, but the basic memory cell has six transistors.

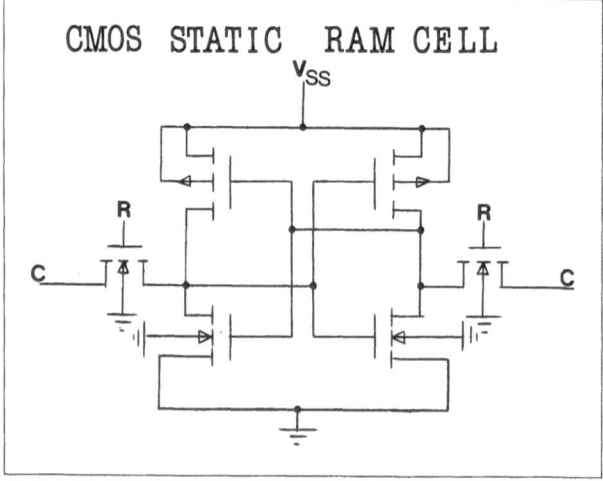

Reduction of current consumption may be obtained by the use of a more complex cell architecture. The basic design of a purely static CMOS cell, i.e. without any valuable quiescent current consumption, needs 6 transistors (Fig. 4).

What is the state of the art in CMOS memory that one could use in a pacemaker? There is a gap of a few years between the appearance of a new unproven semiconductor technology and its application in life support systems. Obviously the reason for this is the need to accumulate sufficient data on the reliability of new components. CMOS microprocessors or microcomputers manufactured in the mid 1970s were used in implantable units only in the early 1980s.

Another difficulty in describing the state of the art is the high rate of progress, characterized mainly by the conductor's required line width reduction. This width reduction (by two) divides the cell memory area by four. During the last decade integrated circuit capacity has doubled each year. This means that each year more electronic functions are engraved on silicon than the sum of all the functions integrated from the beginning.

In 1980 a CMOS memory which could be used in a pacemaker had 4096 bits (4 k) organized in 1024 (1 k) words of 4 bits. A practical version of this chip had a 2 micron line width, for conductors. Today we can find a 2 k × 8 bits memory with a similar size chip, and a capacity increased by 4. This integration level is far from the present technology border: new memories have been released recently on the commercial market with capacities up to 64 k × 1 bit for dynamic CMOS cells and 8 k × 8 bits for static CMOS cells, with a line width for conductors close to 1 μm [8]. Therefore today it is possible to integrate more than 600,000 transistors on a 6 × 6 mm size single chip. Moreover the increasing memory density required a reduction of supply voltage from 5 V in 1980 to less than 2 V now as the insulation distance between adjacent conductors becomes very small. Consequently the power dissipated in the chip does not vary as much as the number of gates integrated, as the consumption of each one is reduced. This last point is very important for a designer as we can look forward to being able to increase ECG time recording without a drastic reduction of pacemaker longevity.

What will the near future bring?

Thanks to the time gap between the existing most advanced semi-conductor technology and its application to pacemakers, the near future is now predictable.

The memory capacity increase will come from:

1. Line width reduction. Present photo lithographic techniques are limited to 1 micron line width. UV lithography allows a 0.75 micron definition, which electron beam or X-ray lithography could allow a reduction in the line width to 0.1 μm. IBM bas announced integrated circuits with 0.5 micron line width. Some laboratories [9] have pro-

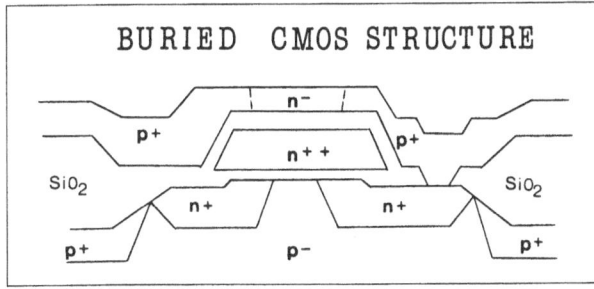

Fig. 5. Three dimensional (3D) CMOS design. In the buried CMOS structure the gate is folded and N and P channels are superimposed, thereby providing reduction of the gate surface area.

51

duced experimental 0.3 micron designs. The enormous cost of machinery to implement these new processes limits high density memory production to a few manufacturers.

2. Interconnection level increase. Standard CMOS technology has three levels. By going from 3 to 6 levels one may increase the percentage of the chip covered by memory cells. This is counter-balanced by the main disadvantage of a reduction of the manufacturing yield.

A more promising solution seems to be the use of 3D (three dimensional) structures. In buried CMOS structure, the CMOS gate is folded and the N channel and P channel are superimposed (Fig. 5). This provides an important reduction in the gate surface area. In addition 3D structures are not sensitive to latch-up phenomena. This might be an efficient protection for integrated circuits from transient reverse voltage applied between bulk substrate and input/output ports.

Conclusion

In 1980 the available technology only allowed a few seconds of endocardial ECG storage. Today it is possible to record a few minutes. We believe that in 1990 it will be possible to integrate 10 million transistors on the same chip, which will then allow storage of several hours.

Nevertheless one wonders whether the energy needed for storing and then reading this permanent data might affect the pacemaker lifetime. It is perhaps more interesting to strictly select the events to be stored and the results' synthetic presentation.

The saved capacity would then lead to a more reliable system and to better defined RAM stored program instructions.

References

1. Edhag O, Vallin H (1978) An implantable bradycardia-indicating pacer. First European Symposium on Cardiac Pacing. London, May, 1978
2. Attuel P, Mugica J, Buffet J (1978) The diagnostic pacemaker. First European Symposium of Cardiac Pacing. London, May, 1978, p 83
3. Mugica J, Coumel P, Attuel P (1981) Holter implantable, concept de stimulation cardiaque avec fonction Holter incorporée. Arguments cliniques. In: Mugica J (ed) Cardiostim 80-SEPFI, Paris, 1981
4. Ripart A, Fontaine G, Mugica J (1984) How should the software pacemaker be programmed during manufacturing and after implantation? PACE 7: 1202
5. Ripart A, Jacobson P (1982) Memory technology and implantable Holter systems. In: Barold S, Mugica J (eds) The third decade of cardiac pacing. Futura Publishing, Mount Kisco, New York
6. Ripart A, Jacobson PM, Dalmolin R (1984) Clinical value of a microcomputer in an implantable pacemaker. In: Quetglas GM et al (eds) The applications of computers in cardiology. Elsevier Science Publishers, Amsterdam
7. Texas Instruments Documentation TIB 0303, Dallas, Texas
8. Nippon Electric Company (1984) New Memory Products Brochure. NEC GmbH, Düsseldorf
9. LETI Rapport d'activité 84. CEN G Grenoble

Authors' address:
A. Ripart
Ela Medical S.A.
100 rue Maurice Arnoux
92120 Montrouge
France

Value and Limitations of the Holter Functions of a Single Chamber Diagnostic Pacemaker

U. J. Winter, D. W. Behrenbeck, Th. Brill, M. Höher, V. Hombach, and H. H. Hilger

Summary: Modern Holter ECG devices offer a whole variety of different recording, analysis and data presentation techniques as well as a high sensitivity. Developments in the field of CMOS technology have increased the memory capacity in implantable pacemakers. Whereas earlier diagnostic pacemakers offered only 1 or 2 diagnostic features (e.g. indication of bradycardias or tachycardias) the recently developed diagnostic pulse generator DPG 1 (Vitatron) has several Holter functions.

The aim of the study was to investigate the clinical reliability of these Holter functions, especially in comparison with external Holter ECG devices. Therefore, 19 patients with symptomatic bradyarrhythmias were treated with the DPG 1 (15 VVI; 4 AAI) and a Helifix lead. The monitored data of the pacemaker were controlled by external 24-hour Holter ECGs (Ela Medical: Anatec). The Holter functions of the pacemaker included counting of stimulations, sensing, sense-to-pace events, bradycardias, tachycardias, premature beats and rate histograms. A 100% precision was found with the counter of stimulations, sensing, sense-to-pace events and bradycardias. Bradycardia counting, which is realized in this pacemaker by means of a negative hysteresis and the sense-to-pace counter, revealed false-positive results with small hysteresis values and false-negative results with large hysteresis values. Due to an inaccuracy of the premature beat and tachycardia counting, these Holter functions were not reliable. A differentiation of the premature beats according to morphology and origin was not possible in the single lead, single chamber device. Prematurity as detection criterion does not seem to be sufficient for a correct arrhythmia recognition. Also, tachycardias cannot be classified. In the DPG 1, the tachycardia counting is related to the use of the automatic underdrive mode. In contrast to external Holter ECG devices, ECG samples cannot be stored due to the limited memory capacity. The rate histogram offers a reliable long-term monitoring tool of cardiac activity, especially in patients with recurrent tachycardias during drug treatment.

In conclusion, the Holter functions of implantable single chamber devices offer new monitoring capabilities in pacemaker patients, but do not represent an alternative to external ECG devices. Holter monitoring in pacemaker patients should be improvable by a separate pacemaker spike recording track.

Introduction

The clinical problems concerning pacemaker patients suffering from obscure syncope or persisting symptoms after implantation led to the inauguration of a diagnostic pacemaker by J. Mugica et al. in 1978 (1). This pulse generator could indicate pauses by hysteresis circuitry. The progress in CMOS technology allowed the construction of software-guided pacemakers with extended memory functions. But until today continuous monitoring of the electrical activity of the heart by an implanted pacemaker, comparable to an external Holter device with recording of ECG samples, could not be realized due to limited space and storage capacity in the pacemaker. Currently available devices are able to count bradycardias, premature beats, tachycardias, the heart rate (rate histogram) and its own stimulations or inhibitions (2; see Table 1).

Table 1. Pacemaker with Holter functions (modified according to A. W. Nathan, see (2)).

Bradycardia indication	Tachycardia indication	Stimulation and sensing counter	Rate and interval analysis
Siemens Dialog P 38	Intermedics Cybertach 60	CPI Command Ultra I	Vitatron DPG 1
Teletronics Bradycardia indicating PM	Vitatron DPG 1	Teletronics Optima MPT	Cardiofrance Lidia 4
Vitatron DPG 1	Cardiofrance Lidia 4	Siemens Dialog 718 and 704	
Cardiofrance Lidia 3		Cardiofrance Lidia 4	
		Intermedics Cosmos	

Objective

The aim of this study was to determine the clinical value and limitations of the Holter functions of an implantable, software-based, single chamber diagnostic pacemaker (DPG1, Vitatron). We wanted to find out whether or not these memory functions in the present state of development are a helpful tool in non-invasive, long-term pacemaker patient follow-up.

General considerations: Holter-monitoring technique and automatic arrhythmia analysis

Ambulatory, long-term ECG recording or Holter monitoring:

Long-term ECG recording from the body surface with external recorders, mainly in English-speaking countries known as Holter monitoring, is now a well established diagnostic tool in clinical cardiology. This technique started with the radiotransmission of the ECG in 1949 (3, 4) and now includes small external recorders and computer-assisted or real-time ECG analysis, different types of data presentations and recording periods of 24 or 48 hours (5).

Holter function of implantable, single chamber devices:

The so-called Holter functions are, besides the analysis functions, diagnostic options of software pacemakers. In currently available pacemakers they include 1. bradycardia recognition (indication of bradycardia or bradycardia counting), 2. tachycardia detection (indication of tachycardia or tachycardia counting), 3. paced and sensed beats counters, 4. premature beat counters, and 5. rate as well as interval analysis with a graphic display as a rate histogram (2). Table 1 shows the different pacemakers with the various diagnostic functions, as they were developed during recent years. The term "Holter functions" has been in clinical use for some time. Despite the fact that the Holter functions of implantable pacemakers and the capabilities of modern ambulatory Holter monitoring are not really comparable in the present state of development, this term will be used in this article for the sake of simplicity.

Automatic arrhythmia analysis:

Modern, software-based arrhythmia monitoring systems in intensive or coronary care units use different arrhythmia recognition criteria in combination, in order to achieve a sufficient arrhythmia detection accuracy: 1. interval analysis; 2. form analysis; 3. cross correlations; 4. noise recognition; 5. Fourier analysis (6). But even with these large systems 100% accuracy could not be achieved.

Memory organisation

Memory organisation in ambulatory long-term ECG devices:

The external recorders use tapes or solid state memories for primary storage.

Memory organisation in the DPG 1:

The DPG 1 is a software pacemaker in which a microprocessor controls the ROM (read only memory) and the RAM (readable adressable memory) (see Fig. 1). The ROM contains the software routines and the fixed parameters. The RAM includes programmed parameters and functions, measurement and Holter data as well as optional software for investigational devices.

Holter functions of the DPG 1

In this study the Holter functions of the DPG 1 (Vitatron) were examined. The modes of function are explained below. The print-out of the telemetered Holter data is shown in Fig. 1.

Bradycardia counting:

In contrast to early bradycardia indicating pacemakers (Siemens-Elema, Teletronics etc.) the DPG 1 uses the programmable hysteresis function and the sense-to-pace counter for the determination of the number of bradycardias. Due to the programmed negative hysteresis (that means that the escape interval is significantly longer than the automatic interval) the spontaneous heart rate can drop to the preselected value before the pace-

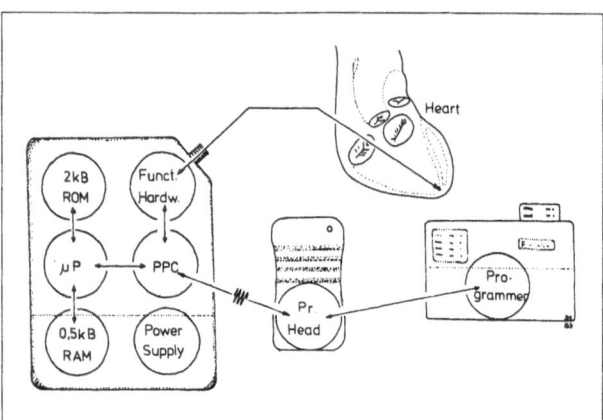

Fig. 1. Memory organisation in the diagnostic pacemaker Vitatron DPG 1 and the HP 85 personal computer.

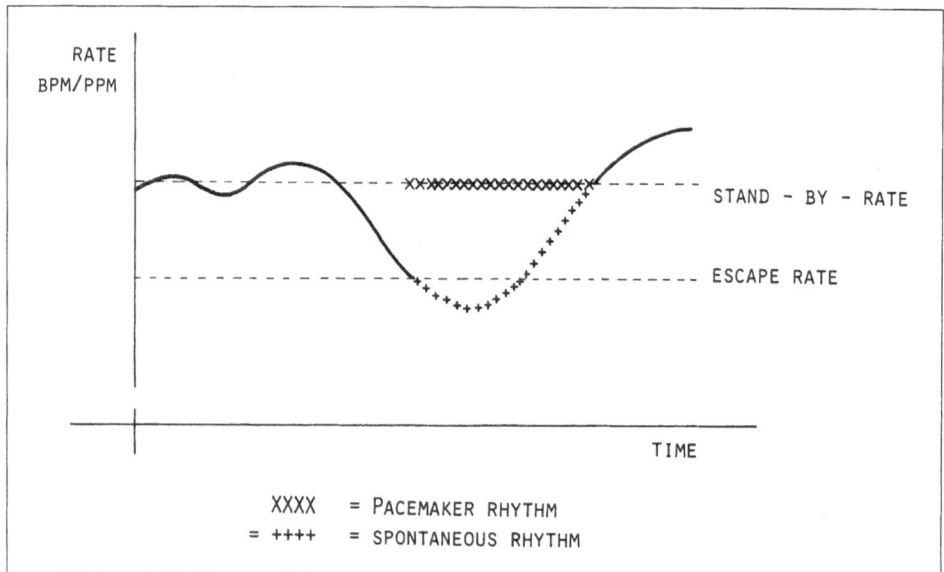

Fig. 2. Bradycardia counting using the negative hysteresis of the pacemaker. If the negative hysteresis is switched on, the spontaneous rate can drop to a preselected value below 70 bpm before the generator starts to pace. (Vitatron DPG 1)

maker starts to pace with the programmed stand-by rate (Fig. 2). The number of sensing and paced events during the observation period indicates the number of bradycardias.

Tachycardia counting/TC:

With the antitachycardia mode "automatic underdrive" switched on the tachycardia counter is set up as 1, if the tachycardia exceeds a preselected rate limit (Fig. 3).

56

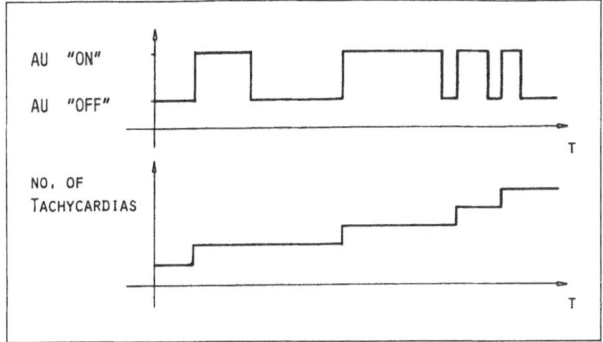

Fig. 3. Tachycardia counting is realized using the automatic underdrive pacing mode. If a tachycardia exceeds a preselected rate limit 1 will be added to the tachycardia counter. (Vitatron DPG 1)

Stimulation – inhibition counter/STIC:

This counter records the number of stimulations and inhibitions of the pacemaker. It reflects the pacemaker dependence of the patient and the energy consumption of the pulse generator.

Sense-to-pace counter/STPC:

The counter within the sensing and stimulation circuit measures the events of sensing and pacing.

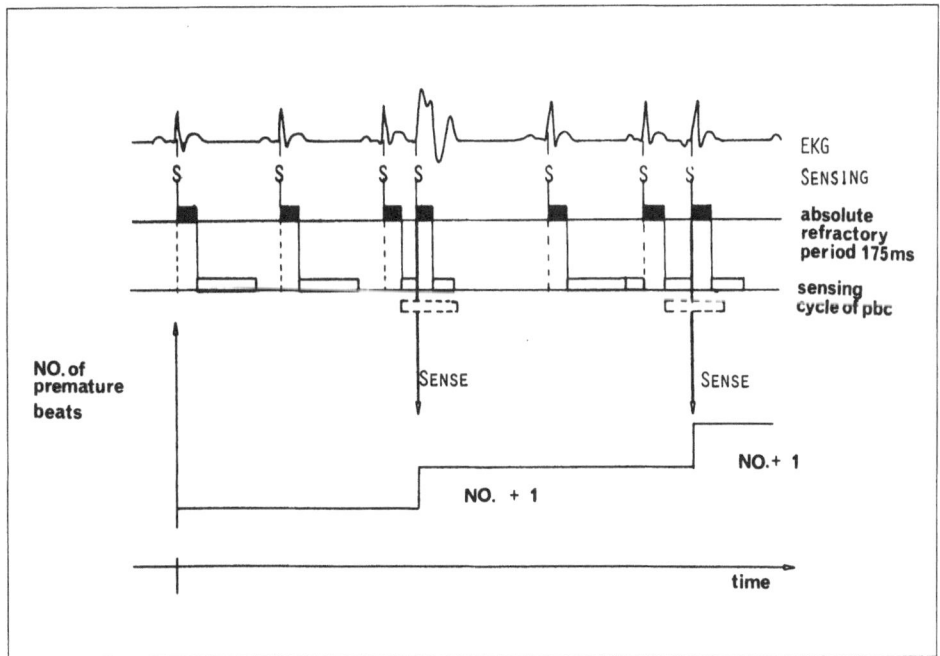

Fig. 4. Working mechanism of the "premature beat counter" in a single lead, single chamber pacemaker using the prematurity criterion. (Vitatron DPG 1)

Premature beat counter/PBC:

Premature beat counting in this pacemaker is a special type of interval analysis (time-window principle). Signals which are detected after a time period which is 12.5 or 25.0% shorter than the preceding R-R interval are classified as premature beats (Fig. 4). The recognition of premature events is highly influenced by the sensing characteristics of the individual pacemaker-lead system. This kind of ES detection is realized in most of the modern single or dual chamber devices.

Interval and rate analysis: heart rate histogram:

Figure 5 shows how the heart rate histogram is obtained. During the monitoring period, each R-R interval is measured and the value designated as 1 in a register which corresponds to 8 preprogrammed classes of heart rate in the rate histogram. Thus, the external HP 85 computer can construct a rate histogram in which the number of beats in each rate register is indicated by its absolute values and is graphically designed by columns. Furthermore an alternating and a continuous histogram can be alternatively performed.

Fig. 5. The heart rate histogram is constructed by entering the determined value of each R-R interval in one of the 8 preselected rate registers. (Vitatron DPG 1)

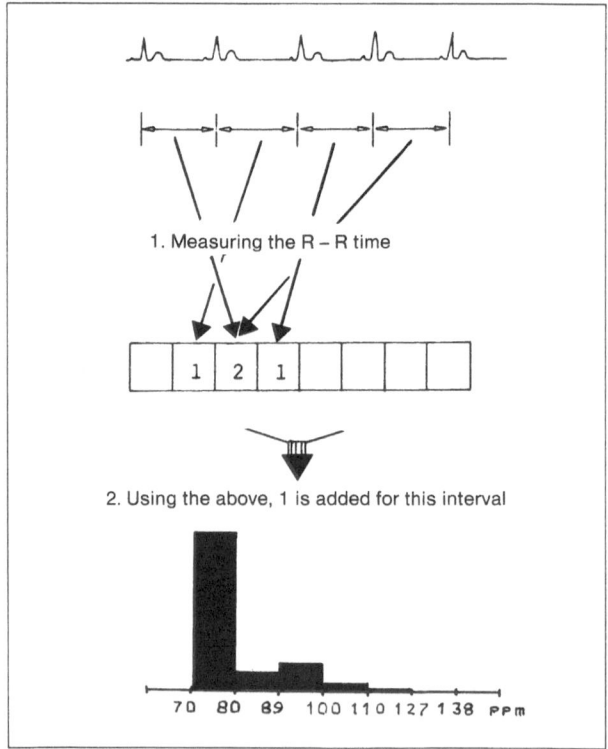

Validation of the pacemaker's Holter functions by a continuous Holter ECG device: methodological considerations

The validation of the pacemaker's Holter functions by an external Holter ECG device is difficult, for several reasons: 1. the arrhythmia recognition is performed in both systems in different ways (Holter ECG: prematurity and morphology; DPG 1: prematurity alone); 2. the signals are detected at different places (Holter ECG: body surface; DPG 1: right ventricular apex); 3. the kind of data storage is different; 4. front end processing in the DPG 1; 5. external Holter ECG devices mainly reach a sensitivity of $\geq 95\%$; 6. different pacemaker spike recognition (DPG 1: stimulation circuit; pacemaker Holter ECG: special spike recognition algorithm). In computer-assisted analysis of continuously recorded 24-hour Holter ECGs the following criteria are used to differentiate arrhythmias: 1. time interval; 2. maximal velocity of voltage change of the R wave; 3. signal width; 4. planimetry of the signal. A systematic recognition of P waves, P-R intervals and T waves is not possible at this time (5). In contrast to the external Holter devices currently available, implantable pacemakers are able to detect extrasystoles only on the basis of prematurity (time interval). Whereas signal recognition from the body surface can be disturbed by noise and artefacts, the endocardial recording site has a high signal-to-noise ratio. Furthermore the Holter functions of pacemakers cannot store real-time ECG samples as the external ones are able to do. Even external Holter ECG devices do not reach 100% precision, since R waves, ventricular extrasystoles, P waves, T waves, muscle potentials and noise, caused by movements of the body, have a similar frequency content (5). As investigated by Höpp and Osterspey (5) even modern continuous Holter ECG devices show significant discrepancies in bradycardia, premature beat, tachycardia etc., recognition. At the time when our study was performed there was no continuous Holter ECG device with special pacemaker spike detection algorithm clinically available. Knowing all these limitations we used the Holter device for continuous, 24-hour tape-recording, audiovisual (1 : 100) and computer-assisted analysis. But also audiovisual control of continuous 24-hour tape recordings do not have 100% accuracy (5).

Methods

Patients:

The DPG 1 (15 VVI, 4 AAI) and a Helifix lead were implanted in 19 patients (56 ± 15 years, 3 female, 16 male) with different bradyarrhythmias in combination with atrial fibrillation and VES, due to CHD.

Holter ECG:

The Holter functions were controlled by recording 24-hour Holter ECGs (Anatec, Ela Medical, n = 48). The tapes were examined visually (1 : 100) and with computer assistance.

Holter functions of the pacemaker:
Bradycardia counting:

The bradycardia counting option of the DPG 1 was investigated in 6/19 patients with bradyarrhythmias. Starting at zero, the value of the negative hysteresis was successively increased by 10 ppm every 24 hours, until the patients showed symptoms due to the low heart rate. The 24 h observation periods were monitored by continuous 24 h Holter ECG (Anatec) and the sense-to-pace counter which was reset to zero before the onset of a new measurement. Thus, the number of sense-to-pace events could be compared with the number of bradycardias identified from the Holter tape by the analysis computer and visual control.

In 1 patient with hypersensitive carotid sinus syndrome we compared bradycardia counting by the DPG 1 with the conventional ECG which was recorded during repetitive carotis sinus massage.

Tachycardia counting:

In 4 patients with the AAI (n = 3) and VVI mode (n = 1) and recurrent supraventricular tachycardias the automatic underdrive mode was switched on. In the case of tachycardia recognition the tachycardia counter was increased by 1. The tachycardia number was controlled by automatic and visual analysis of the Holter tape.

Premature beat counting:

The precision of the premature beat counter with the 25% prematurity criterion was tested in 8 patients, mainly suffering from coronary heart disease (Table 2). The detection of extrasystoles in single chamber, one lead systems based on prematurity is mainly dependent on optimal sensing. The sensitivity was individually adjusted in each patient. All 8 patients had the same, non-traumatic Helifix lead (Vitatron).

Table 2. Patient group for the evaluation of the Vitatron DPG 1 premature beat counter (PBC)

Patients:	n = 8, age 61 ± 11	
	Male: 7; Female: 1	
Underlying diseases:	CHD: n = 7	MVR: n = 1
Arrhythmias:	Atrial flutter / fibrillation	: n = 2
	Stable sinus rhythm	: n = 6
	Stable sinus rhythm + VES	: n = 1
	Stable sinus rhythm + VES/SVES	: n = 5
	Few SVES	: n = 4
	Many SVES	: n = 1
Bradycardias:	Carotid sinus syndrome	: n = 2
	Sinus bradycardia	: n = 1
	Sick sinus syndrome	: n = 1
	Atrial fibrillation with intermittent bradycardias	: n = 1

The patients who were monitored had the following arrhythmias (see Table 2): atrial fibrillation: 2/8; stable sinus rhythm plus VES: 1/8; stable sinus rhythm plus VES and SVES: 5/8. The kind and incidence of the extrasystoles were controlled by 24-hour Holter monitoring.

Stimulation-inhibition counter:

The number of stimulations and inhibitions were controlled by automatic examination of the tape.

Rate analysis and rate histogram:

The 8 classes of heart rates, ranging from 30 bpm to 250 bpm, were individually programmed. After a control period of 24 hours the data of the rate histogram were visualized on the monitor screen (HP 85) and then printed out, containing absolute numbers of the beats and the rate histogram itself. Using the rate trend and histogram feature of the Anatec, the DPG's heart rate histogram was controlled.

8. Results

Bradycardia counting:

In 6/19 patients in whom the bradycardia counting was tested the tolerance of increasing escape intervals was individually different. We found (see Fig. 6) that with large values of negative hysteresis the number of false-negative bradycardia indications increased, whereas small values of hysteresis were followed by an increasing number of false-positive results. With the individually different, "optimal" value of negative hysteresis, 100% cor-

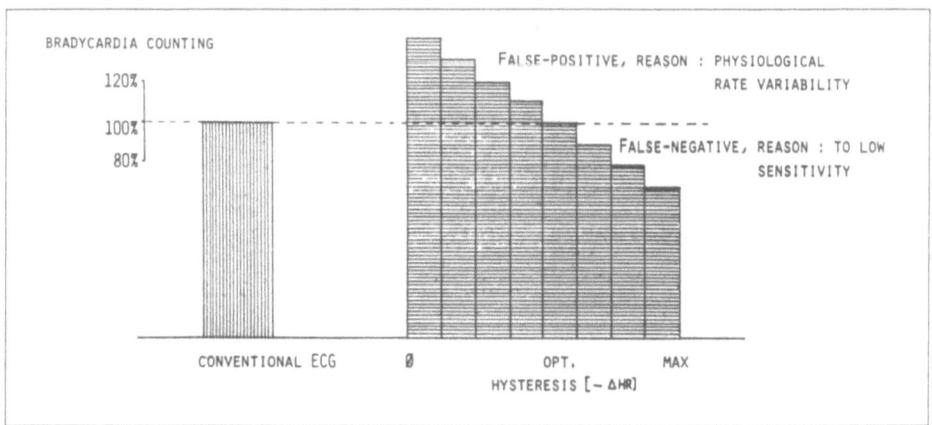

Fig. 6. Large values of negative hysteresis produce an increased number of false-negative bradycardia indications, small values cause many false-positive bradycardia recognitions. (Vitatron DPG 1)

rect bradycardia counting could be achieved. Also, bradycardia indication during carotid sinus massage in one patient with hypersensitive carotid sinus was accurate. In the external Holter ECG device, bradycardia recognition was always misled by baseline shifts.

Tachycardia counting:

Tachycardia counting always revealed false-positive results in 4 patients, since the tachycardia recognition system was always misled by sinus tachycardias (young and active patients). But even supraventricular tachycardias were not always correctly recognized (1 patient with fever and supraventricular tachycardias). According to our experience the single chamber lead pacemaker cannot differentiate sinus, supraventricular and ventricular tachycardias.

Premature beat counting:

Premature beat counting by the VVI pacemakers revealed false-positive data in patients suffering from atrial fibrillation, supraventricular or ventricular extrasystoles. Only in 1/8 patients with stable sinus rhythm and one type of premature beat was sufficient precision achieved. A differentiated extrasystole analysis with respect to origin (SVES – VES) or type (polymorphous-monomorphous salvo couplets) as performed by external Holter ECG devices cannot be obtained with this single chamber lead device.

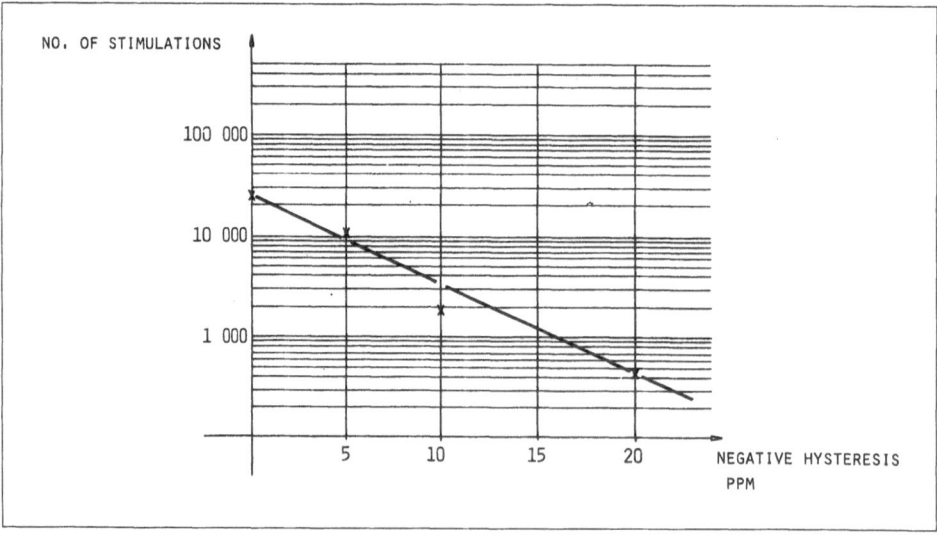

Fig. 7. With increasing value of negative hysteresis a decreasing number of stimulations and thus increasing energy conservation are achieved in a patient with intermittent bradyarrhythmia. (Vitatron DPG 1)

Stimulation-inhibition counter and sense-to-pace counter:

The precision of the STIC and STPC must be assumed to be 100%. Since the Holter ECG device had no special pacemaker spike recognition, the number of pacemaker spikes indicated by the Anatec was mostly too low as compared with the pacemaker's STIC. The STPC and STIC were found to be helpful in adjusting the negative hysteresis for energy conservation. Figure 7 shows the increasing reduction of the stimulation number with rising value of the negative hysteresis in one patient suffering from intermittent bradyarrhythmias (semilogarithmic graphic design). Similar findings were obtained in another 5 patients with bradyarrhythmias.

Rate histogram:

The programmable, 8 classes of heart rate gave sufficient flexibility. The absolute numbers indicated (in the columns of the histogram) gave no clinically important information. Figure 8 shows the repeatedly controlled rate histogram of a patient suffering from recurrent supraventricular tachycardias (VVI pacemaker) during treatment with increasing doses of propanolol. Before the onset of β-blocking drug therapy, the heart rates were between 70 and 110 bpm. During propanolol treatment (2×40 and 2×60 mg p.o.), the mean heart rate was reduced to 70 to 80 bpm. Figure 9 demonstrates the clinical course of a female patient with tachyarrhythmias after successful mitral valve replacement. Combined therapy with quinidine and digitoxin led to a remarkable heart rate decrease until 25. 5. 1983. After this drug treatment was discontinued heart rate increased again until 27. 5. 1983. Figure 10 shows the follow-up of a patient with obesity, coronary heart disease and latent myocardial insufficiency. An intermittently occurring decrease of left ventricular pump function led to a further increase of the mean heart rate from 100 bpm to 120 and 140 bpm. After consequent saluretic therapy heart rate decreased to 100 bpm. The heart rate trends demonstrated above could be confirmed by the heart rate trend analysis of the external Holter ECG device. When the automatic underdrive was switched on, the indicated rate numbers were too high at the rate of active underdrive stimulation and too low at the rates in which the underdrive mode was activated. A comparison of

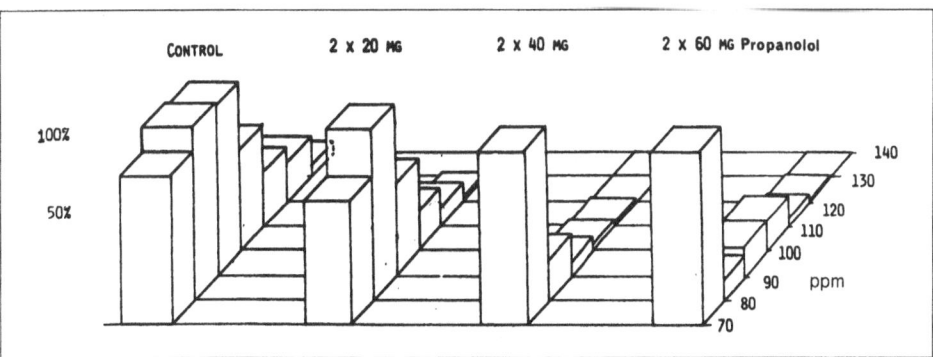

Fig. 8. Therapy control during the treatment of recurrent supraventricular tachycardias by increasing doses of propanolol using a heart rate histogram. (Vitatron DPG 1)

63

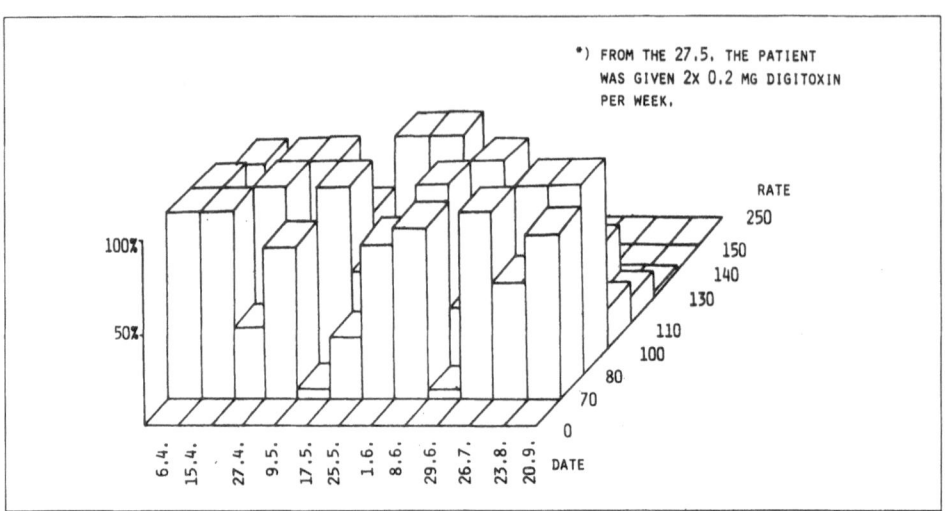

Fig. 9. Therapy control during treatment with quinidine and digitoxin. A remarkable heart rate decrease could be achieved until 25. 5. 1983. But when the patient refused further drug treatment heart rate increased again.

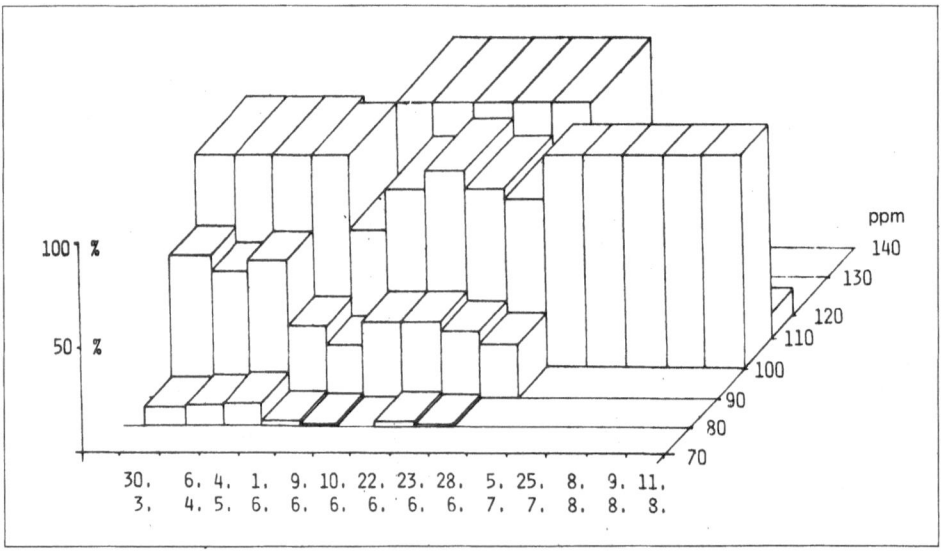

Fig. 10. Heart rate trend in a patient with marginal left ventricular pump function. (Vitatron DPG 1)

the rate histograms in the DPG 1 and the Anatec has been difficult, since the DPG 1 measures and counts rates, whereas the Anatec demonstrates R-R intervals with their relative incidence as histograms.

64

Discussion

Bradycardia counting:

Bradycardia indication, i.e. indication of 1 bradycardia, was performed by early devices, such as the Siemens Dialog P 38 and the Teletronics bradycardia system (2). It is still offered in a recently available pacemaker, the Cardiofrance Lidia III.

It sometimes takes a few days to find out the "optimal" value of negative hysteresis in each patient. In the case of large hysteresis values the sensitivity of bracycardia counting is too low. Small values of hysteresis cause false-positive results due to the physiological rate variability. Bradycardia counting with the help of hysteresis was the first diagnostic option inaugurated by J. Mugica et al. (1). The "optimal" value of negative hysteresis for bradycardia counting in our series was the lowest possible (only discrete symptoms like dizziness) rate plus 10 bpm. The detection of bradyarrhythmias in pacemaker patients can also be performed by Holter ECG or pacemaker Holter ECG devices. The recognition algorithms in these analysis machines are sometimes fooled by baseline shifts or artefacts (5, 7) with the consequence of false-positive indication of bradycardias or asystolic pause. Since Holter monitoring is limited mainly to observation periods of about 24 hours bradycardia counting in symptomatic pacemaker patients could be realized during long observation periods with this method. According to our experience patients with programmed long escape intervals (large value of negative hysteresis) should be monitored in parallel with pacemaker Holter ECGs in order to be able to distinguish pauses (due to the long escape interval) from failure to sense, if a sudden increase in pauses in the sense-to-pace counter is to be seen.

Tachycardia counting:

Tachycardia recognition by single chamber, single lead devices is still an unresolved problem. Introduction of multiple recording sites and electrodes as well as additional tachycardia parameters may improve tachycardia detection in future pacemakers.

Premature beat counting:

At the present state of development premature beat counting cannot be recommended. Future technological progress, such as dual chamber recognition, and extrasystole detection by means of mechanical or biochemical parameters, will perhaps improve premature beat counting.

Stimulation-inhibition counter and sense-to-pace counter:

The stimulation-inhibition counter and sense-to-pace counter are helpful and accurate in the follow-up of pacemaker patients, for instance allowing the control of energy conservation effects of hysteresis. Hysteresis can save energy, but also needs energy for driving the circuitry (8).

Furthermore an individual adjustment of the value of negative hysteresis is necessary since not all patients tolerate long escape intervals.

65

Rate histogram:

The capability of rate histogram recording over different time intervals is a clinical useful tool. Heart rate trend recording is possible for periods of about 24 hours. In contrast rate histogram recording with the implanted devices can be performed for several days or weeks. In the latter case discrimination naturally decreases. As shown in the figures a more dynamic approach of the graphic design makes heart rate trend analysis easier.

Time relation of the heart rate histogram and extrasystoles:

Digital data storage and limited memory capacity in the implantable unit lead to a condensation of all monitored parameters, such as heart rate, extrasystoles, sensing and pacing events etc., to numerical data. Physicians who are used to examining EGGs or rate trend etc. have some difficulty in managing the large amount of figures on the print-out. Furthermore a time related display of the rate histogram or the extrasystoles as shown by the Holter ECG print-out would lead to increased understanding of the figures.

Proposed technical improvements

Pacemaker functions:

In order to achieve a further increase of the internal storage capacity we propose either to expand the memory capacity of the RAM or to reduce the amount of stored data to an understandable and manageable level. Increased storage capacity would allow to store "snapshot" electrograms for better arrhythmia differentiation and a time indication of important stored data. RAM with a size of 1 k byte for example would perhaps allow morphological analysis or arrhythmias. Bhatt and Schober found that 20 M bytes are necessary for a 24-hour ECG storage with a band width of 100 kHz (9). Furthermore time indication of the arrhythmia events, improved extrasystoles and tachycardia differentiation should be realized.

Monitor program of the HP 85:

Programming should be easier and quicker using condensed software menus and EPROMs. A data storage facility should be available for each controlled patient in the HP 85.

Conclusions

As described above bradycardia counting (with the help of negative hysteresis and sense-to-pace counter), stimulation and sense-to-pace counting and rate histogram are accurate (precision: 100%) and helpful tools for the non-invasive follow-up of pacemaker patients. The advantages of the bradycardia counting functions compared to external Holter ECG are: 1. better signal-to-noise ratio, 2. less false-positive diagnosis due to baseline shifts or artefacts, 3. longer monitoring periods.

Furthermore it is understandable that any pacemaker has a better recognition of its own sensing and pacing than an external device can ever achieve. The monitoring of the heart rate can be performed during long periods, which is more cost-effective and practicable than the external Holter ECG system.

Tachycardia and premature beat counting cannot be recommended at the present state of technological development. But significant improvements will be realized in the foreseeable future.

The advantages and disadvantages of currently available, implantable Holter devices are listed in Table 3.

Table 3. Advantages and disadvantages of implantable Holter devices.

Advantages	Disadvantages
Less noise (intracardiac recording)	Limited storage capacity; therefore no storage of real-time electrogram
Immediate detection of sensing and pacing	No time relation of the recorded events
Monitoring periods > 24 hours easily performable	No data control due to front-end processing
Cost reduction	Recognition of extrasystoles only based on interval analysis (prematurity) and only in one chamber

References

1. Mugica J, Thornander H (1982) An experimental implantable "Holter". In: Feruglio GA (ed) Cardiac Pacing. Piccin Medical Books, Rome, pp 1311–1314
2. Nathan AW (1985) Comparison of different pacemakers with Holter functions. This volume
3. Holter NJ, Gengerelli JA (1949) Remote recording of physiological date by radio. Rocky Mt Med J 46: 747
4. Holter NJ (1957) Radioelectrocardiography: a new technique for cardiovascular studies. Ann NY Acad Sci 65: 913
5. Höpp HW, Osterspey A (1984) Long-term electrocardiography: basics and practical importance (Langzeit-Elektrokardiographie: Grundlagen und praktische Bedeutung). Boehringer Mannheim Study Series: Cardiological diagnostics. Boehringer, Mannheim
6. Meyer J (1983) Automatic arrhythmia analysis (automatische Arrhythmieanalyse) In: Schaper W, Gottwik MG (eds) Proceedings of German Society for Heart and Circulation Research, Vol 47 (Verhandlungen der Deutschen Gesellschaft für Herz- und Kreislaufforschung, Bd 47). Steinkopff Verlag, Darmstadt, pp 34–44
7. Shaw DB, Kekwick CA, Whistance A (1983) Bradycardia detecting pacemakers, scope in diagnosis. VIIth World Symposium on Cardiac Pacing, Vienna, PACE 6/3 (Part II): A-153
8. Berman ND, Dickson SE, Walker BM, Lipton IH (1982) Documenting the value of rate hysteresis. In: Feruglio GA (ed) Cardiac Pacing. Piccin Medical Books, Rome, pp 597–599
9. Bhatt S, Schober RC (1982) Holter monitoring using implanted pacemakers. In: Barold S, Mugica J (eds) The third decade of cardiac pacing. Futura Publishing company, Mount Kisco, New York, pp 333–343

Authors' address:
U. J. Winter, M.D.
Medizinische Universitäts-Klinik III, Kardiologie
Joseph-Stelzmann-Str. 9
5000 Köln 41
West Germany

Pacemaker Holter ECG: Value and Limitations in Follow-up of Pacemaker Patients

M. Höher, U. J. Winter, D. W. Behrenbeck, E. Vonderbank, H. W. Verhoeven, V. Hombach, and H. H. Hilger

Summary: Conventional Holter ECG devices have no separate track for the pacemaker spike recording. Thus, an exact differentiation of the underlying rhythm, pacemaker rhythm, background and pacemaker-related arrhythmias or pacemaker dysfunctions (failure to sense; failure to output; failure to capture) is not possible. This seems however to be important since several investigators found that up to 30% of pacemaker patients were symptomatic. The aim of the study was to investigate the clinical reliability of three different pacemaker Holter ECG devices (Del Mar Avionics: Trendsetter, Pacerecorder; Reynolds: Pathfinder; Ela Medical: Anatec). Therefore we performed 24-hour pacemaker Holter ECG recordings in 157 consecutive pacemaker patients (47 female; 83 male, age: 63 ± 12 years). The patients had 119 VVI, 5 AAI, 13 DDD, 5 DVI, 1 VAT and 14 rate adaptive pacemakers. In each patient a careful exploration of the anamnesis and symptoms was performed. A good signal quality can be achieved by careful electrode position and cable fixation, avoidance of high amplitude artefacts and electrostatic interference. An automatic analysis of the tapes is technically possible in VVI and AAI pacemakers. An additional visual control of the tapes should nevertheless be performed in each case. We found a high sensitivity combined with a high number of false-positive events. A differentiation of the rhythm, arrhythmias and pacemaker reactions was easily possible. Pacemaker dysfunctions could be separated according to type and incidence (I°: no dysfunctions; II°: 1 dysfunction per hour; III°: 1 to 30 dysfunctions per hour; IV°: 30 dysfunctions per hour). In some pacemaker Holter ECG devices, the differentiation of fusion beats from failure to sense is not always performed correctly. Failure to sense detected mainly in patients with premature ventricular beats, tachyarrhythmia and bundle branch blocks. Failure to output is often the consequence of false inhibition by noise. According to our data pacemaker patients at high risk are the following: patients with AV-block III° and increased ventricular vulnerability (VES Lown III°, IV°) or ≥ 1 pacemaker dysfunctions per hour.
In conclusion, the pacemaker Holter ECG is a time consuming technique, but a powerful diagnostic tool in pacemaker patient follow-up.

Introduction

Pacemaker (PM) patients are reported to have heart-related symptoms after PM implantation in about 10 to 30% (1–4). Several investigators proposed conventional Holter ECG as a useful differential diagnostic tool (1–4). But accurate follow-up of pacemaker patients with background arrhythmias, PM dysfunctions, unexplained discomfort and complex PM systems, such as rate responsive or antitachycardia PMs, is only possible with special PM Holter ECG devices (5, 6).

Objective

The aim of the study was to find out the clinical reliability of three different, currently available pacemaker Holter ECG devices. Furthermore, we wanted to look at the incidence of background arrhythmias and PM dysfunctions in consecutive PM patients of our PM surveillance clinic.

Method and patients

In newly developed PM Holter ECG devices the PM spikes are recorded additionally to the ECG signals from the body surface. They are electronically modified (rectangular impulses) and than stored on the second recording channel, allowing better PM spike detection. *157 patients,* 83 male, 47 female, aged 63 ± 12 years, with *47 different PM types* from 9 companies (119 VVI, 5 AAI, 13 DDD, 5 DVI, 1 VAT, 14 rate responsive VVI) were investigated 23 ± 25 (0.1–115) months after the implantation. Twenty-four hour pacemaker Holter ECGs were recorded using *3 different devices* (D: Del-Mar-Avionics 53, Pacerecorder; R: Reynolds, Pathfinder II 47; E: Ela-Medical, Anatec 57). The tapes were investigated by automatic and visual analysis (D 1 : 240, R 1 : 60; E 1 : 100). The *mean heart rate per hour and the percentage of paced beats were displayed.* The *PM dysfunctions* were classified as failure to sense (FTS) (Fig. 1), failure to capture (FTC) (Fig. 2) and failure to output (FTO) (Fig. 3).

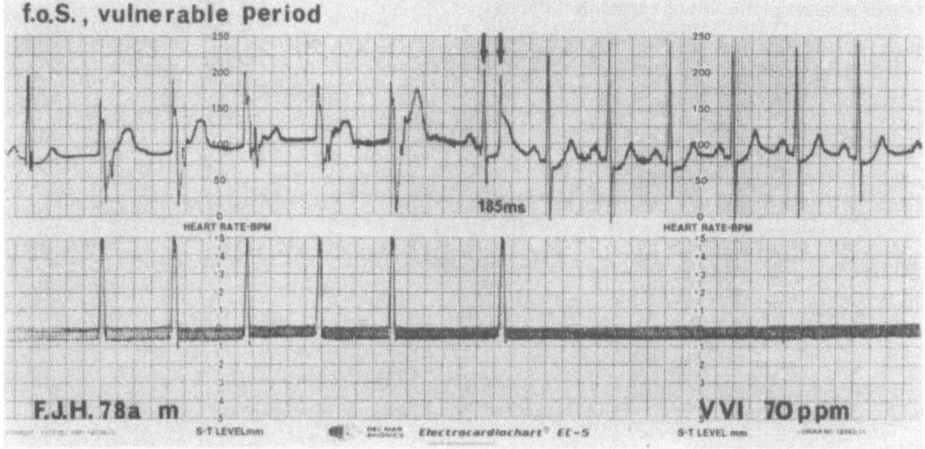

Fig. 1. In a 78 year old male patient a failure to sense led to a spike delivery (see the second channel with the pacemaker spike) in the vulnerable period.

Pacemaker dysfunctions

Failure to sense (FTS)

FTS may be due to 1. reduced signal amplitude and/or slew rate as well as bundle branch block, 2. electrode displacement, fracture or insulation defects, and 3. long technical refractory period of the pacemaker, defect of the sensing circuit or non-adjusted sensitivity. Sometimes FTS also causes FTO.

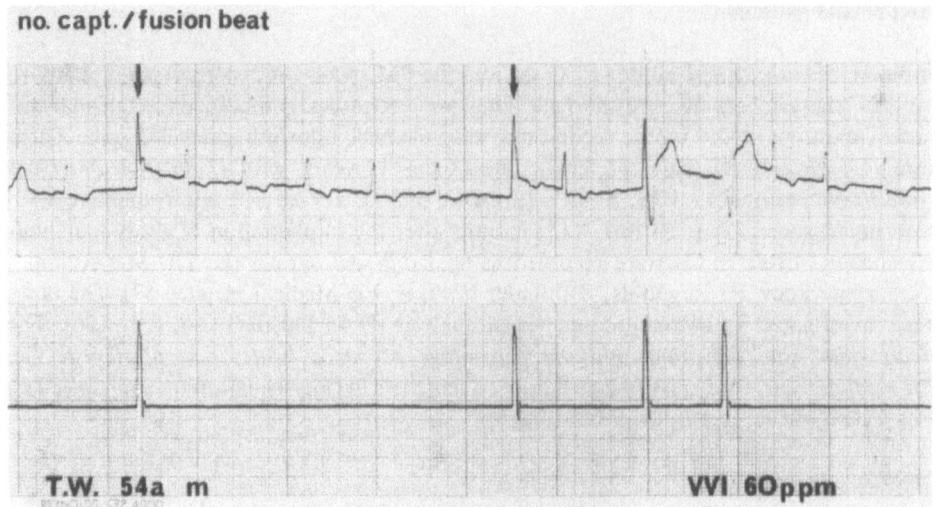

no. capt. / fusion beat

T.W. 54a m

VVI 60ppm

Fig. 2. The 24-hour pacemaker Holter ECG revealed several failures to capture. In a few cases a differential diagnosis from fusion beats was difficult.

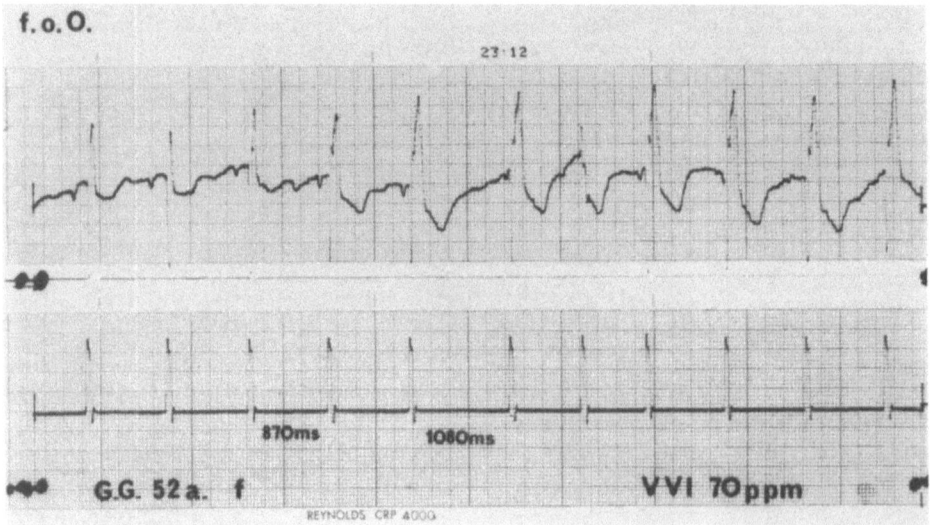

f.o.O.

23·12

870ms   1080ms

G.G. 52 a. f

VVI 70ppm

REYNOLDS CRP 4000

Fig. 3. During a sequence of regular pacing (interval of 870 ms) a sudden prolongation to 1080 ms occurs. The reason for this failure to output is not completely clear (T-wave sensing).

Failure to capture (FTC)

FTC may have the following reasons: 1. an increase of the pacing threshold; 2. appearence of leakage currents due to insulation defects or lead fractures; 3. impulse delivery during the refractory period of the myocardium as a consequence of FTS.

70

Failure to output (FTO)

Inhibition of the impulse delivery in demand pacemakers (by spontaneous cardiac activity, VES and tachyarrhythmias, muscle potentials, and by electromagnetic interference and artefacts) or a technical defect of the impulse delivery may be the reasons for FTO.

Entrance and exit block

According to previous nomenclature, FTS was termed entrance block, whereas FTC and FTO were termed exit-block.

Results

Signal quality

This could be significantly increased by choosing recording positions with a high signal-to-noise ratio on the body surface, low noise electrodes, avoiding electrostatic discharges (Figure 4) and excluding insulation defects of the wires.

Automatic analysis

This analysis is possible only in VVI and AAI PMs. A high sensitivity (95%) is combined with a high number of false-positive events, depending on the duration of the time windows taken for the analysis algorithm and QRS triggering (in the analysis device), on the stability of the tape velocity and on the signal-to-noise ratio in the recorder. Therefore *a visual control* of the events is necessary.

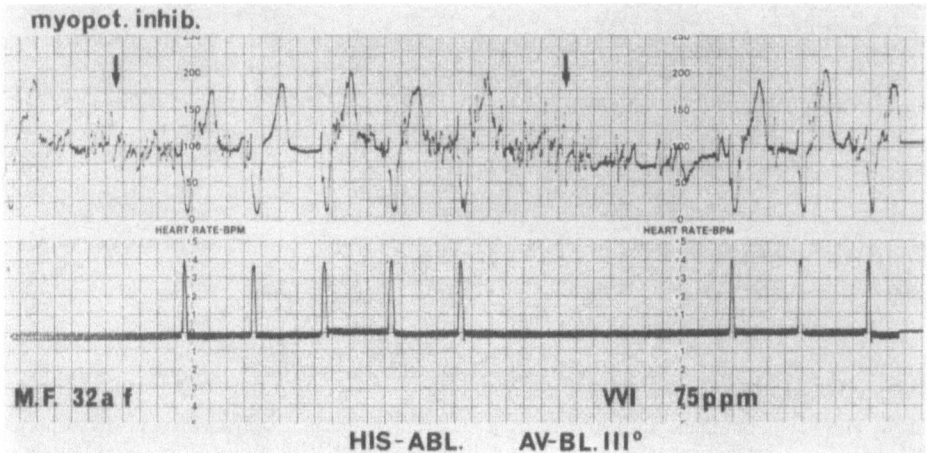

Fig. 4. This young nurse with AV-block III after His bundle ablation had multiple failure to output incidents due to myopotential inhibition.

Pseudo pacemaker spikes

Spikes which resemble pacemaker spikes without being such spikes are named *pseudo pacemaker spikes*. These spikes may be initiated by marker impulses of the pacemaker, may be due to a moving surface electrode, a crushed tape or a dirty recording head (Fig. 6). Furthermore they can be mimicked by muscle potentials, electromagnetic interference and high amplitude artefacts (Fig. 5).

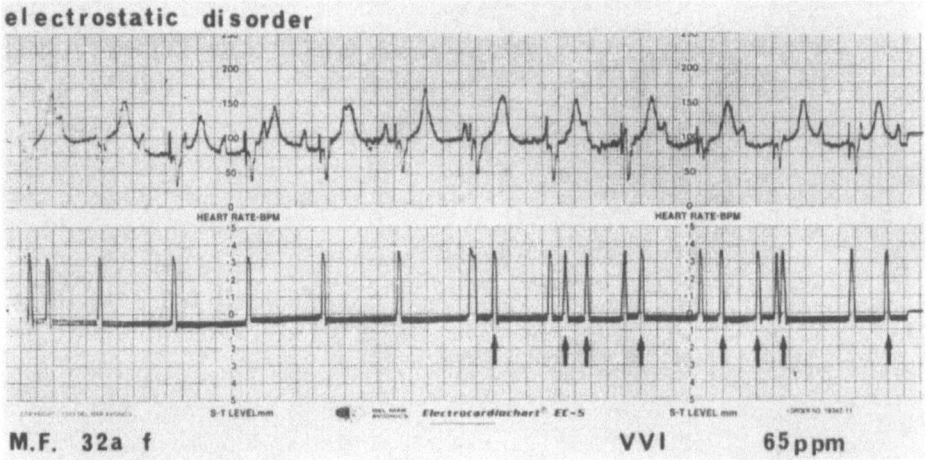

Fig. 5. In this young nurse complete AV-block could be achieved by His bundle ablation due to recurrent supraventricular tachycardias. The second channel of the recording showed many ,,spikes". Since telemetry of the software pacemaker demonstrated normal pacemaker function the signals between two spikes are electrostatic discharges.

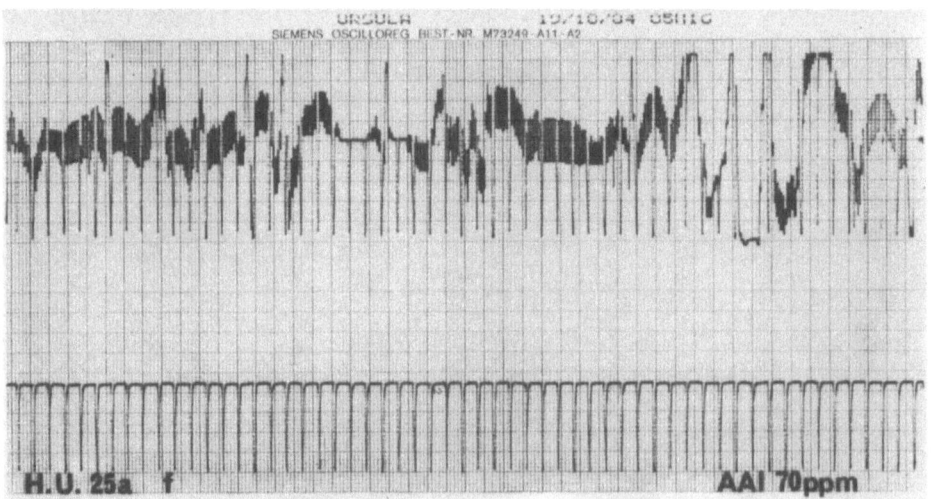

Fig. 6. This young physiotherapist suffered from recurrent ventricular tachycardias. It was suspected that the AAI pacemaker, switched to atrial overdrive pacing for VES suppression, could initiate or maintain the tachycardias. The high frequency signals in the second channel are caused by a moving surface electrode and thus mimic a pacemaker-mediated tachycardia.

Fusion beats

These are a combination of a spontaneous QRS complex and a pacemaker spike. They may reflect an interference of physiological and pacemaker-induced cardiac depolarisation, a non-synchronisation of the channel recordings, an incorrect position of the recording head, or an entrance and/or exit block.

Atrial and ventricular spikes in bifocal pacemakers

An automatic analysis of tapes from pacemakers with bifocal stimulation is not yet possible with today's technology, since a differentiation between atrial and ventricular spikes cannot be performed and since the refractory period of the detection system has a duration of up to 200 ms with AV delays between 10 and 220 ms.

Heart related discomfort

During intensive questioning 124/157 (79%) patients reported *heart related discomfort* in spite of clinical improvement after implantation (Table 1).

Table 1. Reported, heart-related discomfort in 157 consecutive PM patients.

Dyspnoe on exertion	55/157	(35%)
Dizziness	47/157	(30%)
Malleolar edema	39/157	(25%)
Angina pectoris	31/157	(20%)
Tachycardias	27/157	(17%)
Palpitation	15/157	(9%)
Eye glittering	10/157	(6%)
Syncope	5/157	(3%)

Underlying rhythms

These were: sinus rhythm in 82/157 patients, continuous atrial fibrillation in 32/157 patients, intermittent atrial fibrillation in 6/157 patients, AV-nodal-rhythm in 2/157 patients and 100%-pacemaker-rhythm in 35/157 patients.

Pacemaker-dependent arrhythmias

Pacemaker-mediated tachycardias were observed in 1, pacemaker-mediated VES in 3, and pacemaker tachycardias in 4 patients.

73

Table 2. Background arrhythmias in 157 consecutive PM patients.

SVES	18/157
SV tach	8/157
VES < 1/min	24/157
VES > 1/min	18/157
Lown I + II	18/157
III	16/157
IV	8/157
pauses ≥ 2.5 s	8/157

Background arrhythmias

These arrhythmias are pacemaker-independent, mostly correlated to the underlying disease. These background arrhythmias were detected in 118/157 patients (Table 2):

Bradycardias and tachycardias

We found that real sinus bradycardias or bradyarrhythmias, and also intermittent lead displacement with consecutive FTO, hysteresis and baseline shifts (indicated by the Holter analysis device as bradycardia or asystolic pauses) can initiate a bradycardia indication during the tape analysis.

Tachycardias may reflect real sinus, supraventricular or ventricular tachycardias (in pacemakers without run-away protection), but also one loose surface electrode, muscle potentials or electromagnetic interference can lead to a false-positive indication of tachycardia.

Pacemaker dysfunctions

PM dysfunctions which did not trigger additional arrhythmias were observed in 97/157 patients (Table 3).

Table 3. PM dysfunctions in 169 consecutive patients.

Class	Incidence	FTS	FTO	FTC
I	0	67/169 (40%)	77/169 (46%)	138/169 (82%)
II	1/h	61/169 (36%)	52/169 (30%)	23/169 (14%)
III	1–30/h	27/169 (16%)	33/169 (19%)	6/169 (4%)
IV	> 30/h	17/169 (10%)	6/169 (4%)	2/169 (1%)

Discussion

Special efforts have to be undertaken in order to obtain *sufficient signal quality* with the 3 recording systems, since the 3 devices have different PM spike detection algorithms. So far, *automatic analysis* has been reliable in single – chamber PM recordings, but should be visually controlled, especially in cases of arrhythmias, PM dysfunctions or complex PM systems. In our unselected PM patient population intensive questioning revealed *heart-related discomfort* in nearly 80% of the PM patients.

Our data show a much higher incidence than in recently reported studies (2, 3). The intensity of questioning greatly influences the kind and number of reported symptoms (Kennedy, H. L., personal communication). However, there were *no significant correlations* between arrhythmias or PM dysfunctions and the severity or incidence or the reported discomfort (same experiences: 6). As shown in Table 3, many of the PM patients had *PM dysfunctions.* According to the Lown gradation for VES were propose a similar *classification for the incidence of FTS, FTO and FTC.* In future it will perhaps be possible to define a subgroup of PM *patients at special risk* (Tables 3 and 4).

Table 4. Pacemaker patients at particular risk.

– CHD patients with VES ≥ Loww III°
  (→ SCD)

– Patients with high ventricular vulnerability and failure to sense
  (→ arrhythmias)

– Pacemaker dependent patients
  and failure to output   (1–30/h; > 30/h)
  and failure to capture   (1–30/h; > 30/h)
  and false inhibition   (over-, undersensing)

To this patient group which needs repeated controls belong:
1. Patients with coronary heart disease and Ves ≥ Lown III (danger of sudden cardiac death);
2. Patients with increased ventricular vulnerability and FTS (danger of arrhythmias);
3. Pacemaker dependent patients (i. e. patients with a preautomatic pause > 6.0 sec) with FTS (incidence: 1–30/h; > 30/h), FTC (incidence: 1–30 h; > 30/h) and over or undersensing.

Limitations of the pacemaker Holter ECG

Technically caused recording of many pseudopacemaker spikes, of many incidences of false-positive FTS, which are really fusion beats, and indications of baseline shifts such as bradycardias or asystolic pause may be a limitation of the clinical reliability.

Conclusion: Improvement of non-invasive pacemaker patient follow-up

The development of bidirectional telemetry, including analysis, Holter functions and marker impulses, and pacemaker Holter ECG during recent years has led to a significant improvement of the non-invasive pacemaker follow-up (Table 5). But nevertheless further technical improvement will have to be made for the sake of more simplicity and accuracy.

Table 5. Improvement of non-invasive pacemaker patient follow-up.

Bidirectional telemetry	
Analysis functions	– Programmed parameters
	– Battery and output status
	– Intracardiac electrogram or signal amplitude
	– Pacing threshold
	– Lead impedance
Holter functions	– Bradycardia counting
	– Stimulation / sensing / inhibition counting
	– Rate histogram
Marker impulses	– Sensing
	– Stimulation
	– Refractory periods
Pacemaker Holter ECG	– Pacemaker dependence
	– Underlying rhythm
	– Arrhythmias
	– PM dysfunctions

The ability to perform continuous PM Holter ECG recordings allows new insights into PM function after implantation. This new technique will probably induce questions about the quality standards in PM technology and PM function in vivo.

References

1. Bleifer SB, Bleifer GJ, Hausmann DR, Sheppard JJ, Karpmann HL (1974) Diagnosis of occult arrhythmias by Holter electrocardiography. Prog Cardiovasc Dis 16: 569
2. Burkhardt D, Hoffmann A, Jost M, Pfisterer M, Burkhart F (1984) Persistent symptoms despite permanent pacing. Chest 85: 207–210
3. Höpp H-W, Osterspey A (1984) Long-term electrocardiography: basics and practical importance. Boehringer Mannheim Study Series
4. Kennedy HL (1984) Ambulatory electrocardiography including Holter recording technique. Lea & Febiger, Philadelphia

5. Kennedy HL, Redd RM, Wiens RD, Buckingham TA, Romano GL, Joynes VE (1984) Ventricular arrhythmias in a pacemaker population. Eur Heart J Vol 5 A (Suppl I): 1124
6. Kunz G, Raeder E, Burckhardt D (1977) What does the symptom "palpitation" mean? – Correlation between symptoms and the presence of cardiac arrhythmias in the ambulatory ECG. Z Kardiol 66: 138–141

Authors' address:
M. Höher, M.D.
Medizinische Universitätsklinik III, Kardiologie
Josef-Stelzmann-Straße 9
5000 Köln 41
West Germany

Prevention and Improved Detection of Pacemaker Dysfunctions

U. J. Winter, D. W. Behrenbeck, M. Höher, Th. Brill, and H. H. Hilger

Summary: The studies presented in this paper demonstrated that the telemetry of the analysis functions in diagnostic pacemakers and the pacemaker Holter ECG are accurate and reliable, non-invasive methods for pacemaker control, and the adjustment and therapy of pacemaker dysfunctions. The clinical value and the differential diagnostic aid of the telemetry functions in implantable pacemakers are shown, discussing special case reports.

Introduction

Increasing health costs around the world led to a discussion about the necessity and value of different clinical diagnostic and therapeutic approaches. Enormous technological progress in computer technology enabled the pacemaker manufacturers to build demand pulse generators of acceptable size with complex functions. This increased complexity also made it more difficult to understand and handle these pacemakers. It was often questioned whether these extended capabilities could also improve therapy and diagnosis for pacemaker patients.

Objective

The aim of this contribution is to define the present and future clinical value of the pacemaker Holter ECG and the diagnostic pacemaker functions for the prevention, differential diagnosis and therapy of pacemaker dysfunctions. The performance of a controlled study concerning the clinical importance of both techniques is rather difficult since not all patients suffering from pacemaker dysfunctions have a diagnostic pacemaker with special analysis and Holter options, and were applied to a pacemaker Holter ECG recording. The number of implanted diagnostic pacemakers is still limited due to the higher cost and the complexity of functions.

The three different pacemaker Holter ECG devices which were used to perform the study are at present only available for special centers and are generally expensive. Furthermore the concrete cost-effect relationship of diagnostic pacemakers can only be determined after follow-up periods of at least 5 years.

Pacemaker dysfunctions: definitions

Pacemaker dysfunctions are classified as failure to sense, failure to capture and failure to output:

Failure to sense/FTS
If the pacemaker, i.e. the sensing circuit, cannot sense (detect) the intrinsic heart signals for demand pacing this situation is named failure to sense or entrance block.

Failure to capture/FTC
When the pacemaker spike is not followed by a myocardial depolarisation this is termed a failure to capture or exit block.

Failure to output/FTO
Failure to output or exit block means that the pulse generator does not deliver any pacemaker spike.

Pacemaker dysfunctions: pathogenesis and detection by pacemaker Holter ECG (PHE) and pacemaker telemetry

Failure to sense
FTS may be due to the following reasons:

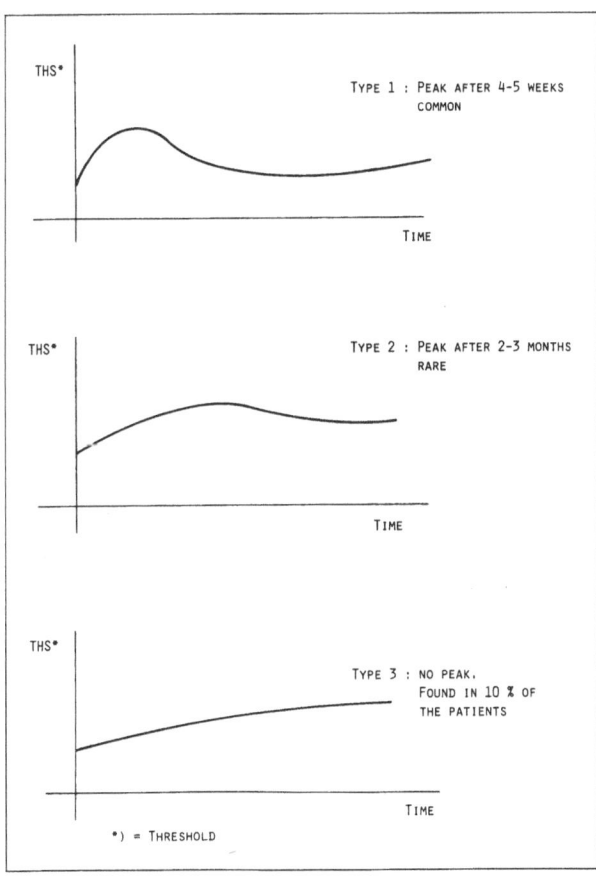

Fig. 1. Three types of threshold behaviour after implantation.

1. reduced signal amplitude and/or slew rate (telemetry of the intra-cardiac electrogram) as well as bundle branch block (ECG, PHE);
2. electrode displacement, fracture or insulation defects (telemetry; X-ray examination of the chest);
3. long technical refractory period (telemetry);
4. defect of the sensing circuit (telemetry);
5. non-adjusted sensitivity (telemetry).

Failure to capture
FTC may be due to:
1. constant increase of pacing threshold (type 3, see Figure 1) due to anoxia or electrolyte imbalance (telemetry);
2. leakage currents following insulation defects or lead fractures (telemetry);
3. delivery of the impulse during the myocardial refractory period due to FTS (telemetry, ECG, PHE);

Failure to output
FTO as a consequence of an impulse delivery inhibition may occur in demand pacemakers in the presence of intrinsic cardiac activity (telemetry), VES (ECG, PHE), tachyarrhythmias (ECG, PHE), muscle potentials (ECG, PHE), electromagnetic interference or artefacts (ECG, PHE), or technical defect of the impulse delivery (ECG, PHE).

If the *"End of Life"* criteria are reached the magnet test shows a significant ($\geqslant$ 10%) drop of the magnet rate, and the telemetry of the battery and output status a reduction of the battery output and an increase of the battery impedance. In contrast, a *leakage at the battery, a short circuit and an insulation fracture of the electrode* lead to a rise of the current drain, whereas a lead fracture or a displacement of the electrode cause a decrease of the current drain.

Pacemaker dysfunctions due to alterations at or of the electrode: pathogenesis and detection by PHE and pacemaker telemetry

An *unstable electrode position* is characterized by largely differing ($\geqslant$ 50%) pacing threshold values, as measured on 4 consecutive days. Sometimes, a differentiation from a normal, steep threshold increase in the early postimplantation period (type I) is difficult.

Table 1. Differential diagnosis of pacemaker dysfunctions with the help of pacemaker telemetry.

Measured parameter	Insulation defect of the electrode	Electrode fracture	Electrode dislocation
Threshold	$=/\uparrow$	$=/\uparrow/\uparrow\uparrow$	$\uparrow$
R-wave amplitude	$=/\downarrow$	$\downarrow\downarrow$	$\uparrow/=/\downarrow$
Lead impedance	$\downarrow$	$\uparrow$	$=/\uparrow$

80

In the case of an *electrode displacement* (Table 1) sometimes the morphology in the surface ECG has changed. Furthermore, mechanically induced VES can be detected. Additionally an abrupt threshold increase as well as varying R-wave amplitude and lead impedance (floating electrode) are observed.

An *electrode fracture* (Table 1) leads to a loss of sensing, to a significant threshold increase, to a remarkable decrease of endocardial signal amplitude and to an increase of the lead impedance.

In contrast, an *insulation defect of the electrode* (Table 1) is characterized by FTS, varying threshold and R-wave values as well as a decrease of the lead impedance.

Clinical value of pacemaker Holter ECG for the detection and differential diagnosis of pacemaker dysfunctions

As demonstrated in another of the contributions in this volume (Höher et al.: Pacemaker Holter ECG: Value and Limitations in Follow-up of Pacemaker Patients) pacemaker Holter ECG (Del Mar Avionics, Pacerecorder Reynolds Pathfinder; Ela Medical Anatec) was found to be reliable in 169 consecutive patients for the detection of the nature and incidence of pacemaker dysfunctions. The following ECG samples may underline the clinical value (Figures 2 to 4).

Clinical value of analysis and Holter functions for the detection and differential diagnosis of pacemaker dysfunctions

De Jongste et al. and Winter et al. (see the contributions in this book) demonstrated the clinical reliability, accuracy and variability of the different diagnostic pacemaker

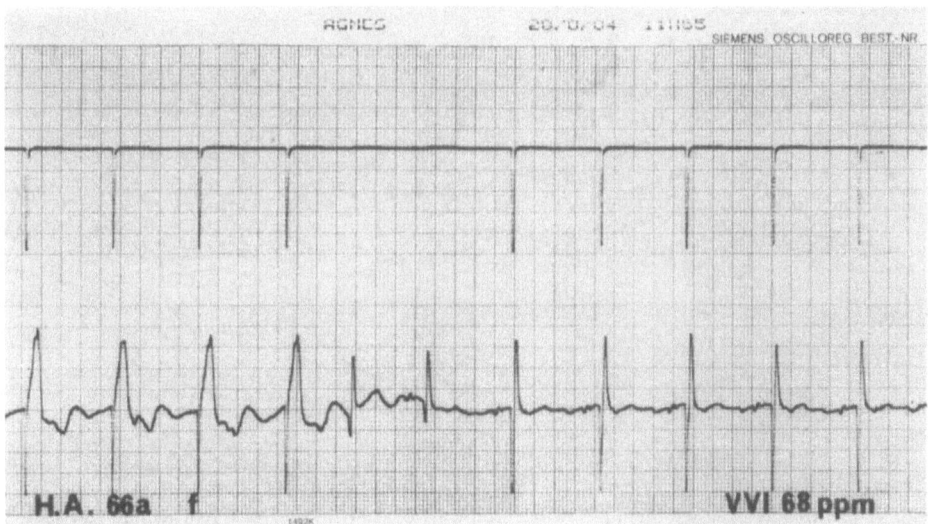

Fig. 2. Combination of paced beats (left part of figure; see pacemaker spikes which are visualised in the separate channel), spontaneous rhythm and fusion beats (right part of figure) in a 66 year old woman with normal VVI pacemaker function (Ela Medical: Anatec).

Fig. 3. This recording shows a failure to output due to myopotential inhibition (left part of the first and fourth channel) which is followed by a failure to sense (see arrows) in a VVI pacemaker. In each case the top channel shows the surface ECG, the bottom one the pacemaker spike (Reynolds: Pathfinder).

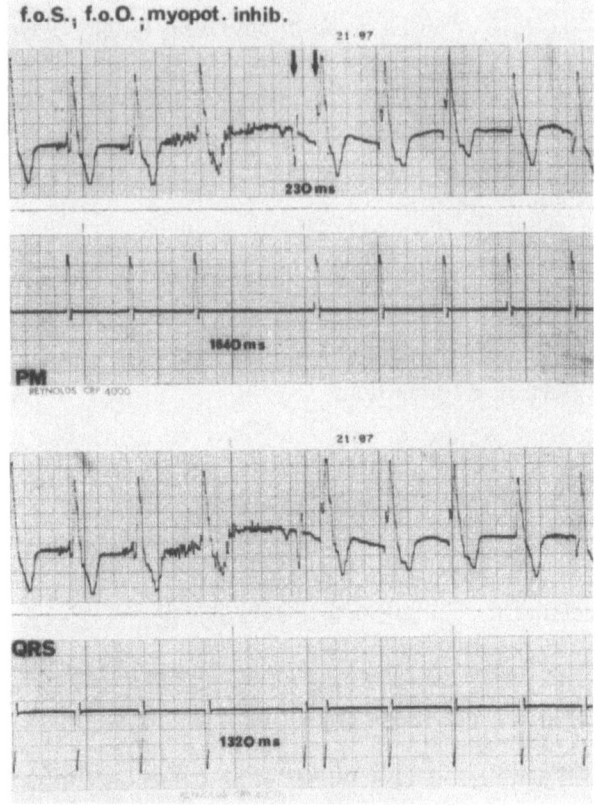

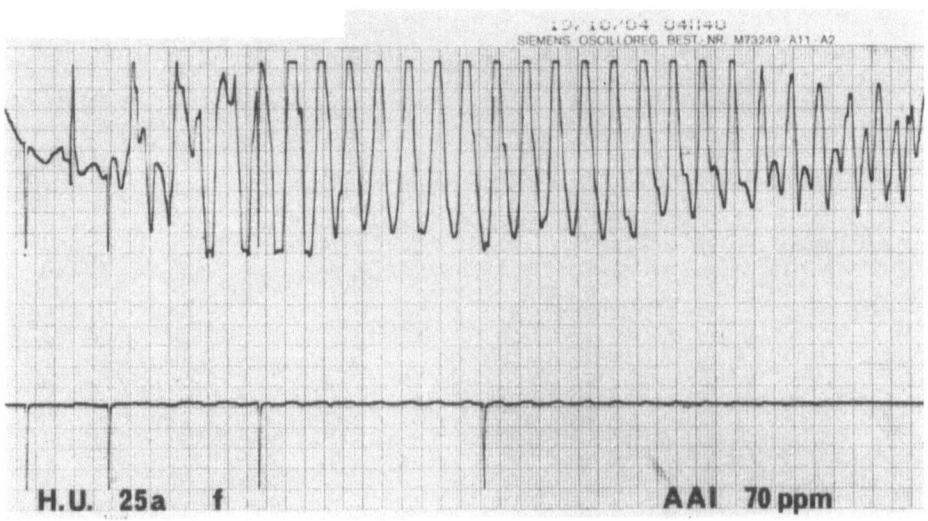

Fig. 4. In this young physiotherapist with chronic myocarditis, recurrent ventricular tachycardias and ventricular "torsade de pointes" tachycardias were observed. Atrial overdrive (AAI pacemaker) led to a significant suppresion of VES. The pacemaker Holter ECG revealed a pacemaker spike induced "torsade de pointes" tachycardia during permanent atrial "overdrive which was hemodynamically very well tolerated. (Ela Medical: Anatec)

options. In order to show the important differential diagnostic help of the pacemaker telemetry, special clinical courses of patients from our DPG study group are reported and explained here.

Case 1: O., M., 50 a, m.

Unexplained dizziness and reduced physical capacity after the implantation of VVI pacemaker

The patient received a VVI pacemaker because of carotid sinus syndrome and brady-cardias, especially if the head was abruptly turned. After several months of well-being he reported dizziness and reduced physical capacity. Conventional pacemaker control showed a regular function of the pacemaker. The telemetry of the analysis parameters revealed a programmed hysteresis of 20 ppm. Interrogation of the Holter functions of the pacemaker (negative hysteresis and stimulation-inhibition counter; rate-histogram) showed persisting bradycardias up to 30 bpm and spontaneous rates of mainly 90 to 100 bpm, indicating persisting carotid sinus syndrome and the beginning of myocardial insufficiency. It was now understood that the bradycardias and the longer escape inter-val led to the reported dizziness. After a saluretic treatment, an increase of the stimula-tion rate to 90 ppm, and programming of the hysteresis to zero ppm, the patient felt well again.

Case 2: H., H., 54 a, m.

Unexplained septic temperatures

This patient received a VVI pacemaker because of sinus bradycardia due to complex antiarrhythmic drug therapy of complex and multiple VES associated with CHD. After an initially regular clinical course, the patient came back to our hospital with un-explained septic temperatures, which could not be successfully treated by the family doctor. Telemetry of the pacemaker showed regular function of the pacemaker lead system. Thus, the suspected infection of the pacemaker lead could be excluded with a very high certainty. The rate histogram revealed heart rates mainly in the range of 90 to 100 ppm/bpm, associated with the septic desease.

Case 3: F., J., 63 a, m.

Bacterial infection of the battery pocket

The 63 year old patient came to our pacemaker surveillance clinic with febrile tem-peratures. Clinical examination revealed an infection of the battery pocket with im-minent decubitus. The telemetry of the analysis parameters showed a regular function of the pacemaker-lead system. A battery leakage could definitely be excluded, since the current drain remained constant. Antibiotic therapy and implantation of a lead and pacemaker solved the problem.

Cases 4 to 6: H., V., 71 a, m; F., H., 63 a, m; F., J., 63 a, m.

Decompensated myocardial insufficiency during dynamic overdrive stimulation

In these 3 male patients with coronary heart disease, myocardial failure occurred during long-term ventricular dynamic overdrive stimulation. The telemetry of the analysis para-meters gave no information about the possible reasons for the myocardial insufficiency. The saluretic therapy was performed in the hospital. An imbalance of the electrolytes, leading to a threshold increase, was not observed. The Holter functions of the pacemaker (stimulation counter; rate histogram) indicated long-term high-rate ventricular stimulation. Programming either to VVI pacing mode or a lower "upper rate limit" led to a recompensation during saluretic therapy.

Case 7: S, I., 41 a, f.
Displacement of the middle part of the atrial electrode in the right ventricle
A 41 year old woman reported extrasystoles and palpitations during dynamic overdrive and automatic underdrive stimulation by an AAI pacemaker. Conventional pacemaker control (ECG) showed an increase of the extrasystoles after an initial drug- and electrically induced significant decrease. The repeated telemetry of the analysis parameters revealed correct function of the pacemaker and electrode but in a Holter ECG recording, an increased number of PVCs could be seen. Finally, the X-ray examination of the chest showed a dislocation of the middle part of the atrial electrode throughout the

Fig. 5. In a patient with latent myocardial insufficiency and suspected myocarditis the R-wave amplitude decreased and finally became unmeasurable (< 1.0 mV). The lead impedance did not change significantly. The determined threshold values showed large deviations during subsequent days. Clinical diagnosis: insulation defect.

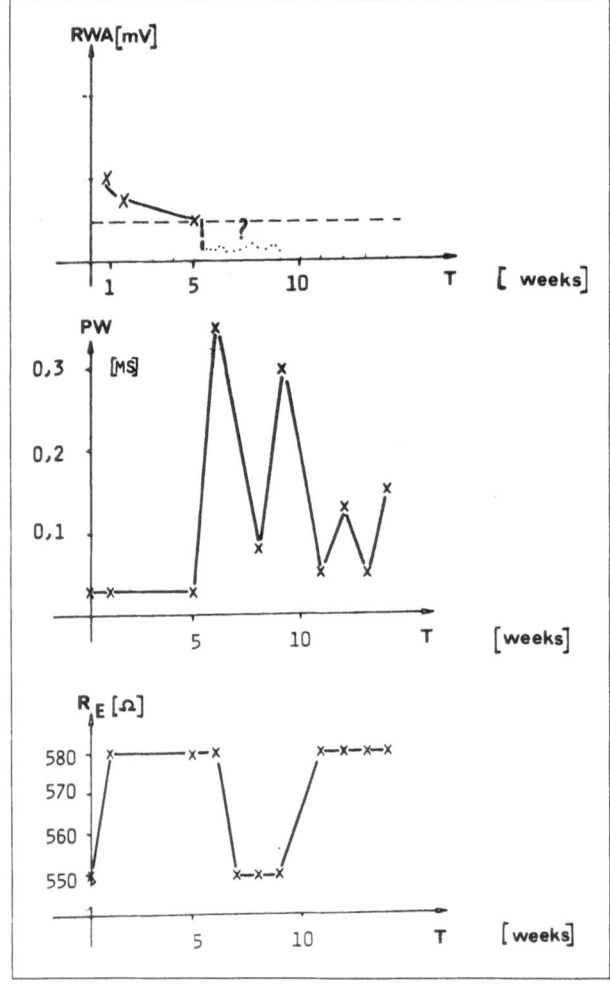

tricuspid valve into the right ventricle. Thus, the ventricular extrasystoles were mechanically induced by the displaced electrode.

Case 8: H., E., 72 a, m.
Loss of sensing due to a fracture of the electrode insulation
This 72 year old man felt well after the implantation. During the early follow-up period a slowly decreasing R-wave amplitude was detected (Fig. 5). During regular pacemaker telemetry in the 6th week after the implantation an unmeasurable R-wave amplitude was observed. In parallel the pacing threshold showed a significant increase, followed by significant changes of the values in subsequent days. Furthermore the lead impedance was decreased (Fig. 5). Conventional and 24-hour Holter ECG showed multiple FTS. As suggested from the telemetered data the X-ray examination of the chest revealed a defect of the lead close to the adapter. It was assumed to be either mechanical damage or breakage of the lead. When the lead was revised, it turned out to be an insulation defect.

Case 9: S., B., 43 a, m.
Loose contact at the adapter
In this patient with a temporary atrial electrode connected to the DPG 1, working as an AAI pacemaker, a loose contact at the adapter caused an increase of the lead impedance from 620 to 730 Ω, a non-measurable P-wave amplitude, which was evaluated before to be 2.5 mV, and an increase of the pacing threshold.

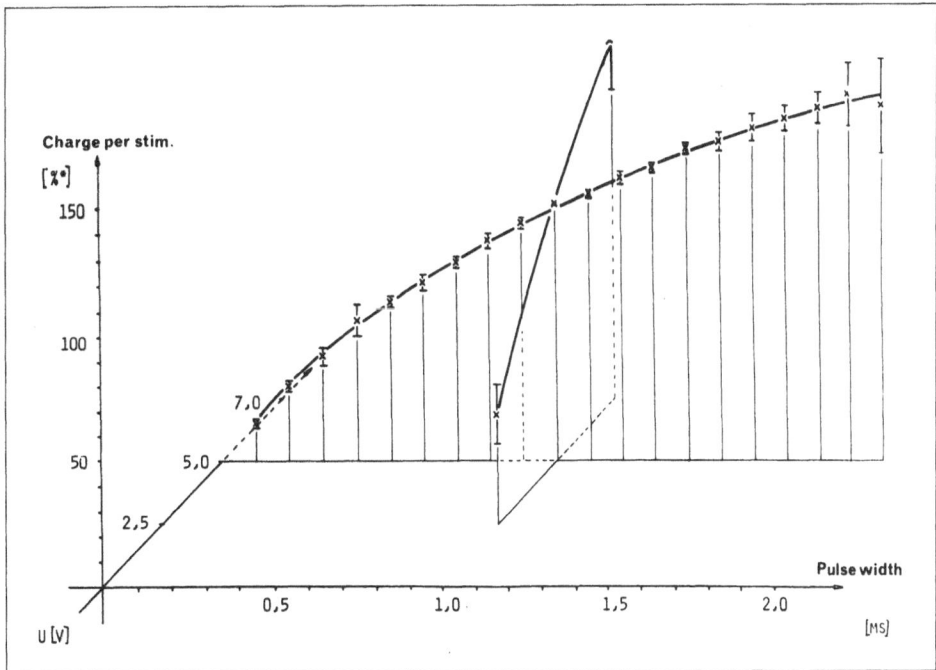

Fig. 6. Dependance of the charge per stimulus as percentage of the values at 5.0 V and 1.0 ms on impulse duration and output voltage, measured in 8 VVI pacemakers ($\bar{x} \pm$ S.D.; Vitatron DPG 1).

Cases 10 and 11: G., F., 58 a, m: W. H., 53 a, m.
Diaphragmatic pacing
At the regular pacemaker control 8 weeks after implantation two patients reported troublesome diaphragmatic pacing. After the measurement of the pacing threshold at 3 different voltages and impulse widths, the output voltage could be reduced to 2.5 V, thus leading to a termination of diaphragmatic pacing without losing a pacing safety margin. The effects of voltage and impulse duration on the energy consumption are demonstrated in Figure 6.

Discussion and conclusion

As pointed out earlier the follow-up period for diagnostic pacemakers is too short and the development stage of pacemaker Holter ECG too early to come to a final conclusion concerning the clinical value of both methods. But it can be said already at this stage that with the combination of both non-invasive methods, pacemaker control and adjustment, as well as treatment of pacemaker dysfunctions become significantly improved. Even the prevention of pacemaker dysfunctions seems to become realistic with both these techniques. As reported in the previous papers increasing technical capabilities also lead to more difficulties in the understanding and handling of these devices. Furthermore, future studies should try to determine the final cost reducing effects of fully adaptable pacemakers and pacemaker Holter ECG during a longer follow-up period. Pacemaker telemetry helps to follow up each individual pacemaker patient, to find its own "fine tuning" and to prevent pacemaker dysfunctions at an early stage. Pacemaker Holter ECG might become a screening method for larger populations, without having direct preventive effects.

Authors' address:
U. J. Winter, M.D.
Medizinische Universitätsklinik III, Kardiologie
Joseph-Stelzmann-Straße 9
5000 Köln 41
West Germany

Physiological Pacing and Biological Rate Adjustment

E. Alt and A. Wirtzfeld

Summary: In recent years pacemaker therapy has changed from a mainly life preserving therapy towards a therapy to improve quality of life. Hemodynamic aspects have become more and more important. The beneficial effect of atrioventricular synchrony has been studied with respect to different influencing factors such as heart rate, AV interval, presence or absence of retrograde ventricular-atrial conduction, heart failure and exercise. The results of such studies performed at our clinic are presented and discussed.

Special interest is directed towards the factor of heart rate increase under exercise condition on cardiodynamics. A truly physiological pacemaker system takes account of both features of the healthy heart: AV synchrony and rate responsiveness. While for resting hemodynamics the avoidance of consistently mistimed atrial contractions following retrograde conduction is of great importance, an increase in exercise hemodynamics is mostly determined by the ability to adjust heart rate according to the metabolic needs of the exercising body. For patients in whom a rate increase with exercise cannot be accomplished by AV synchrony, atrial independent pacing systems are currently under development or clinical investigation.

We report on the measurement of right ventricular temperature for rate control of a physiological pacemaker system that is under evaluation at our institute at present.

Hemodynamic aspects have become more and more important in recent years, especially for the indication of so-called physiological pacing systems, which are supposed to yield better hemodynamic results than the former ventricular stimulating systems. These ventricular stimulating pacemakers may prevent syncopes and achieve a longer lifetime, but marked hemodynamic improvements, however, cannot generally be obtained. Sometimes even a hemodynamic deterioration, the so-called pacemaker syndrome, is seen during ventricular stimulation. The cause of this situation, besides an eventual heart failure, is the unphysiological working mode of these VVI systems. They provide neither atrioventricular synchronization nor rate adjustment during physical exercise. Therefore in recent years physiological pacing systems have become more and more important.

Physiological pacing systems are those that preserve atrioventricular synchronization, i.e. the AAI, DVI, VAT, VDD and DDD pacemakers. While all these systems preserve atrioventricular synchronization, only the dual-chamber systems VAT, VDD and DDD allow a rate adjustment during physical exercise. The prerequisite for this is a normally working sinus node. As the vast majority of patients with an implanted physiological system fail to achieve sufficient rate adjustment during exercise, currently available physiological systems can only improve hemodynamics at rest, not during physical activity.

These considerations led to the development of rate adjusting pacemakers on the basis of measurement of biological parameters. Therefore a real physiological system should result not only in atrioventricular synchronization, but also in rate adjustment during physical exercise. In the following the hemodynamic fundamentals and determinants of physiological pacing are presented.

Fig. 1. Simultaneous registration of ECG, left ventricular filling pressure (L.V.) and pressure in the brachial artery (B.A.) in a patient with aortic stenosis. If the P-wave (vertical arrow) happens to appear before the ventricular complex, the end-diastolic pressure is elevated (oblique arrow). When atrioventricular synchronization is missing there is a decrease in end-diastolic pressure and therefore a decrease in left ventricular systolic and brachial artery pressure.

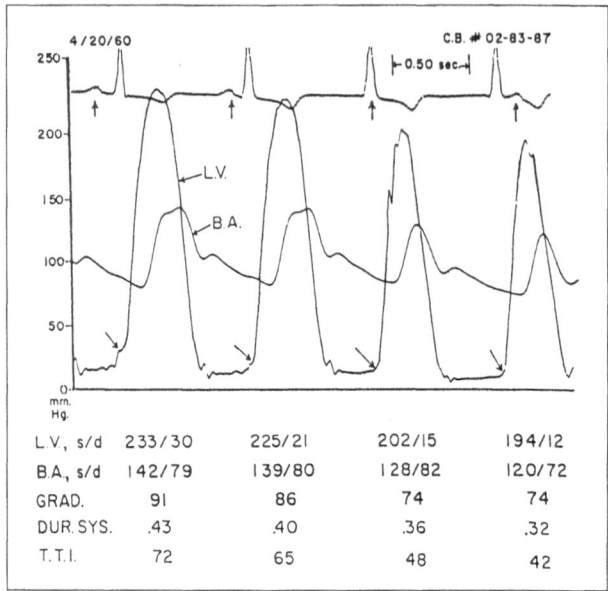

L.V, s/d	233/30	225/21	202/15	194/12
B.A, s/d	142/79	139/80	128/82	120/72
GRAD.	91	86	74	74
DUR.SYS.	.43	.40	.36	.32
T.T.I.	72	65	48	42

Importance of atrial systole

The importance of the atrial systole for ventricular filling is well known. If in an AV-dissociation the P-wave happens to precede the QRS complex with a physiological interval, the positive influence on the ventricular parameters of contractility and the peripheral blood pressure will be distinct (Fig. 1). These results are reasonable when considering the normal hemodynamic events in the heart. After ventricular depolarization the ventricles begin to contract and advance a certain stroke volume during systole. According to the Frank-Starling mechanism the output is determined by the end-diastolic stretching of the myocardial fibers which is correlated with the end-diastolic pressure. In early diastole which begins approximately at the end of the T-wave in the ECG the blood flows passively from the atria to the empty ventricles and fills them up. At the end of diastole the normally atria contract, recognizable by the P-wave in the ECG. This atrial contraction results in an additional blood flow into the ventricles and thus in an increase of the end-diastolic ventricular pressure. Therefore, according to the Frank-Starling mechanism the stroke volume will normally be enhanced. This positive influence of atrioventricular synchronization during normal sinus rhythm becomes lost during ventricular stimulation. Thus in recent years it could be shown that during physiological pacing the cardiac output rises between 6 and 43% compared to mere ventricular stimulation. The question, however, of which patients during which conditions profit most by an atrioventricular synchronization, is still contested in the literature. While some older studies lay stress on the importance of atrioventricular synchronization in patients with heart failure, some other studies deny this importance.

The influence of atrial systole on ventricular function is a complex procedure which is influenced by heart rate, ventricular filling pressure, timing of atrial contraction, course of

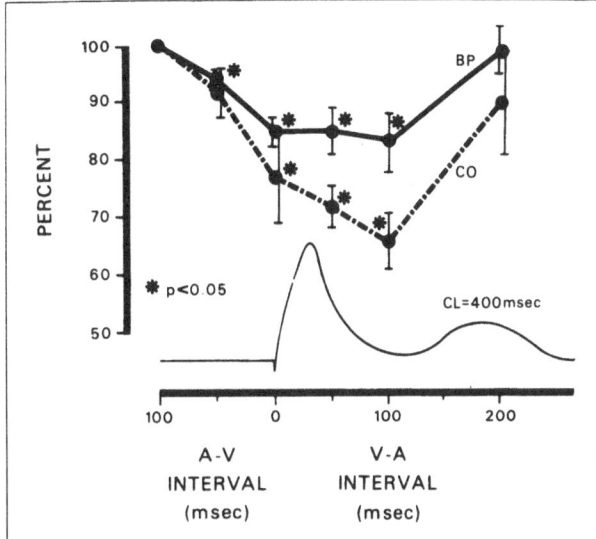

Fig. 2. Decrease (in percent) in blood pressure (BP) and cardiac output (CO) in relation to the AV interval. In particular when the atria are depolarized 100 ms after the ventricular stimulation (VA interval 100 ms) there is a decrease in cardiac output of more than 30%, whereas the fall in blood pressure is stopped by peripheral reflex mechanisms.

the individual Frank-Starling curve, atrial filling pressure, contractility of the atria and peripheral resistance.

The timing of atrial contraction plays an important role in this. Figure 2 shows the influence of different AV-intervals on peripheral blood pressure and cardiac output in an animal experiment. One can see that the best hemodynamic results are obtained with an AV-interval of 100 ms. If atrial stimulation follows ventricular stimulation, i.e. the atria contract against the closed AV valves, an additional drop in blood pressure and cardiac output results. This experiment corresponds to the presence of retrograde ventricular-atrial conduction in clinical practice, where the atria also contract against the closed AV valves. Diminished early diastolic filling is the result, as at the beginning of the diastole the atria are less filled. Additionally the late diastolic filling is reduced, as atrial contraction in time before the beginning of the systole is omitted.

We studied the clinical relevance of these hemodynamic results observed in the animal experiment in 50 patients of our hospital, who had pacemakers because of a constant sinus bradycardia of about 50/min due due to sick sinus syndrome. We studied the cardiac output and the stroke volume during intrinsic rhythm, during ventricular and during atrial stimulation (Fig. 3). We found that during ventricular stimulation, in spite of a rise in heart rate from 50/min to 70/min, the cardiac index dropped 4% due to an overproportional decrease in stroke volume. Only by atrial stimulation could an increase in cardiac index from 2.9 1 during intrinsic rhythm to 3.4 1 during atrial stimulation be achieved. A detailed analysis showed that patients who had a retrograde conduction with the atria contracting against the closed AV valves were particularly concerned in this drop in cardiac index during ventricular stimulation (Fig. 4). Whereas in patients without retrograde atrial conduction there was nearly no change in cardiac index during intrinsic rhythm and during ventricular stimulation and an increase of 19% during atrial stimulation, in patients with atrial conduction the cardiac index dropped by 12% during ventricular stimulation compared to the value during intrinsic rhythm. Only by atrial stimula-

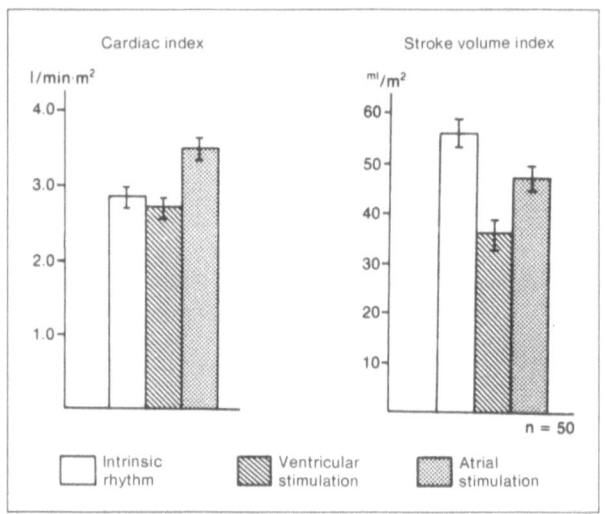

Fig. 3. Cardiac index and stroke volume index in 50 patients during intrinsic rhythm (sinus bradycardia 50/min), ventricular stimulation (70/min) and atrial stimulation (70/min).

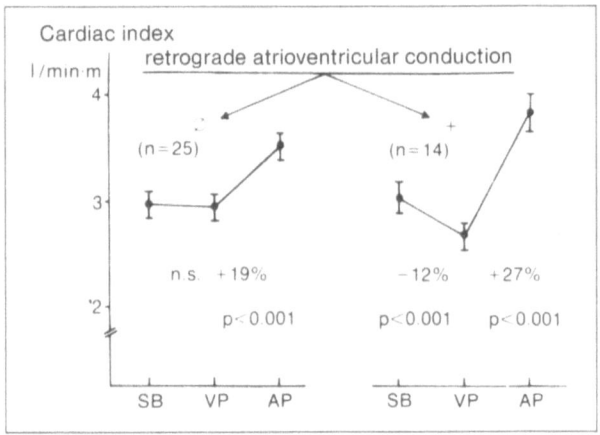

Fig. 4. Cardiac index in patients with and without retrograde atrial conduction during sinus bradycardia (SB), ventricular pacing (VP) and atrial pacing (AP).

tion could a hemodynamic benefit of 27% compared to sinus bradycardia be obtained. When these patients are paced, in some untoward cases a drop in blood pressure occurs, so that a collapse or even a syncope may follow (Fig. 5). This seems not only to be due to a decrease in stroke volume, but also to a reflex drop in peripheral resistance.

Influence of myocardial parameters of contractility on the effectiveness of atrioventricular synchronization

Besides the timing of the atrial contraction myocardial factors play an important role in the effectiveness of the AV synchronization. Apart from ventricular filling pressures and left ventricular compliance the course of the individual Frank-Starling curve is of importance. Figure 6 shows Frank-Starling curves in the case of enhanced contractility, e.g. a

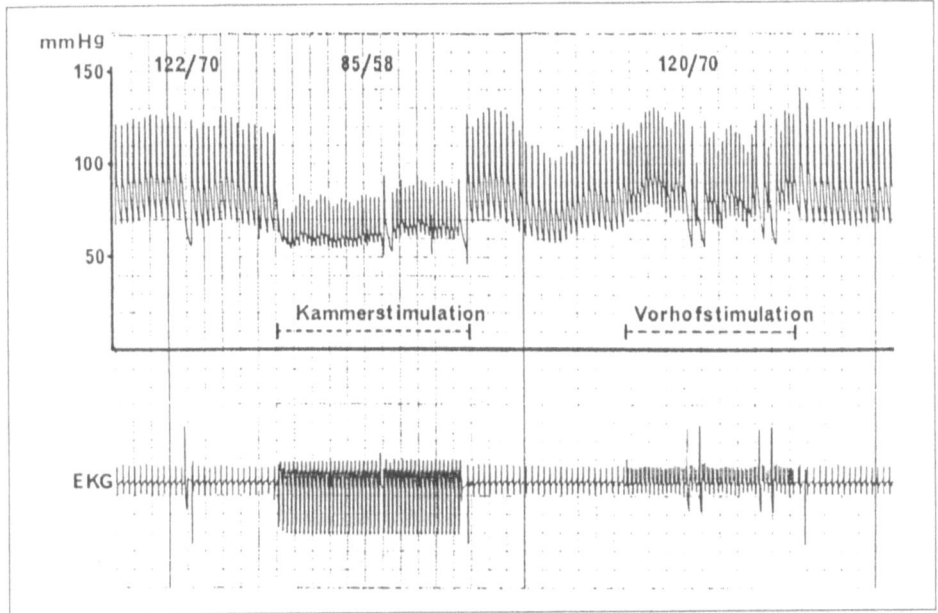

Fig. 5. Blood pressure drops from 122 mm Hg (systolic) to 85 mm Hg (systolic) during ventricular pacing, whereas during atrial pacing it is kept constant. This so-called pacemaker syndrome has been seen particularly in patients with sick sinus syndrome and retrograde atrial conduction.

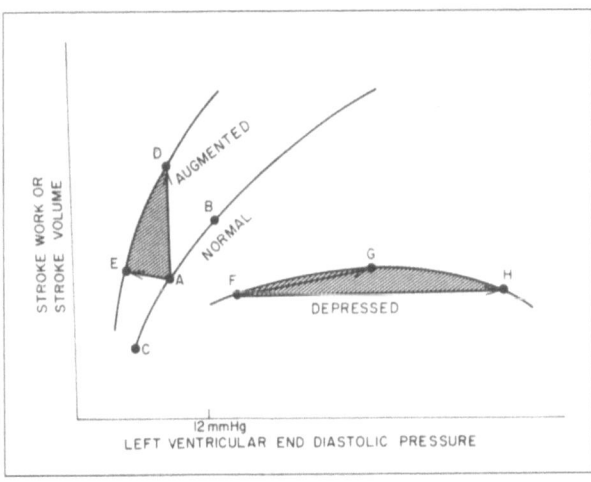

Fig. 6. Stroke volume index in relation to pulmonary wedge pressure, the indirect measurement of left ventricular filling pressure (Frank-Starling curve). The stroke volume index rises much more in patients with augmented (1) or normal (2) contractility than in those with depressed contractility (3).

well trained sportsman, of normal contractility and of reduced contractility, as is often seen in pacemaker patients. One can see that the well trained or normal myocardium responds to an increase in the end-diastolic filling pressure with an increase in the stroke volume. In the healthy heart this curve is steep, i.e., an increase in filling pressure such as this is caused by atrial contraction at the end of diastole (from A to B), is leading to an enhanced stroke volume, whereas the ventricle with reduced contractility presents a flat

91

curve (from F to G). Thus, in these patients a further increase in filling pressure is not accompanied by an adequate increase in stroke volume, and beyond an upper value of filling pressure a further enhancement brings about no increase in contractility (from G to H), and sometimes even a decrease in cardiac performance. So it is understandable that the results of physiological pacing in comparison with ventricular stimulation are rated differently in the literature. In particular in patients with a damaged myocardium, such as in most pacemaker patients, the level of the filling pressure seems to decide whether physiological pacing is of hemodynamic benefit compared to ventricular pacing. There is some evidence that beyond an upper limit of filling pressure, such as in patients with a distinct heart failure, physiological pacing is of only little benefit. On the other hand, however, it is understandable that a drug therapy which reduces the filling pressure is capable of restoring the effectiveness of a physiological pacemaker.

Influence of atrioventricular synchronization and rate adjustment on the hemodynamics during physical exercise

In 14 patients with a VDD pacemaker system we studied the importance of AV synchronization and rate adjustment during physical exercise in the hemodynamics of pacemaker patients. All patients had a III° AV block with a normally working sinus node.

The cardiac ouput was measured by thermodilution at rest and during different levels of exercise, in each case at three modes of pacing: ventricular pacing at a rate of 70/min (VVI 70), atrial triggered pacing (VDD) and ventricular pacing at a rate equal to that during VDD pacing at the particular level of exercise.

Fig. 7. Hemodynamics at rest and during exercise with ventricular pacing at 70/min (VVI 70), VDD pacing and ventricular pacing with a rate adjusted to that during VDD pacing.

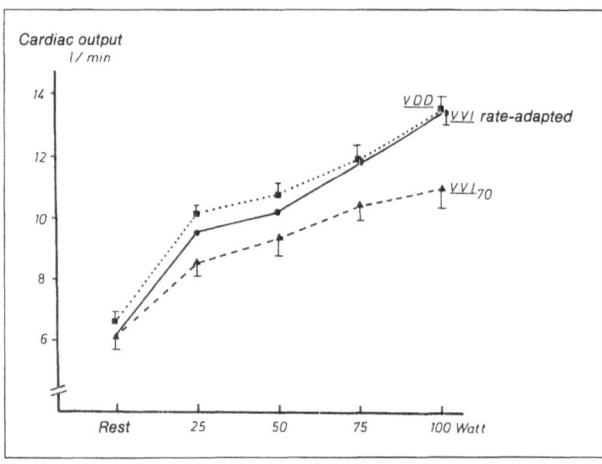

Figure 7 shows that the increase in cardiac output during exercise is mainly caused by the rate adjustment and only in part by the atrioventricular synchronization.

In another study with the same design, however, we found that patients with a good ventricular function had much more hemodynamic benefit from atrioventricular synchronization during exercise than patients with a ventricular malfunction. The latter patients

92

are supposed, especially during physical work, to have filling pressures that are closed to the peak of the Frank-Starling curve.

As expected, only in those patients who retained good contractility did a further enhancement of the end-diastolic pressure by atrial contraction lead to a positive hemodynamic result. However, there are definitely quantitative differences between patients with a slightly or markedly reduced myocardial function, also dependent on the level of exercise.

Clinical results

The results of a follow-up examination, which we performed on all patients who had received a physiological pacemaker since 1977, corresponded to these hemodynamic considerations and studies. We found that the functional results relating to symptoms of dizziness, syncopes and palpitations were dependent on the pacemaker, whether it was an AAI, DDD or VDD/VAT system, and therefore dependent on the patients, whether they had sick sinus syndrome, binodal disease or III° AV block. Concerning the functional results relating to physical capacity we classified the pacemaker patients according to the New York Heart Association Classification (Table 1). It has been shown that physical capacity had been improved by cardiac pacing in 59% of the patients with an atrial pacemaker, in 70% of patients with a DDD pacemaker and in 93% of patients with a VDD pacemaker. The difference between AAI and VDD systems was significant ($p < 0.01$). Table 1 shows that 86% of patients who were postoperatively in NYHA Class I had received such a pacemaker due to III° AV block, so that they could raise their heart rate during physical work. In contrast to this, only 48% of patients with an atrial pacemaker were in NYHA class I postoperatively. This is understandable, since patients with a VAT or VDD pacemaker also benefit from their physiological pacemaker during exercise, as it raises the pacing rate, whereas patients with an AAI pacemaker exceed their pacing rate during exercise in 90% of the cases, but not to an adequate extent due to their sinus node malfunction. This shows that in patients with a sinus node malfunction the pacemaker mainly improves the hemodynamics at rest, but it has no or only slight influence on the hemodynamics during exercise.

Table 1. Functional results.

	Preoperative	Postoperative	Preoperative	Postoperative
NYHA I	27%	48%	0	86%
NYHA II	33%	43%	36%	14%
NYHA III	20%	7%	29%	0
NYHA IV	20%	0	36%	0
Pacemaker	AAI		VAT/VDD	

Rate adjusting pacemakers

These findings lead to considerations of how patients with an inadequate rate enhancement during exercise can also be given the opportunity of physiological rate-adapted

Table 2. Physiological parameters for the control of rate adjusting pacemakers.

Blood pH value	(Cammilli 1973)
Respiration rate	(Funke 1975, Ionescu 1980, Rossi 1982)
Blood temperature	(Csapo 1976, Alt 1984)
Oxygen saturation of mixed-venous blood	(Wirtzfeld 1978)
QT time	(Rickards 1981)
Average atrial rate	(Goldreyer 1981)
Physical activity	(Anderson 1983)

pacing. Therefore for some years several endogenous biological parameters were examined for controlling the rate of a pacemaker (Table 2). Whereas the blood pH value, which had been suggested by Cammilli as a control parameter in 1973, has since been abandoned pacemakers whose rates are controlled by respiration rate or QT interval are now being clinically tested. A pacemaker which operates by registering physical activity by means of a built-in microphone which perceives muscle sound, and another which works by measuring the oxygen saturation of mixed-venous blood, are also being tested clinically.

At our clinic we are concerned with the mixed-venous blood temperature that had first been suggested as a control parameter by Csapo and Weißwange in 1977.

The physiological foundation of this principle consists in the exact heat regulation of the body. It is also a physiologically sensible mechanism that the temperature of the interior of the body fluctuates in a circadian rhythm about 0.5 °C with a minimum in the early morning and a maximum in the afternoon.

Man as a homotherm being is provided with a precise heat regulation in order to balance exogenous and endogenous influences on the body temperature. Thermogenesis consists in the oxidation of fats, amino acids and carbohydrates, with 4.9 kcal metabolic energy resulting from one liter oxygen that is used for oxidation. The distribution of the energy produced by oxidation into heat and high-energy substrates is equal in all human beings. The first law of thermodynamics means that the sum of all forms of energy is constant in a closed system, and the second law says that in every transformation from one form of energy into another there is an increase in entropy, i.e. in the part of free heat. Accordingly in man the oxidation of food and the production of ATP results in about 50% heat, the same value as in the transformation of chemical energy (ATP) into mechanical energy (physical work); thus the efficiency of mechanical work is about 23%. This is not much, but the production of thermic energy is a reasonable mechanism in order to maintain in man as a homothermic being the body temperature that is nearly always higher than the temperature of the environment. Normally the production of ATP is linked to the oxygen uptake, the so-called coupling. Only in hyperthyreosis is there a so-called decoupling, i.e. the thermogenesis increases at the expense of a reduced production of high-energy phosphates. In the conditions of physical work, however, heat production is strictly linked with oxygen uptake. As the oxygen uptake during physical work is directly correlated with the heart rate in a individual, dependent on his fitness, in the

94

particular individual there is a strict correlation between oxygen uptake, heart rate, physical work and heat production. As the blood serves as a carrier for the heat, the mixed-venous blood temperature is the parameter that rises first with an enhancement of the body temperature.

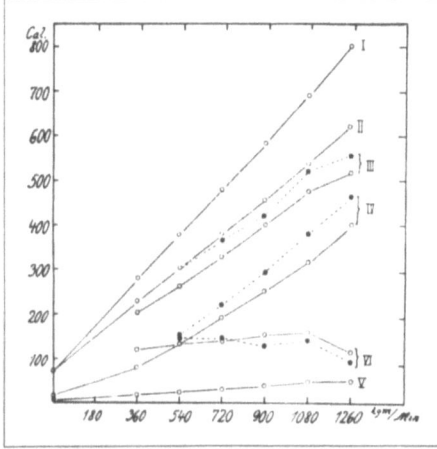

Fig. 8. Calories per hour in relation to the work intensity in kgm/min. I Total expenditure of energy; II Total heat production; III Total heat release; IV Heat release by evaporation (skin and lungs); V Heat release by evaporation (lungs); VI Heat release by convection and radiation.
Continuous line = from the entire work period (0–60 min), dotted line = determinations from 40–60 min work.

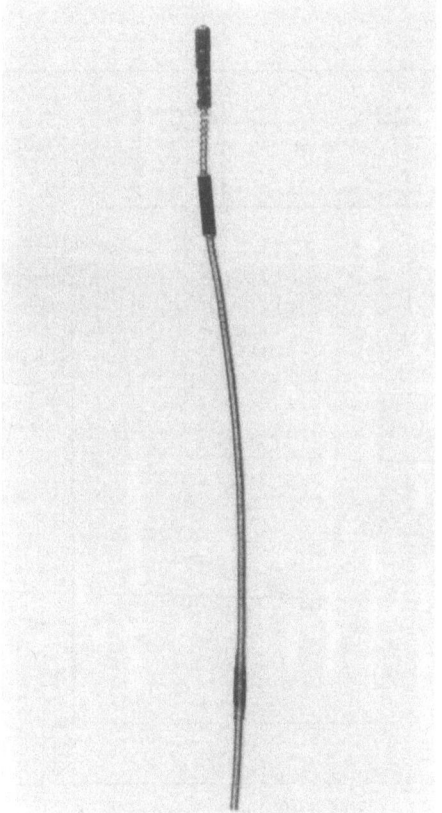

Fig. 9. Electrode with built-in thermistor inside the polyurethane insulation.

Heat regulation

Normally heat production is equal to heat release. The body has different mechanism of heat release:
- radiation (infrared heat rays)
- conduction (in solids)
- convection (in liquids and gases)
- evaporation.

These mechanisms keep the body temperature at a certain level. The individual regulation results from numerous thermoreceptors which are in veins, skin, mucosae, museles, carotid artery, spine marrow and hypothalamus and whose afferent signals are processed in the hypothalamic and pre-optic area. Efferent signals regulate heat production by enhanced thermogenesis and vasoconstriction, heat release by vasodilation and sweating.

The principle of heat regulation was explained for the first time by Nielssen in 1938. Up to this time it was thought that an increase in body temperature during physical work corresponded to a failure of heat regulation. Nielssen, however, demonstrated (Fig. 8), that every level of exercise corresponds to a new nominal value of heat production, and that therefore an increase in body temperature during physical work represents a reasonable mechanism. At a constant level of exercise for a prolonged period this new nominal value, which is achieved within 3 to 4 minutes, is kept at this level by an enhanced heat

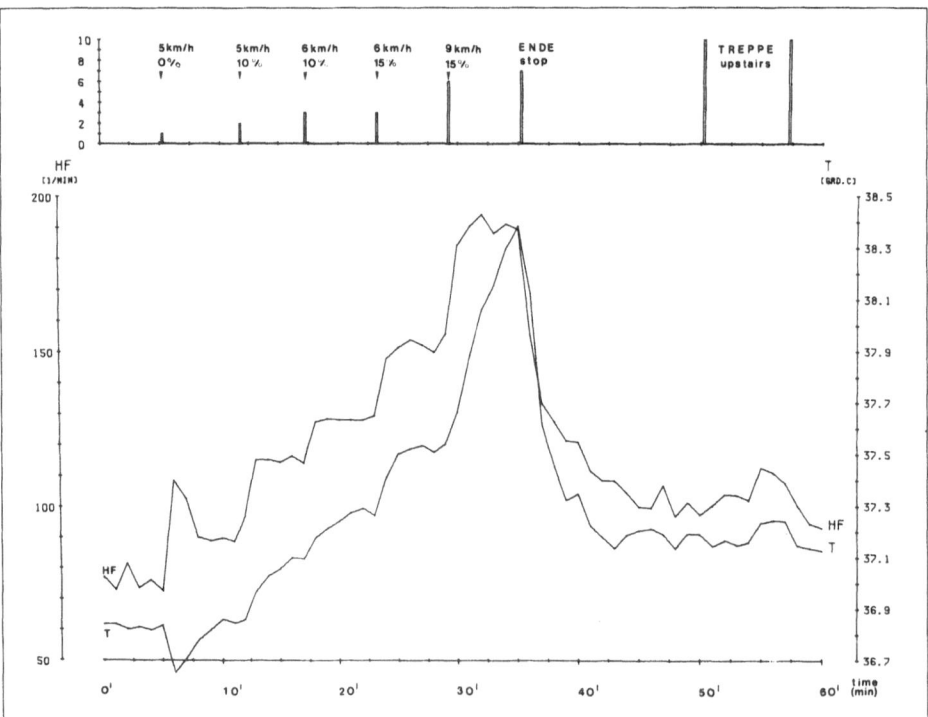

Fig. 10. Increase in mixed-venous blood temperature in a volunteer during treadmill exercise.

96

release. Only a further increase in physical work leads to a new increase in body temperature. Apart from the locally enhanced muscle temperature the blood temperature is the fastest responding parameter, whereas the oesophagus and rectal temperature rises considerably later. At higher levels of exercise the heat release by radiation and convection is no longer sufficient, so that then the new level of temperature must be maintained by evaporation. The storage heat amounts to about 10 to 12% of the total metabolic energy; thus the body temperature rises by this percentage.

Methods and results

On the basis of these considerations and results we constructed a bipolar electrode with a built-in thermistor which is located 5 cm before the lead tip (Fig. 9). The electrode has a diameter of 1.7 mm, is insulated by polyurethane and is placed in the right ventricle, with the thermistor near the AV valves where good mixing of the blood takes place. The electrode is of the multifilar type, very flexible, and can be placed in the particular location by means of an introducible guide. The resolution of the thermistor is very high with an accuracy of 0.01 °C.

Data of temperature, heart rate and respiration were registrated continuously by means of a portable external store with a 28 k microprocessor and were plotted graphically and numerically by a computer evaluation method.

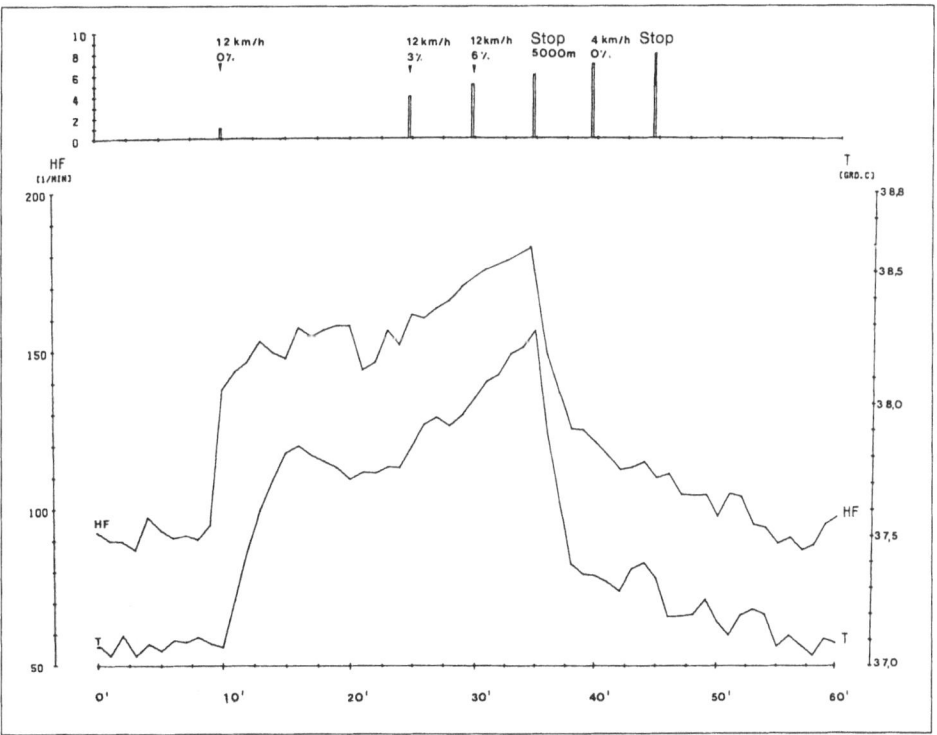

Fig. 11. Increase in mixed-venous blood temperature during initially heavy exercise.

Up to now we have obtained data of 14 volunteers and 17 patients during different forms of physical work. Figure 10 shows the increase in mixed-venous blood temperature during treadmill exercise. The heart rate rises at first overshootingly before balancing out after 2 minutes, while the temperature presents an initial short drop for half a minute, and then a continuous rise that is nearly parallel to the increase in heart rate. After the exercise there is a fast drop in heart rate as well as in temperature.

We obtained similar results during initially heavy exercise (Fig. 11). The rise of the body temperature correlates with the extent of physical work, the higher the initial exercise, the faster the temperature rises up to a new nominal value. This is accomplished after 3 to 4 minutes, while the rise in heart rate lasts 1 to 2 minutes. As exercise goes on, heart rate as well as temperature are kept approximately constant. A new increase in physical work leads to a further rise in heart rate and temperature. As exercise has finished temperature and heart rate decrease quickly.

From these data we developed an algorithm that enables the rate to be adjusted by means of the mixed-venous blood temperature. It could be shown that during physical work particularly in patients with sick sinus syndrome and a conventional physiological pacemaker (DDD) a higher heart rate can be achieved, thus being in good accordance with the normal reaction of rate (Fig. 12).

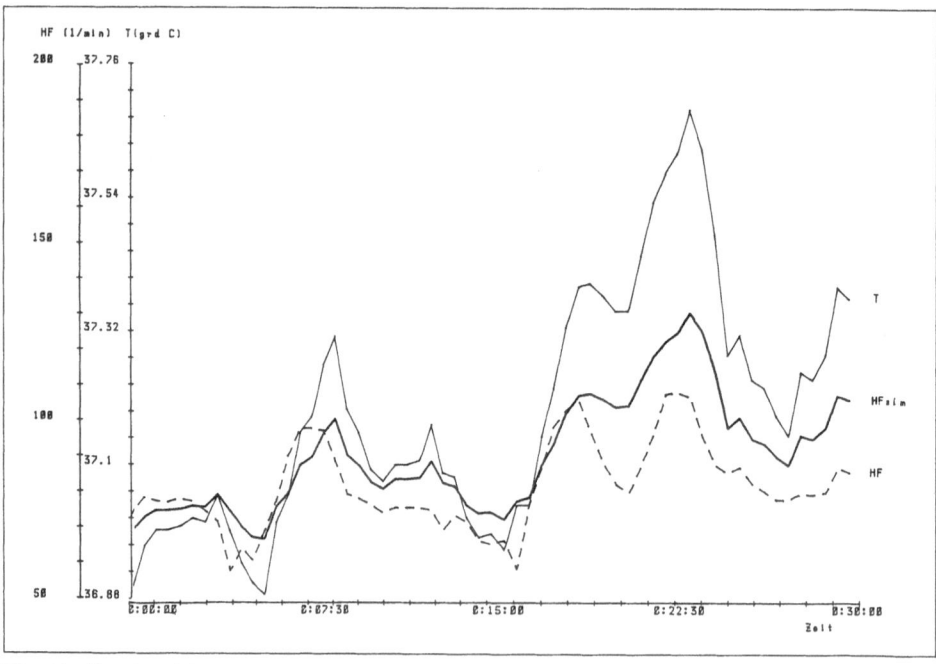

Fig. 12. Simulated heart rate (HFsim) compared to the heart rate during DDD pacing (HF). The simulated heart rate is controlled by blood temperature (T). The patient (63 years) had received the pacemaker 2 years previously. The figure represents the course of heart rate and temperature when climbing stairs at a normal speed.

Besides this advantageous influence on heart rate during exercise an additional benefit of rate control by temperature is physiological rate reduction during sleep, what is not possible with the conventional pacemakers.

Authors' address:
E. Alt, M.D.
I. Medizinische Klinik rechts der Isar
Technische Universität
Ismaninger Straße 22
8000 München 80
West Germany

Rate Responsive Pacing – Initial Experience with the QT(TX/Quintech) and Biorate Pacemakers

B. Maisch and H. Steilner

Summary: Physiological stimulation can be achieved by either bifocal or rate responsive pacing. The latter pacemakers adapt the heart rate to physical activity by biological signals. From many possible approaches only 3 pacemaker systems for rate responsive pacing are available: the QT pacemaker (TX or Quintech), the respiratory Biorate pacemaker and the activity detecting Activitrax. First experiences with 96 QT and 35 Biorate pacemakers from 11 centers are reported. The Biorate pacemaker functions without any problems, its disadvantage being limited programmability. With the TX pacemakers failing frequency adaptation is found more often, mostly due to voltage polarization at the tip of the electrode.

Physiological stimulation can be achieved by either bifocal or rate responsive pacing. In bifocal pacemakers the ventricular stimulus is triggered after atrial potentials are sensed in patients with 2nd or 3rd degree atrioventricular block. This pacemaker should be used in patients with sinus rhythm only. Its hemodynamic benefit persists (1). The rate responsive device adapts heart rate according to physiological demands. It should be used in patients with bradyarrhythmia or with sinus bradycardia and inadequate rate adaptation during exercise.

Atrial contraction or frequency – their relative contributions to the cardiac index

The cardiac index is the product of frequency and stroke volume index. At rest frequency accounts for 50%, left ventricular filling or pulmonary wedge pressure for 30 to 40% and atrial contraction for 10 to 20% of it (2). With increasing frequency heart rate becomes a more prominent factor (3, 4, 5) probably due to the increased filling pressure (6) in most of the patients investigated so far who suffered from more or less overt heart failure. The stroke volume index is influenced by left ventricular filling (filling pressure and atrial contribution) and intrinsic contractility (or inotropism) (7, 8). Karlöf et al. (3) and Fananapazir et al. (9) compared the atrial contribution to the mere frequency adaptation at rest and at exercise in the same patients and concluded that the atrial contribution during exercise is of less importance than at rest, when compared to frequency dependent alterations of the cardiac index. Therefore caution should be exercised with respect to the reliability of several non-invasive methods for the assessment of cardiac function (8, 10). Nevertheless a combination of both rate adaptive pacing in the atrium by means of a biological sensor and the maintenance of AV-synchrony would compose the ideal rate adaptive bifocal pacemaker, which can be expected to be introduced to the market very soon.

100

Rate responsive pacing

Rate responsive pacing can be achieved by various principles, which are listed in Table 1. So far only the first 3 methods have been applied to use in humans:

1. The QT pacemaker, which regulates heart rate by alterations of the stimulus –T interval (Tx/Quintech (Vitatron)).
2. The Biorate (Alpha), which uses respiratory rate as biological signal.
3. The Activitrax (Medtronic), which detects muscle noise due to activity induced muscle motions by a crystal microphone.

Table 1. Rate responsiveness – theoretical and practical possibilities and application.

Principle of rate responsiveness	Examples	References
1. QT interval (catecholamine determined)	Quintech, TX (Vitatron)	Rickards (11) Donaldson (12)
2. Muscle activity (by crystal microphone)	Activitrax (Medtronic)	Anderson et al. (13) Humen et al. (2) Ryden et al. (14)
3. Respiratory control	a) intrapleural pressure	Funke (15)
	b) Biorate RDP (Biotec/Alpha)	Krasner (16) Rossi et al. (17, 18)
4. Central-venous oxygen saturation	(experimental)	Wirtzfeld et al. (19)
5. Central-venous temperature	(experimental)	Griffin (20) Laczkovics et al. (21)
6. pH	(experimental)	Camilli et al. (22) Peterson et al. (23)
7. End-systolic volume	(experimental)	
8. Pressure (P)	(experimental)	
9. dp/dt	(experimental)	
10. Chemical sensors a) ISFET = ion-sensitive field effect transistors, e.g. electrolyte concentration b) fiberoptics	(experimental)	Peterson et al. (23)
11. Threshold (falls during exercise)	(experimental)	
12. Atrial frequency	all DDD-, AAI- and VAT-pacemakers	

QT Pacemakers

In healthy persons the QT interval is dependent on both heart rate and physical activity (= catecholamine concentration). According to Rickards and Norman (11) and Donaldson (12, 24) the QT interval is reduced linearly during physical exercise and mental stress. Thus the reduction of the QT interval (Δ-QT) is a feasible indicator of an expected rate increase. Figure 1 demonstrates that in the QT pacemaker this principle is employed, but due to technical reasons the pacemaker can detect the QT interval of a stimulated heart beat only, the so-called stimulus-T interval (25). To prevent the condition that only the polarisation voltage at the tip of the electrode is detected as T wave the newer systems use a filter combination and a small adverse impulse. The stimulus-T in-

Fig. 1. Detection of the T wave in Quintech pacemakers: the maximum of the deflection of the T wave (first derivative) is the end-point of the stimulus-T interval. Filters and windows help to avoid the measurement of the polarization voltage following ventricular depolarization by the stimulus (modified according to (7)).

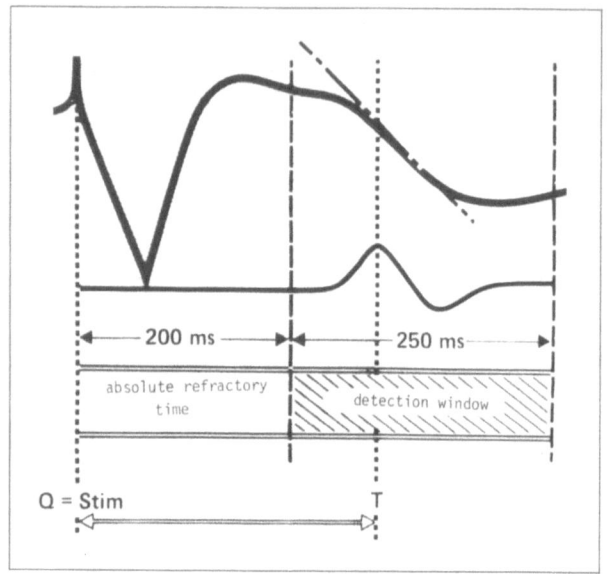

terval sensed by the pacemaker is measured from the pacemaker spike to the maximal deflection of the T wave (first derivative). Alterations of the stimulus-T interval can be transformed to different slopes of rate adaptation. The principal advantage of the QT system is that only one lead (in place or to be implanted) is necessary. Its present theoretical disadvantage is that the QT interval is influenced by a number of drugs and that mental distress may result in unwanted "pacemaker tachycardia".

Figure 2 demonstrates frequency adaptation during hand grip in a patient with a Quintech pacemaker. Whereas we could achieve frequency adaptation in both of our patients with a Quintech pacemaker, TX pacemakers failed to increase stimulation frequency due to polarisation voltage measured at the tip of the electrode in all 6 cases. In these patients a reduction of the stimulation voltage to 2.5 V and changing of the detection window did not solve the problem. With new software now available, one of the TX pacemakers functions properly. One patient, however, demonstrated rate responsiveness only during mental stress and during walking, not during bicycle exercise testing in the supine posi-

Fig. 2. Hand grip in a patient with a QT pacemaker. Rate responsiveness can be demonstrated: 1. sinus rhythm, 2. start of hand grip with rate increase; 3. maximum rate achieved by this Quintech system. In the early devices (TX system) in 6 of 8 of our own patients polarization measurement prevented the detection of an adequate stimulus-

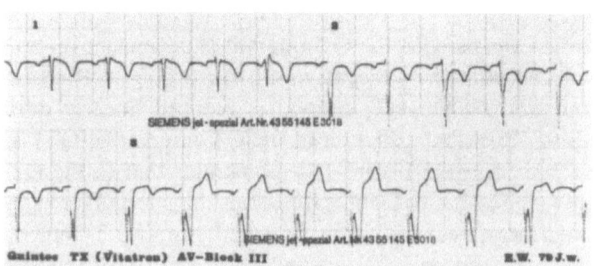

T interval, thus preventing frequency adaptation.

tion. In this case the measured stimulus-T intervals were reduced during exercise but a rate increase did not occur. In this patient, however, nightly tachycardias were observed that were experienced as nightmares.

To ensure objectivity in judging the new rate responsive pacemakers a telephone survey including 11 hospitals implanting rate adaptive devices was carried out[1]. Ninety-five QT pacemakers were implanted, 74% of which showed rate responsiveness (Table 2). In 26%, mostly due to measuring a polarization voltage, as in our patients, no frequency adaptation was achieved. "Pacemaker tachycardias" due to mental stress were observed in 7 cases. In one patient, a hard working wood-cutter, the slope of frequency adaptation seemed to be insufficient: after starting to work he had to wait some seconds until the cardiac output had reached the amount necessary to continue working. From the experience of the 11 centers some additional information could be derived: 1. Before permanently programming the pacemaker recently implanted electrodes should have healed in: so some 4 weeks may pass. 2. Porous or carbon tip electrodes gave fewer polarization voltage measurements and thus a better T wave sensing. 3. Stimulation amplitudes should not exceed 2.5 V, whenever possible (26).

Table 2. Survey rate responsive pacemakers, TX and Quintech (Vitatron) and Biorate RDP (Alpha/Biotec) (n = 131).

	TX and Quintech (n = 95)		Biorate (n = 36)	
	n	%	n	%
Perfect rate responsiveness	70	74	36	100
Not working or explanted	25[1])	26	1[2])	3
Pacemaker induced tachycardias	7	7	0	0
Latency period too long	3	3	0	0
Indication modified	3	3	1	3

[1]) one of these a Quintech TX
[2]) increase in threshold

Respiration and activity controlled pacing

The pacemaker with respiratory control adapts the ventricular pacing rate to respiration frequency. In 1975 Funke (15) first described a pacemaker whose intrapleural sensor detected pressure gradients due to respiration. This signal was used for frequency adaptation in dogs only.

Only one respiration controlled system is in clinical use, the Biorate RDP (Biotec/Alpha).

---

[1]) Contributions were made by the following centers and their doctors, whom I should like to thank for their collaboration: Chirurg. Univ.-Klinik Frankfurt (Mr. Kreuzer), Krankenhaus Hagen (Dr. Kunze), Krankenhaus Krumbach (Dr. Otter), Krankenhaus Lohr (Dr. Dammermann), Städt. Krankenhaus Mannheim (Dr. Kollmeyer), Maria-Theresien-Klinik München (Prof. Schaudig), Klinikum Rechts der Isar (Dr. Alt), Klinikum Passau (Dr. Luckner), Schwabinger Krankenhaus (Dr. Kronski), Krankenhaus Schweinfurt (Prof. Gattenlöhner).

Respiration is measured by the Biorate RDP as changes of the impedance between the pacemaker and a second subcutaneous electrode which incorporates a radiofrequency system (17, 18). The relationship between the frequency of respiration and of stimulation can be programmed individually for each patient. If the biorate rhythm is working the surface ECG demonstrates rheography spikes. The frequency profile of a patient with a respiration controlled device when lying, walking, sitting and during bicycle supine exercise (75 watts) and a final provocative hyperventilation can be seen from Figs. 3 and 4. Hemodynamic measurements with the thermodilution method demonstrated a twofold increase of the cardiac index during exercise (Fig. 4). If the patient is paced at baseline frequency and the same exercise test is performed, inadequate frequency adaptation resulted in a much lower cardiac index. In contrast, forced hyperventilation without stress or activity induced catecholamine release resulted in an identical stimulation frequency during the biorate mode of 120/min without any increase of the cardiac index when compared to the index at rest.

Fig. 3. Frequency profile of a patient with a Biorate pacemaker: During rest and exercise prompt frequency adaptation could be observed.

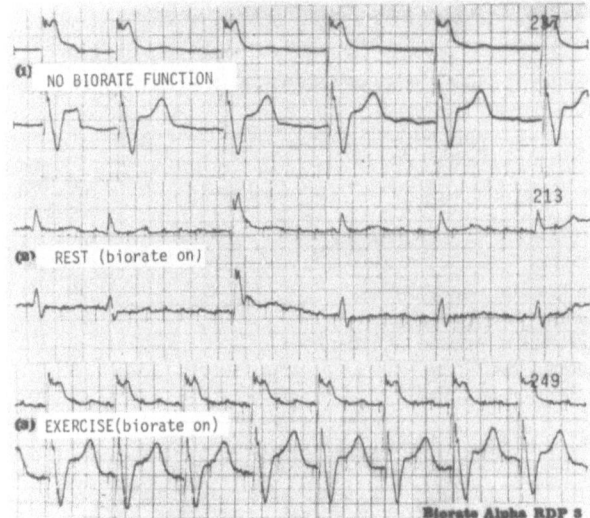

Fig. 4. Hemodynamic evaluation of a patient with a respiration controlled rate responsive pacemaker (Biorate) during rest, bicycle exercise with and without biorate mode and forced hyperventilation.

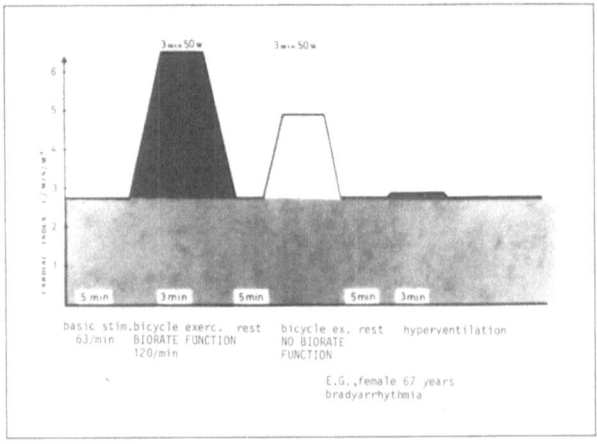

104

By analysing the Biorate in our patients its prompt frequency adaptation, its easy handling and fast programmability were much appreciated (26). Possible disadvantages at present are the use of an additional (respiratory) electrode, which can be implanted very easily, however. The first model of the Biorate only offers 2 baseline frequencies; all other features of a standard multiprogrammable pacemaker are still missing. Our personal impression of the Biorate was validated by the survey conducted (Table 2): all 36 pacemakers functioned properly. In one patient the device was explanted due to an increase in the stimulation threshold, a problem that may also arise in other pacemakers. In the case of the Biorate, however, it could not be solved by increasing stimulation voltage or impulse width, since these parameters are not yet programmable.

Experience with the new activity controlled Activitrax (Medtronic) (13) is rare in Europe. Only Ryden et al. (14) have implanted and published 3 devices. The sensor of the Activitrax is a piezo-crystal on top of a modified Enertrax system. The Activitrax can be used to stimulate both chambers. Ryden found the frequency adaptation reliable and was impressed by the easy handling of the new device. Since the sensor is localized on the pacemaker no second electrode is necessary. Possible disadvantages may arise from some interference with external noise, e.g. traffic or airplanes. In most cases filters seem to restrict this interference satisfactorily, which is also the case in our first 2 implants of an Activitrax (26).

References

1. Kruse I, Amman K, Conradson TB, Ryden L (1982) A comparison of the acute and long-term hemodynamic effects of ventricular inhibited and atrial synchronous ventricular inhibited pacing. Circulation 65: 5
2. Humen DP, Anderson K, Brumwell D, Huntley S, Klein GJ (1983) A pacemaker which automatically increases its rate with physical activity. In: Steinbach K et al (eds) Cardiac Pacing. Steinkopff Verlag, Darmstadt, p 259
3. Karlöf J (1975) Hemodynamic effect of atrial triggering versus fixed rate pacing at rest and during exercise in complete heart block. Acta Med Scand 197: 195
4. Koretsune J, Kodama K, Nauto S, Ischikaira K, Toniurer K, Mishima M, Inone M, Abe J (1983) The effect of pacing mode on external worker and myocardial oxygen consumption. In: Steinbach K et al. (eds) Cardiac Pacing. Steinkopff Verlag, Darmstadt, p 183
5. Samet P, Bernstein WH, Nathan DA (1965) Atrial contribution to cardiac output in complete heart block. Am J Cardiol 16: 1
6. Greenberg B, Chatterjee K, Parmeley WW (1975) The influence of left ventricular filling pressure on atrial contribution to cardiac output. Am Heart J 198: 742
7. Knapp K, Gmeiner R, Hammerle P, Raas E (1977) Der Einfluß der Vorhofkontraktion auf das Schlagvolumen bei Schrittmacherstimulation. Z Kardiol 65: 783
8. Maisch B, Ertl G, Eiles Ch, Gerhards W, Knoblauch J, Kochsiek K (in press) Cardiac function during VVI- and DVI-Pacing at different rates. A comparative study using one and two dimensional echocardiography, gated single photon emission computerized tomography (GASPECT) and thermodilution
9. Fananapazir L, Bennert DH, Monks P (1983) Atrial synchronized pacing: Contribution of the chronotropic response to improved exercise performance. PACE 6: 601
10. Maisch B, Kochsiek K (1983) Underestimation of stroke volume (SVI) and cardiac index (CI) by TM-echocardiography during ventricular pacing. In: Steinbach K et al (eds) Cardiac Pacing. Steinkopff Verlag, Darmstadt, p 193
11. Rickards AF, Norman J (1981) Relation between QT interval and heart rate. New design of a physiologically adaptive cardiac pacemaker. Br Heart J 45: 56
12. Donaldson RM, Fox K, Rickards AF (1983) Initial experience with a physiological, rate responsive pacemaker. Br Med J 286: 667

13. Anderson K, Humen D, Klein GJ, Brumwell D, Huntley S (1983) A rate variable pacemaker which automatically adjust for physical activity. PACE 6 A – 12
14. Ryden L, Smedgard P, Kruse J, Anderson K (in press) Rate responsive pacing by means of activity sensing. Stimucoeur
15. Funke H (1975) Ein Herzschrittmacher mit belastungsabhängiger Frequenzregelung. Biomed Technik 20: 225
16. Krasner J (1966) A physiologically controlled Pacemaker. JAAMS 1 (3): 476
17. Rossi P, Plicchi G, Canducci G, Rognoni G, Aina F (1983) Respiratory rate as a determinant of optimal pacing rate. PACE 6: 502
18. Rossi P, Plicchi G, Canducci GC, Rognoni S, Aina F (1984) Respiration as a reliable physiological sensor for controlling cardiac pacing rate. Br Heart J 51: 7
19. Wirtzfeld A (1982) Central Venous Oxygen Saturation for the Control of Automatic Rate Responsive Pacing. PACE 5: 829
20. Griffin J (1983) Central Body Temperature as a Guide to Optimal Heart rate. PACE 6: 498
21. Laczkovics A, Schlick W, Losert U, Simbrunner G (1983) The use of central venous blood temperature (CVT) as a guide for rate control in pacemaker-therapy. PACE 6: Abstr 46
22. Camilli L (1972) A new pacemaker autoregulating the rate. Proceedings Cardiac Pacing, 5th International Symposium Excerpta Medica, p 414
23. Peterson JI, Goldstein SR, Fitzgerald RV (1980) Fiberoptic pH probe for physical use. Anal Chem 52: 864
24. Donaldson RM, Rickards AF (1983) The ventricular endocardial paced evoked response. PACE 6: 253
25. Gebhardt-Seehausen U (1984) Der frequenzadaptierbare Tx-Schrittmacher. Herzschrittmacher 4: 94
26. Maisch B, Steilner G (1985) Praktische Herzschrittmachertherapie. Perimed Verlag

Authors' address:
Prof. Dr. B. Maisch
University Hospital of Internal Medicine
Josef-Schneider-Str. 2
D-8700 Würzburg, F.R.G.

Problems with the Slope Adjustment and Rate Adaptation in Rate Responsive Pacemakers: Oscillation Phenomena and Sudden Rate Jumps

U. J. Winter, D. W. Behrenbeck, B. Candelon*, M. Höher, Th. Brill, J. Missler, and H. H. Hilger

Summary: The recently developed rate-responsive pacemakers are a clinical alternative to dual chamber devices. Patients who are treated by these pulse generators have different underlying diseases and exercise profiles. The aim of the study was to investigate how the adjustment of the slope and rate adaptation can be improved individually by means of repeated exercise tests. The TX pacemaker and Helifix lead (Vitatron, The Netherlands) were implanted in 5 patients with AV-block III° or sinus bradycardia. Using different bicycle exercise tests in the sitting position (stepwise increase of the work load; exercise at a high work load; short and long-term exercise) we tried to imitate the daily activity profile.

In subsequent stress tests, a normalisation of the respiratory and hemodynamic parameters as well as stim.-T interval has to be achieved in order to avoid a delayed heart rate increase. If the pacemaker slope was programmed to > 80% of the theoretical value measured at rest (= 100%), sudden rate jumps were observed ("oscillation phenomenon"). Sudden rate jumps also occurred in patients with exercise-induced AV-block II° in whom the 'tracking mode' was not used. During the inhibition of the pacemaker by the rate increase, this mode decreases the stimulation interval in parallel. A "drift mode" slowly reduces the increased pacing rate in the case of elevated plasma catecholamine levels associated with myocardial failure.

Conclusion: Although technical improvements have increased the reliability T-wave sensing, slope and rate adjustment to suit individual needs still remains a problem. The TX algorithm should allow repetitive and long-term exercise with adequate rate adaptation.

Introduction

The TX pacemaker is a rate responsive pacemaker in which a biosensor senses the indicator QT (Fig. 1). The pacemaker's TX algorithm causes a heart rate increase if the QT duration shortens. The system works as an open loop. This contribution deals especially with the adjustment of the slope and the rate adaptation (Fig. 1). Based on the experiences of nearly 800 TX implantations world-wide from summer 1982 to December 1984 many technical improvements were made to the TX pacemaker. The primary pacemaker version, the TX 1, showed failure to sense of T-waves in about 10%, mostly due to afterpolarizations at the electrode. Furthermore sudden rate reduction or too fast drift were detected (1). The revised version, the Quintech TX, contains new hardware, improved software, a new TX algorithm including the tracking mode and better T-wave sensing (2).

---

* Vitatron Medical BV, Dieren (NL)

Fig. 1. In rate responsive pace-makers the implanted sensor measures the indicator. Changes of the indicator lead to a modification of the resting value. The slope 'α' determines the degree of heart rate increase during exercise.

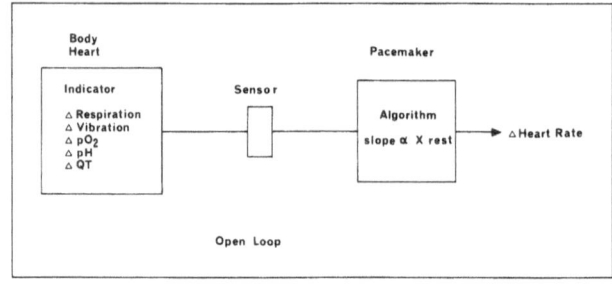

The latter could be achieved due to a lower band width of the T-wave sensing channel and a faster recharge impulse (< 300 ms). The rate of failure to sense of T-waves dropped from about 10% to 3.6% (1, 2).

Objective

The aim of the study was to:
1. find a reliable method to control heart rate adaptation during exercise after the slope determination;
2. investigate if a slope, higher than the calculated pacemaker slope (100%), can improve the exercise performance of the patients;
3. control the problems of long-term rate responsive pacing.

Individual adjustment of the TX pacemaker

The individual adjustment of TX pacemakers includes the "tuning" of the VVI pacemaker (threshold and sensitivity-guided pacing) and of the rate responsive pacemaker (adjustment of the sensor: T-wave sensing, sensing window, and the response: upper rate limit, mode, slope).

Adjustment of the VVI pacemaker

Threshold adjustment:

The measurement of the threshold is performed in the pacemaker by automatically reducing the impulse width at 5.0 and 2.5 V output, until the point of no capture is reached (threshold value). Reducing the output voltage from 5.0 to 2.5 V in the sense of threshold-guided pacing also ameliorates the T-wave sensing. A lower voltage for stimulation also decreases the after-polarization on the electrode after the impulse delivery. High threshold values with the consequence of high voltage stimulation made TX pacing difficult in 35/200 (14.5%) cases (3).

108

R-wave sensing adjustment:

Although the TX pacemaker realizes rate responsive pacing by means of T-wave sensing, a correct sensing of the R-wave is a necessary prerequisite for the sufficient function as demand (VVI) pacemaker. The measurement of the endocardial R-wave amplitude helps to adjust the sensitivity.

Adjustment of the rate responsive pacemaker

Adjustment of the sensor:

T-wave sensing and T-wave sensing window

The T-wave sensing in the TX pacemaker (Fig. 2) is realized by a second, T-wave sensing circuit, which has a different filtering charateristic, working in a lower frequency range than the R-wave sensing circuit (10 Hz compared to 22 Hz). After an absolute refractory period of 200 ms a T-wave detection window is opened. During this "window" the evoked T-wave can be sensed, based on the T-wave amplitude and stimulus-T interval measurement. The T-wave should be measured at 2.5 and 5.0 V output voltage. The end

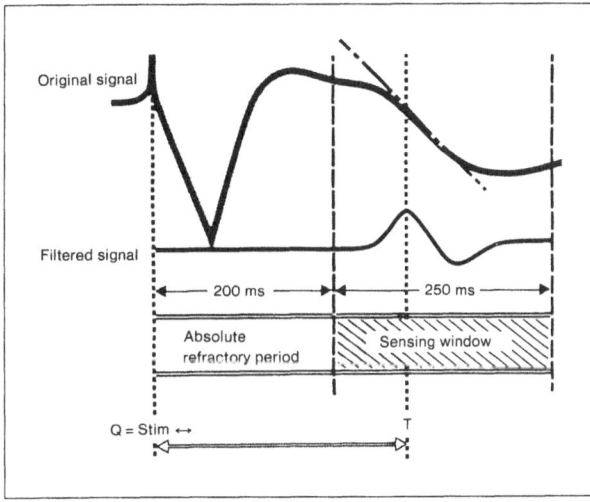

Fig. 2. Principle of T-wave measurement in the TX pacemaker. During a (programmable) T-wave sensing window the filtered evoked T-wave is measured with respect to amplitude and stim.-T interval.

Table 1. Limitation of the maximal stimulation rate by the value of the T-wave sensing window.

T-wave sensing window (ms)	Maximal stimulation rate (ppm)
250–400 ms	140
250–430 ms	130
250–450 ms	125

of the T-wave sensing window is programmable up to 450 ms. As a clinical rule, the end of the T-wave sensing window is derived from the stimulus T-wave interval in ms at the programmed lower rate limit (LRL) plus a 20 ms safety time. The end of the window also limits the maximal stimulation rate (see Table 1). At 400 ms the maximal rate is 140 ppm, at 430 ms it is 130 ppm and at 450 ms it is 125 ppm. The percentage of sensed T-waves should be close to 100% at the programmed T-wave sensitivity.

Failure to sense of the T-waves:

A failure to sense of the T-waves may be caused by the following:
1. a reduced signal amplitude (e.g. myocardial infarction);
2. after-polarization at the electrode (pacing with 5.0 V; recharge impulse 300 ms after the stimulus delivery);
3. an increase of the lead impedance;
4. a competitive spontaneous rate during the stim.-T measurement.

Adjustment of the response:

Adjustment of the upper rate limit

As mentioned before, the upper rate limit is influenced by the T-wave sensing window. Long-term ventricular stimulation with a rate $\geq$ 120 ppm should be avoided in patients with latent coronary heart disease or critical left ventricular performance (4, 5). Many hemodynamic investigations during the 1960s and 1970s revealed a remarkable augmentation of the cardiac index if the heart rate was significantly increased in patients with bradyarrhythmias and AV block III°. Thus, the "rate jump" between the maximal spontaneous rate during exercise and the programmed upper rate limit should be not too low.

Programming of the stand-by rate or lower rate limit (LRL)

The value of the programmed stand-by rate is directed by the symptoms of the patient during day and night (palpitations? tachycardia? etc.) and the spontaneous rate.

Determination of the pacemaker slope

The QT duration is influenced by the heart rate and catecholamines (Fig. 4). The determination of the slope α, i.e. the angle of the linear relationship between heart rate and stimulation-T-interval, is performed at rest in the supine position (Fig. 3). An increase of the stimulation rate (e.g. 70 to 100 ppm) leads to a significant decrease of the stimulus-T interval. In order to control the linear relationship several stimulation rates should be investigated. The quotient (slope α) is calculated by dividing the rate difference (Δ f) by the difference of the stim.-T interval (Δ StimT). The unit of the slope is ppm per 1 ms.

110

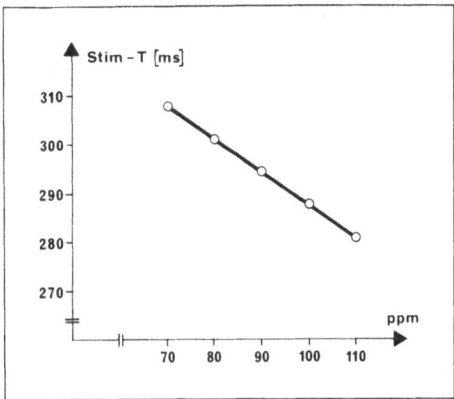

Fig. 3. Measurement of the stim.-T interval at different pacing rates reveals a linear relationship.

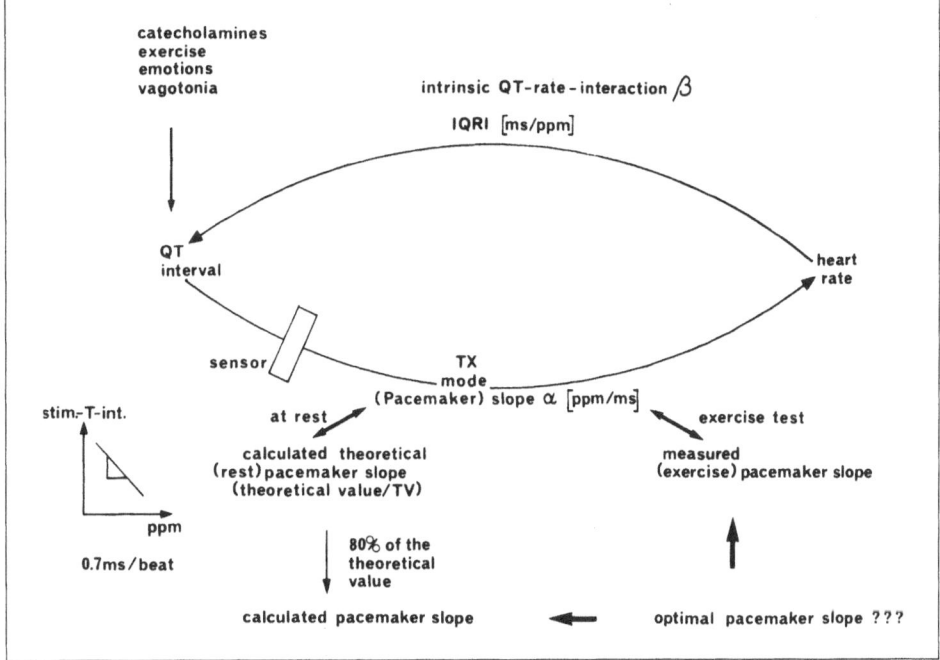

Fig. 4. The intrinsic QT rate interaction 'β' describes the relationship between QT interval and heart rate. The pacemaker slope 'α' can be obtained either by calculation at rest (calculated theoretical pacemaker slope) or measured during exercise test (measured pacemaker slope).

Table 2. Measured slope too high.

1. Measured not at complete rest
   (especially after repeated exercise tests)

2. Measurement of the stim.-T interval too early after a rate change

3. Measurement and calculation of the quotient based on a larger rate range

4. Measurement in a patient with modified drug treatment

Fig. 5. After a sudden change of the pacing rate the stim.-T interval needs 2.5 to 3.0 minutes to reach a plateau phase in which the value should be determined.

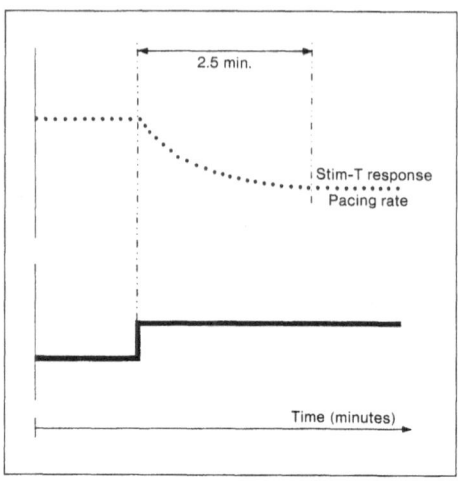

Pitfalls of slope measurements

If the patient is not at complete rest after an exercise test the measured slope is too high due to the output of catecholamines. During exercise the slope is higher (by about 10%) than that at rest. The quotient must always be derived from the same rate range, otherwise the slope values are too high. Also changes in the drug regimen lead to a variation of the slope. Furthermore a special equilibration period should be left after each change of the stimulation rate, since the stimulus-T interval needs about 2 to 3 minutes to reach a stable value after a sudden rate change, e.g. from 80 to 100 ppm (Fig. 5).

Slope and interaction: different expressions

The intrinsic QT rate interaction β (IQRI) is the quotient of Δ QT and Δ heart rate with the unit ms per ppm (Fig. 4).
The *pacemaker slope* (α) is the slope programmed in the TX pacemaker.
The *optimal pacemaker slope* can be obtained either by the measurement of the intrinsic QT rate interaction (IQRI) during exercise, i.e., stress testing (measured exercise pacemaker slope α_E) or by calculation, by taking 80% of 1/IQRI (calculated pacemaker slope α_C).

Tracking mode

The rate responsive mode can be programmed to a tracking mode. This special feature in the TX pacemaker enables the device during inhibition to decrease the escape and pacing interval continuously (by 6.4 ms) during exercise-induced increase of the spontaneous rhythm (Fig. 6). After a period of "shadowing" the spontaneous rate increase a period of fusion beats occurs when the spontaneous rate interval and the stimulation interval are equal. The measured stim.-T-interval is then compared with the last stim.-T-

112

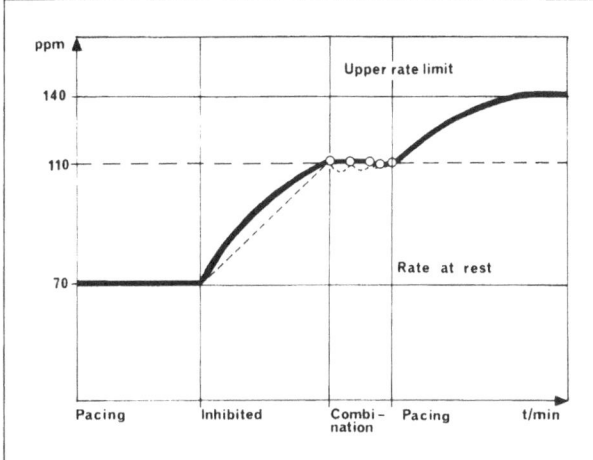

Fig. 6. The "tracking mode" enables the pacemaker to follow the spontaneous, exercise-induced rate increase in spite of inhibition. After a period of no further rate increase and fusion beats the TX mode induces a significant rate increase.

interval value at rest. Based on the programmed characteristics of the TX pacemaker the TX algorithm decides to increase or decrease the stimulation rate.

Stable rate adaptation in the TX pacemaker

The algorithm for the rate adaptation compares the actual stim.-T interval (stim.-T$_2$) with that of the previous cycle (stim.-T$_1$). Stim.-T$_1$ is subtracted from stim.-T$_2$. If this difference is smaller than a defined value Δ T, then the drift mode (continuous reduction of the pacing rate) is initiated. If the difference is larger than Δ T the rate adaptation mode is induced. Stim.-T$_1$ < stim.-T$_2$ leads to a rate decrease, stim.-T$_1$ > stim.-T$_2$ induces a rate increase. The nature and velocity of the rate increase is defined by the pacemaker slope, degree of exercise (catecholamines) as well as original catecholamine concentrations. Figure 2 shows that a catecholamine-induced shortening of the stim.-T interval causes an adequate rate increase. This does not itself induce a reduction of the stim.-T time and thus an unstable rate adaptation.

Methods

The patients were controlled, if possible, every four weeks after the implantation. The control included anamnesis, physical examination, pacemaker telemetry, repeated exercise tests in supine position and 24-hour pacemaker Holter ECG (Del Mar Avionics; Reynolds Pathfinder; Ela Medical Anatec). The tapes were examined visually (1 : 100). The pacemaker adjustment was performed as described previously.

Patients

The TX 1 (n = 1) and the Quintech TX (n = 4) as well as a Helifix lead were implanted in 5 patients (♀ = 1; ♂ = 4; age: 33 to 63 years) suffering from bradyarrhythmias or AV

113

block. The following underlying diseases were present: drug- (sotalol) induced sinus bradycardia and poor left ventricular performance (n = 1); sinus bradycardia and intermittent
AV-block II° and intermittent SA-block (n = 1); Sinus bradycardia and AV-block II° type
2 and right bundle branch block and intermittent SA block (n = 1); AV-block III° after
posterolateral myocardial infarction (n = 1); AV-block II° due to His bundle ablation (n =
1).

Exercise profile of the patients

Two patients are very active and perform many different kinds of sport. One relatively
young woman is a night nurse in a hospital (a great deal of physical work). Two patients
had reduced physical activities due to poor left ventricular performance at rest.

Clinical course

In the female patient the TX mode could not be switched on due to increasing threshold
values. At 5.0 V / 0.5 ms correct T-wave sensing was not possible. In the patient with
AV-block III° after acute posterolateral myocardial infarction intracardiac low signal amplitudes led to a failure to sense. After changing the lead position the sensing problem disappeared. We intend to try the TX mode again. In one patient with drug-induced sinus
bradycardia and poor left ventricular function the TX mode functioned well after we
used the revised Vitatron software.

Fig. 7. Delayed heart rate increase during the second exercise test due to not completely
normalized stim.-T interval.
(Vitatron Quintech TX)

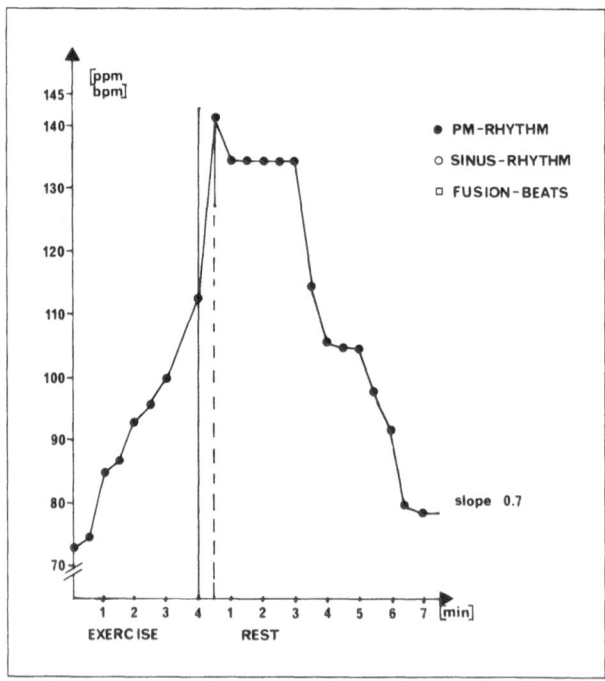

114

Results

Methodological considerations

During "normal" exercise testing the recovery time between two consecutive tests has to be sufficiently long for heart rate, blood pressure and breathing to return to rest condition. Figure 7 demonstrates that during exercise testing of patients with TX pacemakers the stim.-T-interval also has to return to normal values. In this case the patient had a recovery time of about 15 minutes which was sufficient for the normalization of the hemodynamics and respiration, but not for the QT duration. The consequence of the still shortened stim.-T-interval was a delayed heart rate increase during the second exercise test (Fig. 7).

The explanation for this observation is given in Figure 8. The TX algorithm is based on relative changes of the QT interval and the heart rate, namely $\varDelta$ QT and $\varDelta$ HR. To program the algorithm it has to be initialised at defined conditions (rest and the lower rate limit). After an exercise test the drift protection of the pacemaker leads to a slow rate reduction (0.025 microsec/cycle), until the lower rate limit is reached. If the time period between two exercise tests is too short, the TX mode starts at another lower rate limit-related stim.-T-interval. This leads in parallel (to the first exercise test) to the left shifted curve with a delay in reaching the upper rate limit.

Usefulness of the tracking mode in patients without sufficient heart rate increase during exercise testing

Figure 9 shows a case in which the determination of the slope revealed a value of 0.76 ppm/ms and an 80% slope value of 0.62 ppm/ms. The pacemaker slope was programmed to 0.7 ppm/ms. During exercise testing with 100 W (sitting position) the spontaneous heart rate increased from 45 bpm at rest to 100 bpm after 1'30". In spite of the continuation of the stress test, spontaneous heart rate slowly reduced to about 90 bpm, perhaps

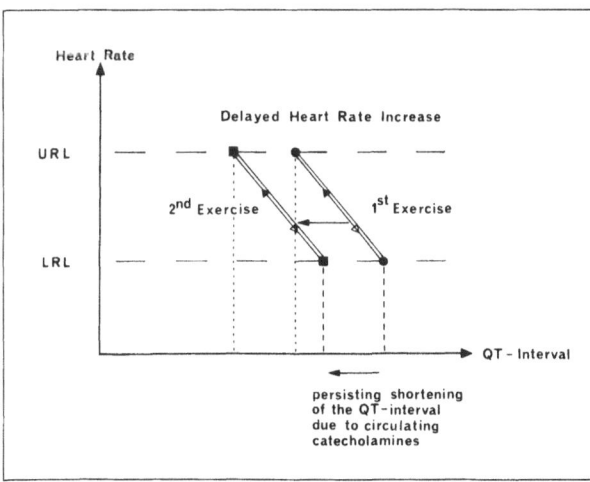

Fig. 8. If a second exercise test is started before the complete normalization of the stim. T interval, a delayed heart rate increase results, since the rate adaptation begins at a different lower rate limit-stim.-T interval relationship. (Vitatron Quintech TX)

115

Fig. 9. The "tracking mode" leads to a significant heart rate increase in the case of exercise induced AV-block II° and / or sinus bradycardia. Without "tracking mode", the pacing rate increases only in the rest period. (Vitatron Quintech TX)

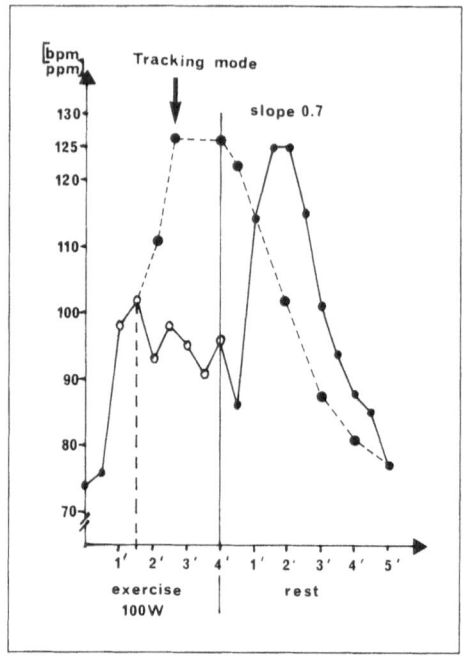

due to hypoxia-induced QT prolongation. During exercise testing the increased heart rate led to an inhibition of the pacemaker. Half a minute after the end of the exercise test, the pacemaker started to pace due to the post-exercise heart rate decrease. Measurement of the stim.-T-interval revealed a significant, catecholamine-induced shortening. This induced a fast rate increase during the rest period, reaching the upper rate limit of 127 ppm at 1'30" after the stress test. The dotted line demonstrates the heart rate course with the tracking mode switched on. At a rate of 100 ppm the pacemaker takes over since no further spontaneous rate increase occurs. In another exercise test the TX mode (pacemaker slope 0.8 ppm/ms) led to a fast rate increase until about 100 ppm. Then the spontaneous rhythm took over for a short while. But due to exercise-induced AV-block II° the intrinsic heart rate "jumped down". At this point the pacemaker took over and induced a sudden rate increase to 127 ppm (upper rate limit). With the tracking mode switched on, no "downward jump" of the heart rate would have occurred.

Slope adjustment

In two patients with many physical activities, the 80% value of the slope was compared with the anamnesis, daily exercise profile and occurrence of emotional tachycardias. In Fig. 10 the same patient as in Fig. 9 was examined by stress testing (100 W, sitting position). This time, the tracking mode was switched on. The determination of the optimal slope revealed a value of 0.5 ppm/ms. Exercise testing showed that this slope was too low since no significant rate increase occurred. After a sufficient recovery time a second stress test was performed, this time with a slope of 0.9 ppm/ms. The graphic shows that

116

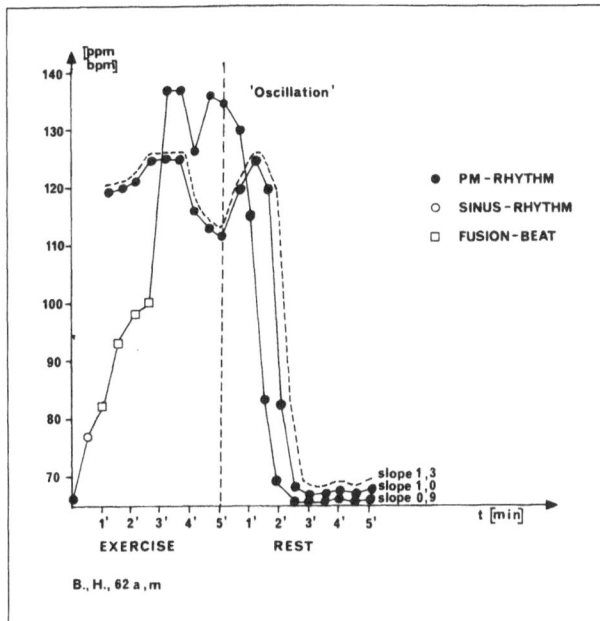

Fig. 10. "Oscillation pheno-menon" of the rate adaptation due excessively high slopes. (Vitatron Quintech TX)

the spontaneous rate increases to about 90 bpm. The tracking mode "shadows" the intrinsic rate increase. At a rate of 100/minute a fast increase of the stimulation rate occurs. But in spite of continuous ergometry the heart rate decreases from 138 ppm (upper rate limit) to 125 ppm. During the rest period the stimulation rate is reduced very quickly. The sudden rate decrease after having reached the upper rate limit can be explained by the fact that the slope was too high and the reaction to QT time variations, either shortening or prolongation, was very powerful. Thus, the exercise test demonstrated that the slope had to be reprogrammed to 0.7 ppm/ms. The patient reported slightly more dyspnea at 0.5 ppm/ms, but no problems at 0.9 ppm/ms. Figure 11 shows a comparable case. This very dynamic sportsman had a slope of 0.833 pm/ms and an 80% value of 0.7 ppm/ms. In order to improve physical performance (e.g. tennis competition, climbing mountains etc.) the pacemaker slope was programmed to 1.0 ppm/ms. As demonstrated in Fig. 6 a very fast heart rate increase in the early beginning of exercise is thus achieved. After 1 minute a heart rate decrease from 138 ppm (upper rate limit) to 130 ppm is observed. Although the exercise test is continued a further drop of the rate down to 110 ppm occurs. Intermittent increase of work load from 100 to 120 W leads to a slow rate increase. As in Fig. 10 the slope was too high.

The usefulness of the drift mode

Figure 12 shows an exercise test (35 W, sitting position) in a patient with sinus bradycardia, coronary artery bypass grafting, anterolateral aneurysmectomy and slowly progressive left ventricular myocardial failure. Due to malignant ventricular arrhythmias the patient was treated by sotalol. This did not affect the TX mode. The 80% value of the slope

Fig. 11. "Oscillation phenomenon" due to a slope which
was about 120% of the calculated theoretical value. Besides a
quick rate increase a fast rate
decrease was also observed. Intermittent increase of the work
load led to a second rate rise.
(Vitatron Quintech TX)

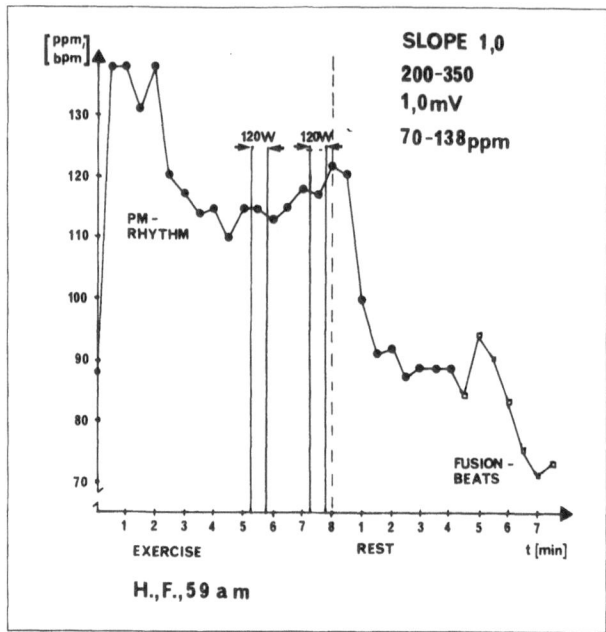

Fig. 12. In patients with elevated plasma catecholamine levels
(e.g. due to myocardial failure)
the "drift mode" helps the normal rate decrease to slowly reduce the heart rate during the
rest period after a stress test.
(Vitatron Quintech TX)

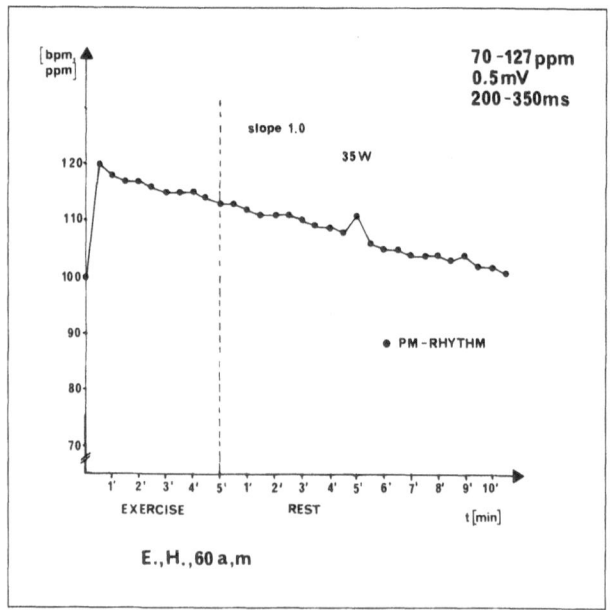

was 1.0 ppm/ms. During exercise testing a fast rate increase was achieved. But already
during the exercise test, heart rate slowly dropped. This slow reduction (about 65
ppm/hour) was continued during the rest period. After 25 minutes the previous rest values were obtained. The slow heart rate decrease was interpreted as an expression of the

normal and drift-induced reduction of the heart rate. This negative drift (65 ppm/hour) is initiated only in a stable rate situation. It is particularly useful in patients with elevated plasma concentrations of catecholamines (myocardial failure).

Discussion

Repeated exercise tests

Our few case reports show that repeated exercise testing in TX patients is an important diagnostic tool to control rate adaptation and slope. As demonstrated in Fig. 7 all parameters, hemodynamic, respiratory and electrophysiological (stim.-T interval) have to return to the rest values before a new exercise test can be performed again. But even different kinds of ergometries (slowly increasing work load; sudden increase in work load; exercise during 10 minutes or longer etc.) are far from imitating the daily exercise profile of active people.

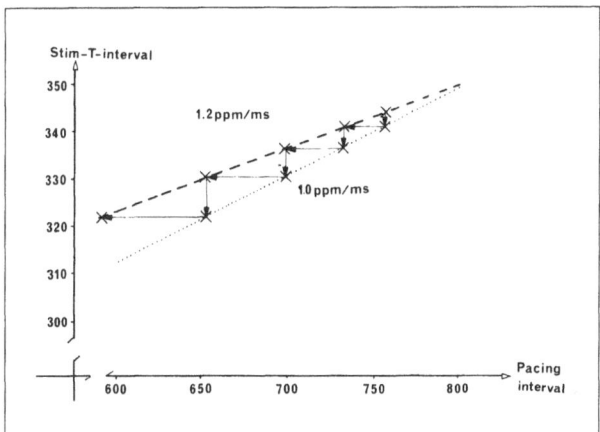

Fig. 13. In the case of excessively high slopes the exercise-induced stim.-T interval shortening is so large that the abrupt rate increase itself reduces QT duration. (Vitatron Quintech TX)

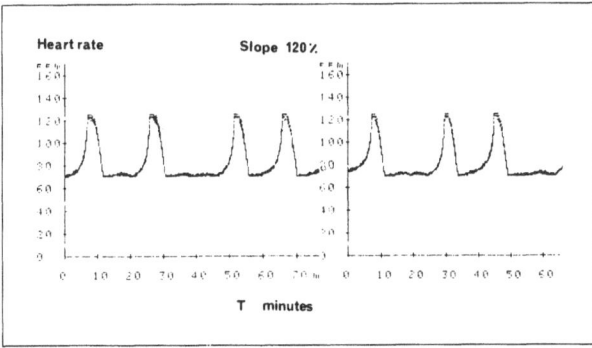

Fig. 14. Computer simulation of the "oscillation phenomenon" using excessively high slopes in the TX mode (HP 85, random generator, TX mode).

Unstable rate adaptation in excessively high slopes: "oscillation phenomena"

Figure 10 demonstrates what happens if the pacemaker slope is programmed to a value higher than the theoretical/calculated value (100%). A shortening of the stim.-T interval due to catecholamine release leads to a significant rate increase, which is so intensive that it itself causes a shortening of the stim.-T interval. This again induces a rate increase and so on (Fig. 13). The self-perpetuating non-linear rate adaptation is only stopped when the upper rate limit is reached. The phenomenon described above may also be explained by rate-induced anoxia with consecutive stim.-T interval prolongation.

Computer simulation of the oscillation phenomenon

In a HP 85 computer the QT rate relationship and the TX algorithm were simulated (Fig. 14). With a random generator, small random variations of the QT interval ($> \pm 3$ msec) could be achieved. As demonstrated in Fig. 14 the TX algorithm showed an oscillation phenomenon between the lower rate limit (70 ppm) and upper rate limit (125 ppm) at a programmed pacemaker slope of 120%. Thus, the unstable rate adaptation could be simulated.

Reasons for sudden rate jumps during rate responsive pacing

During rate responsive pacing sudden downward jumps of the heart rate are detected. The reasons for this phenomenon are the following:
1. pacemaker slope too high (oscillation phenomenon);
2. no tracking mode (exercise-induced increase of the heart rate followed by a sudden rate decrease due to AV-block II° or sinus bradycardia);
3. sudden prolongation of the stim.-T interval due to rate-induced anoxia.

Emotion-induced pacemaker tachycardias in rate responsive pacemakers

With pacemaker slopes of ≥ 1.3 ppm/ms we observed a very fast rate increase during exercise testing, but also very troublesome emotion induced pacemaker tachycardias in 2 patients.

Slope programming

As optimal pacemaker slope, 80% of the calculated/theoretical slope was proposed (A. F. Rickards, B. Candelon, personal communications, 1984). But it is still not clearly defined how to determine the optimal pacemaker slope. Slope programming advice is listed below, based on today's experiences.

Indications for a lower slope (80–15% = 65%)

According to our experience patients with nervousness, a tendency to strong emotional response, elevated plasma catecholamine concentrations (e.g. myocardial insufficiency)

120

and younger people should be programmed to a lower pacemaker slope. This slope represents 60 to < 80% of the theoretical/calculated value of the slope.

Indications for a higher slope (80 + 15% = 95%)

During treatment with β-blocking drugs the pacemaker slope should be programmed to about $80 \pm 15\% = 95\%$ of the theoretical/calculated value of the slope.

Advantages and disadvantages of the TX mode

TX pacing has, according to A. F. Rickards (1) the following *advantages*:
1. TX pacing is possible with a single, unipolar ventricular lead;
2. the TX pacemaker is, in contrast to dual chamber pacemakers, insensitive to atrial arrhythmias;
3. the TX pacemaker has a physiological upper rate limit;
4. the TX pacemaker does not induce reentry tachycardias, as reported from dual chamber devices;
5. rate adaptation during exercise is possible.

The *problems* with TX pacing are:
1. T-wave sensing (now technically nearly completely solved);
2. influence of drugs on the stim.-T interval;
3. T-wave sensing window is different in the lying and standing positions;
4. reduced applicability in patients with bradyarrhythmias;
5. disproportional influences of mental factors on the stim.-T interval;
6. sometimes there is a long latency period between the onset of the exercise and the start of rate adaptation (see Fig. 7);
7. fine tuning of the rate adaptation beside the IQRI with the present algorithm is impossible (oscillation phenomenon);
8. not reliable for endurance exercise (e.g. marathon running);
9. definition and determination of the "optimal" pacemaker slope difficult (Fig. 4).

Proposed technical improvements

Since the TX pacemakers also work as VVI devices additional features (analysis functions: e.g. R-wave determination; Holter functions: e.g. rate histogram) should be incorporated. Furthermore better protection against emotion-induced pacemaker-tachycardias should be integrated. The TX algorithm should also allow physical performances which last longer (e.g. marathon running; walking tour etc.). The drift should be programmable to different values and have the choices of "on/off".

References

1. Rickards AF (1984) Rate responsive pacing. Cardiostim Monaco

2. Wittkampf FWM, Candelon B, Arragon (1984) The importance of software programmable pace-makers: in vivo programming of a prototype device. PACE Vol 7 (Part II): 1207–1212
3. Candelon B (1984) Status report on TX-clinical evaluation. Vitatron Medical, Dieren (NL)
4. Barold SS, Ong LS, Falkoff MD, Heinle RA (1982) Programmable pacemakers: clinical indications, complications and future directions. In: Barold SS, Mugica J (eds) The third decade of cardiac pacing. Futura Publishing Co, New York, pp 27–76
5. Winter UJ, Behrenbeck DW, Brill Th, Höher M, Hombach V, Ebeling H, Hirche HJ, Hilger HH (1985) Hemodynamic and antiectopic effects of long-term dynamic overdrive pacing in implanted VVI pacemakers (this volume)

Authors' address:
U. J. Winter, M.D.
Medizinische Universitätsklinik III, Kardiologie
Josef-Stelzmann-Straße 9
5000 Köln 41
West Germany

Comparison of VVI and QT-Related Rate Adaptive Pacing – Pulmonary Artery Pressure, Pulmonary Capillary Pressure, Heart Rate and Cardiac Output

M. Zegelman, J. Kreuzer, and N. Reifart

Summary: Since October 1983 we have implanted 23 QT-related pacemakers (Vitatron). The problems with the precursor-model TX 1 have been solved except for one case. The Quintech TX 911 exhibited faultless function. The haemodynamic advantage is impressive. Although treatment and follow-up of patients supplied with a QT-related pacemaker needs time and experience we continue to use this device. The manufacturer must take care of further improvements like automatic slope adjustment and slope control and a change of the algorithm for rate adaption.

Introduction

The physiological response to exercise is an increase of both heart rate and stroke volume. A dual chamber pacemaker system can be used to achieve an increase of heart rate under exercise with normal functioning of the sinus node. Patients suffering from sick sinus syndrome, heart block or bradyarrhythmia with atrial fibrillation without sufficient reaction of heart rate can be treated with rate adaptive pacemakers. Up to April 1985 we have implanted 23 Qt-related pacemakers (Vitatron). This single chamber pacemaker is individually rate adaptive by using the actually measured QT- (stimulus-T) interval as an indicator. Full transcutaneous programmability of the pacing and sensing parameters exists with a programmerhead and the Hewlett-Packard Hp 85 computer.

Patients and methods

Sixteen pacemakers of the first generation (TX 1) and 7 pacemakers of the second generation (Quintech TX 911) have been implanted in our center. Until January 1985 11 patients (age 49–87 years, SD 10.44) underwent a follow-up investigation. In a randomized sequence of VVI- or TX-stimulation we examined heart rate, pulmonary artery and pulmonary capillary pressure and cardiac output using the thermodilution technique and oxygen saturation at rest or during submaximal exercise (30–120 watt, 5–8 min) on a bicycle ergometer in the supine position. Five of the patients suffered from heart block, 6 from atrial fibrillation and bradyarrhythmia. The range of the pacing rate was programmed between 70–120 ppm (min.-max.).

Haemodynamic results

We noted no significant change of pulmonary artery and pulmonary capillary pressure under VVI- or QT-related pacing. With exercise the mean heart rate increased from

Table 1. Heart rate and cardiac output on exercise VVI versus TX.

Heart rate on exercise	Cardiac output on exercise

A   VVI 82.8 ppm, SD: 13.3
     TX   123.4 ppm, SD: 10.8
     $\varDelta$ 49% $p < 0.01$
	VVI 8.2 l/min, SD: 3.4
	TX 9.9 l/min, SD: 4.1
	$\varDelta$ 20.7% $p < 0.05$

B   VVI 72.0 ppm, SD: 3.7
     TX   127.9 ppm, SD: 8.4
     $\varDelta$ 77.6% $p < 0.01$
	VVI 7.9 l/min, SD: 3.0
	VVI 10.7 l/min, SD: 3.4
	$\varDelta$ 36% $p < 0.05$

A: n = 11 All patients (including B)
B: n = 7 Patients with absents spontaneous increase of heart rate

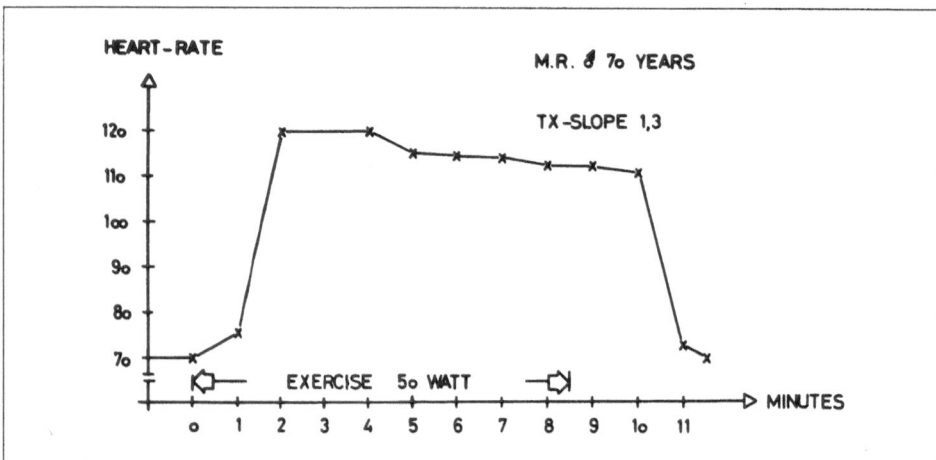

Fig. 1. Behaviour of heart rate during exercise (TX-stimulation)

82.8 ± 13.3 ppm under VVI-pacing to 123.4 ± 10.8 ppm ($p < 0.01$). Mean cardiac output with exercise improved from 8.2 ± 3.4 l/min under VVI-pacing to about 20.7% to 9.9 ± 4.1 l/min under TX-pacing ($p < 0.05$) (Table 1). If the patients with absent spontaneous increase of the heart rate are singled out (n = 7) the increase of cardiac output with exercise VVI versus TX is more impressive (7.89 ± 3 l/min versus 10.73 ± 3.4 l/min) ($p < 0.05$). This fact underlines the contribution of the adaption of heart rate under exercise from 72 ± 3.7 ppm (VVI) to 127.9 ± 8.4 ppm (TX) ($p < 0.01$). The investigations were performed an average of 6.1 months after implantation (Figs. 1–4).

Problems with the TX 1 (precursor-model)

One patient with complete heart block without own heart actions exhibited no adaption of heart rate regardless of a faultless QT-time measurement. Other problems observed were unpleasant nocturnal tachycardias (n = 2) or an undulation of the frequency between

124

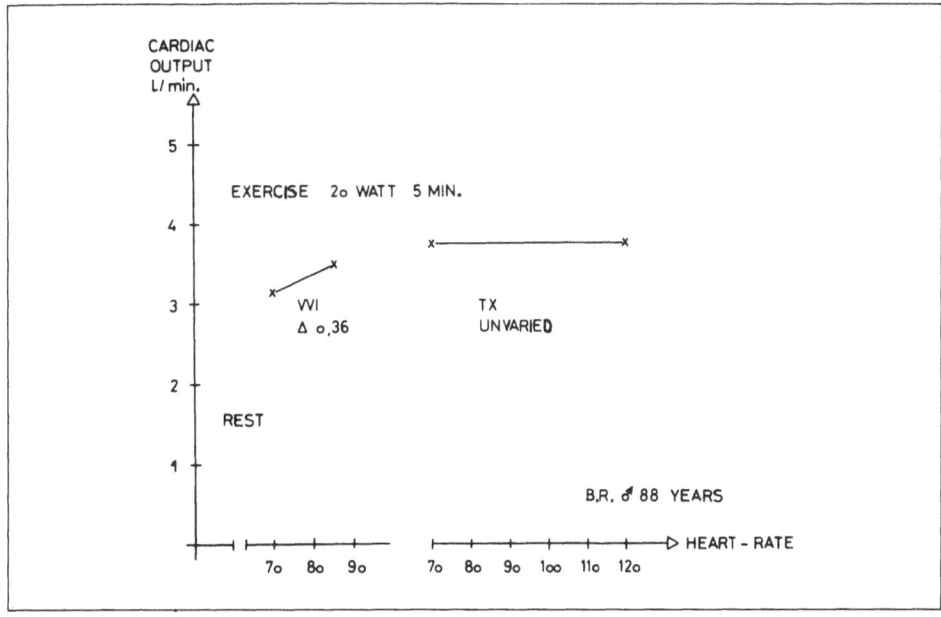

Fig. 2. Patient with severe cardiac insufficiency. No increase of cardiac output under VVI or under TX-stimulation

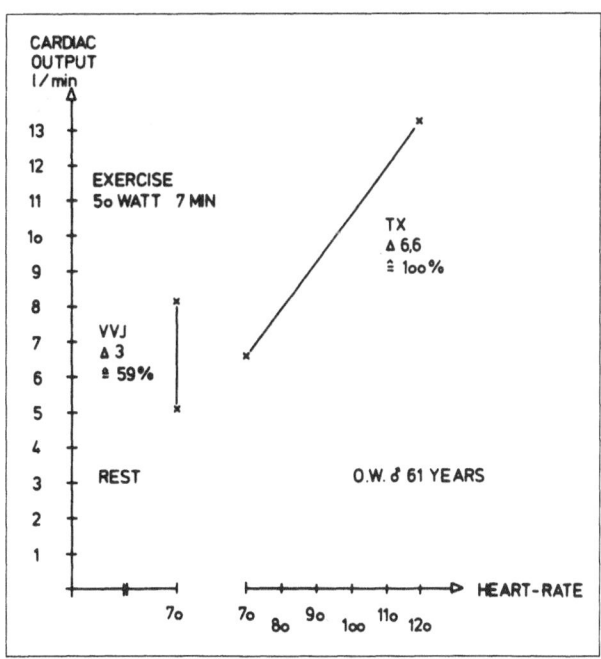

Fig. 3. An impressive improvement of cardiac output under TX-stimulation

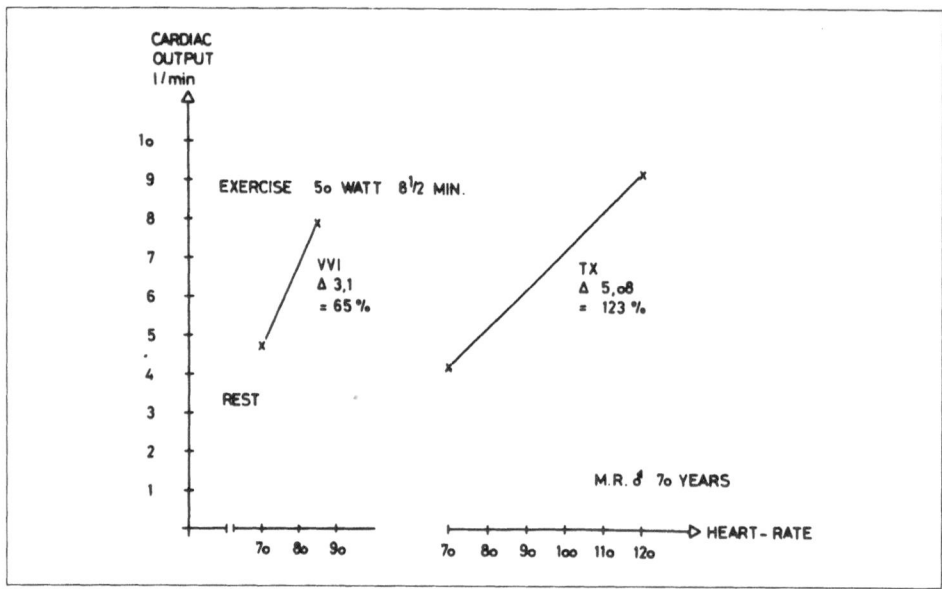

Fig. 4. TX-pacing leads to a considerable increase of cardiac output

the lower and upper rate limits (n = 1) (1). Other difficulties were seen subsequent to the software modification of the previous aggregate to the technically improved Quintech version (TX 1 → TX 2) by routine telemetry during consulting hours (n = 2) (2).

Discussion

In a given case a sufficient improvement of the cardiac output with exercise and VVI pacing is possible by the increase of stroke volume alone. A more economical way seems to be the adaptation of heart rate. This adaptation can be realized by using QT-related pacemakers (3, 4, 5). The problems with the precursor-model TX 1 have been solved except one case (1). The Quintech TX 911 exhibited faultless function without serious technical difficulties, and its haemodynamic advantage is impressive. This justifies an increase in the time spent on repeated clinical controls or adjustments (Holter ECG).

References

1. Zegelman M, Reifart N, Kreuzer J, Koch B (1985) QT-gesteuerte frequenzadaptierende Ventrikel-stimulation – Standortbestimmung nach 15 Monaten (Abstract). Herzschrittmacher 5 (1985) Abstracts 6. Jahrestagung Deutsche Arbeitsgemeinschaft Herzschrittmacher eV, Freiburg, p 8
2. Zegelman M, Kreuzer J (1985) Probleme während der klinischen Erprobung software-gesteuerter Herzschrittmacher – Datenanalyse und Datenkorrektur über Modem Herzschrittmacher 5: 41–43
3. Donaldson RM, Rickards AF (1983) Frequenzangepaßte Stimulation nach dem Prinzip der evozierten QT-Zeit-Messung. Eine physiologische Alternative zu vorhofsynchronisierten Herzschrittmachern. PACE 6: 1344–1349

4. Zegelman M, Kreuzer J, Reifart N (1984) QT-Related Rate Responsive Pacemaker – Improvement of Cardiac Output during Exercise. RBM, vol 6-N 3: 263
5. Zegelman M, Beyersdorf F, Kreuzer J, Reifart N, Happ J (1984) Adaption of Heart Rate to Exercise. Comparison of QT-Related and Respiratory Dependent Pacemakers. Progress in Clinical Pacing, Rome 104–110

Authors' address:
Max Zegelman, M.D.
Division of Thoracic and Cardiovascular Surgery
University Hospital
Theodor-Stern-Kai 7
6000 Frankfurt/Main 70
West Germany

Clinical Experiences with the Respiratory Rate Responsive Pacemaker

P. Rossi, F. Aina, G. Rognoni, and M. D. Prando

Summary: The rate responsive respiratory dependent pacemaker has been implanted in 26 patients. This pacemaker uses breathing frequency and tidal volume as the indicators of physiological demand.

Stimulation rate was strictly related to oxygen uptake. The assessment study was comprehensive, consisting of dynamic electrocardiographic monitoring, and tolerance to treadmill exercise with either fixed rate or rate responsive pacing.

The follow-up time was 217 patient-months. Respiratory dependency of pacing rate was maintained in all patients. The work capacity was significantly higher with rate responsive than with fixed pacing rate. The fluctuations in the ventricular paced rate during various daily activity confirmed appropriate responses to exercise.

Introduction

Recently we described a rate responsive pacemaker that uses the respiration rate as an indicator of metabolic demands. In previous reports we have shown:

1. a satisfactory relationship between breathing frequency and heart rate in normals and in patients with restrictive or obstructive ventilatory insufficiency (1);
2. respiration rate is a valid and stable physiological parameter upon which to control the stimulation rate (2).

Our device consists of a cardiac pacemaker in which pacing rate is controlled by a certain algorithm from sensing of the breathing rate, which is monitored by impedance variations in the respiration. The impedance variations are detected between the pacemaker casing and an auxiliary lead placed in the subcutaneous layer of the thoracic region through the pocket of pulse generator by an introducer with a very simple technique.

The respiratory dependent rate responsive pacemaker increases the pacing ventricular rate during exercise without maintaining A-V synchronization.

Patients and methods

In this presentation we report the first clinical and functional evaluation of a rate responsive respiratory dependent (RD) pacemaker (PM). To date in Novara a respiratory dependent PM has been implanted in 28 patients of a mean age of 64, range 22–88 years, 23 patients received rate responsive ventricular pacing (VVI-RD), 5 patients received rate responsive atrial pacing (AAI-RD), with a total follow-up of 217 patient-months, range 3–24 months.

The respiratory sensing of the implanted unit was assessed by telemetry and converted to an acoustic signal by an external receiver. The level of respiratory sensing remained stable in each patient for the entire observation period.

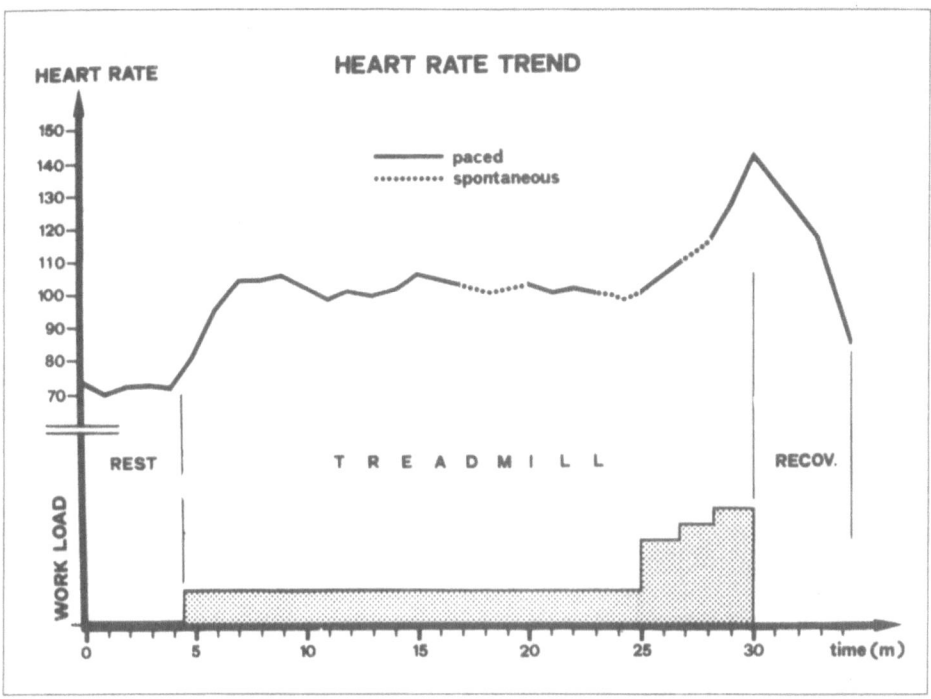

Fig. 1. Treadmill stress testing with work loads of varying duration to show the relationship between the respiration dependent pacing rate and the long-short term activities. A spontaneous rhythm emerges during exercise and the spontaneous rate is in the same range as the paced rate.

A special protocol of stress testing was devised to represent some daily activities, as shown in Figure 1. During this exercise testing with short time and long time work loads, the pacing rate is related to the performed work. Figure 2 shows the electrocardiogram at rest, during dynamic exercise with the increasing pacing rate and during recovery.

The assessment study was comprehensive:

1. 24 hours of Holter monitoring every three months;
2. tolerance to treadmill exercise performed according to the Bruce protocol on two separate occasions with either fixed rate or rate responsive pacing in 23 patients (Table 1).

The fluctuations in the ventricular paced rate during various daily activities were documented by ambulatory monitoring. The daily activities were grouped in mild and moderate and rest or sleepy periods; comparison with the patients' diaries permitted confirmation of appropriate responses to exercise. The predominantly basal rate of 70–80 bpm during overnight rest is also shown.

Results

During treadmill exercise testing with rate responsive pacing the progressive adaptation of ventricular rate was strictly related to the oxygen uptake. Maximum pacing rate coinciding with peak exercise work load attained the peak values of the selected regression

129

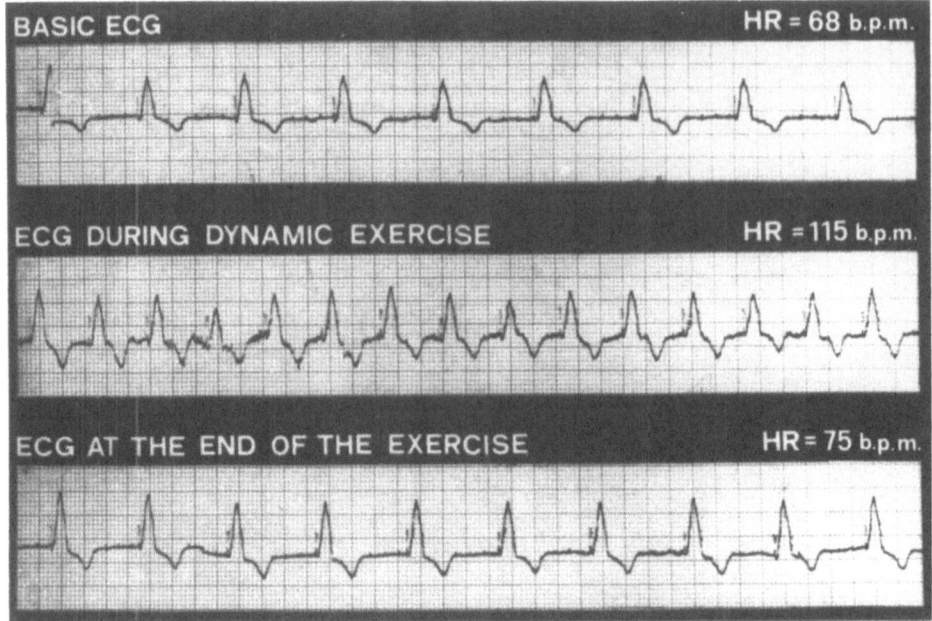

Fig. 2. Patient with VVI-RD pacemaker. Electrocardiogram at rest, during dynamic exercise with increasing pacing rate and during recovery.

line in individual patients. The mean value of the maximum pacing rate was $125 \pm SD$ 17, range 118–155 bpm.

To rule out bias induced by non comparable reasons for stopping exercise we have chosen the determination of anaerobic threshold as an objective means to assess aerobic capacity. All our patients attained the anaerobic threshold in exercise testing with a fixed pacing rate.

In the exercise testing with rate responsive pacing the work time to attain the anaerobic threshold was expanded and the oxygen uptake was significantly higher (Table 1) ($p < 0.01$).

Table 1. Treadmill test (23 patients). Evaluation of respiratory dependent pacemakers (RDP) achieved by ECG and VO_2 monitoring during multistage treadmill test (Bruge protocol), comparison with fixed rate pacing (VVI-AAI).

		Work time (min)	Mets	Anaerobic threshold time (min)	Heart rate (bpm)
V	VVI	7.7 ± 1.8	4.4 ± 1	5.9 ± 1.6	78 ± 5
(18 pts)°	RDP₃ VVI	$10.2 \pm 2.5*$	$6 \pm 1.5*$	$8.1 \pm 2.6*$	$125 \pm 17**$
A	AAI	7.8 ± 3.5	5.2 ± 0.6	7.2 ± 2.9	97 ± 33
(5 pts)	RDP₃ AAI	$9.8 \pm 3.1**$	5.8 ± 1.3	8.2 ± 2.5	$137 \pm 10**$

$* p < 0.0005; ** p < 0.05$.

The essential advantages of selecting respiratory rate as a control parameter for rate responsive pacing are that the sensor is of simple design, is very stable, wastes little energy (less than 3 μA), shows excellent longevity, with the open loop regulation it makes use of the human body computer to select the proper rate with very quick response and then maintains it, and finally it can be adapted very easily to the individual patient. Therefore this principle works for short-term activities like climbing stairs, as well as for long-term activities like walking uphill.

Conclusions

1. During treadmill exercise testing with rate responsive pacing the progressive adaptation of ventricular rate was strictly related to O_2 uptake.
2. The present data show that physical working ability is significantly prolonged in rate responsive respiratory dependent pacing without A-V synchronization.
3. With single chamber ventricular pacing or when sino-atrial function is abnormal the rate responsive respiratory dependent PM consistently improves quality of life.

References

1. Rossi P, Plicchi G, Canducci GC, Rognoni G, Aina F (1984) Respiration as a reliable physiological sensor for controlling cardiac pacing rate. Br Heart J 51: 7–14
2. Rossi P, Plicchi G, Canducci GC, Rognoni G, Aina F (1983) Respiratory rate as a determinant of optimal pacing rate. PACE 6: 502–507

Authors' address:
Professor P. Rossi
Department of Cardiology
Ospedale Maggiore Della Carita
Novara, Italy

Respiration Dependent Pacemakers

F. Beyersdorf[+], J. Kreuzer[+], and J. Happ[*]

During exercise cardiac output rises due to an increase in stroke volume as well as an increase in heart rate. In untrained persons as well as in patients with myocardial insufficiency a rise in cardiac output is mainly due to an increase in heart rate.

Patients with VVI mode pacemakers can increase their cardiac output only while raising their stroke volume. During severe physical stress and especially in patients with myocardial failure and absolute arrhythmia an increase in stroke volume is not possible. This latter group of patients can raise their cardiac output only by increasing their heart rate.

Thus there was a need to develop pacemakers which are able to increase the heart rate according to the metabolic requirements of the individual patient.

For these rate-responsive pacemakers one can use as a reference quantity either stroke volume, blood pH, central blood temperature, arterial O_2, QT interval, P wave or respiratory rate.

Fig. 1. Increase in heart rate during exercise (50 W) in a patient with a respiration dependent pacemaker.

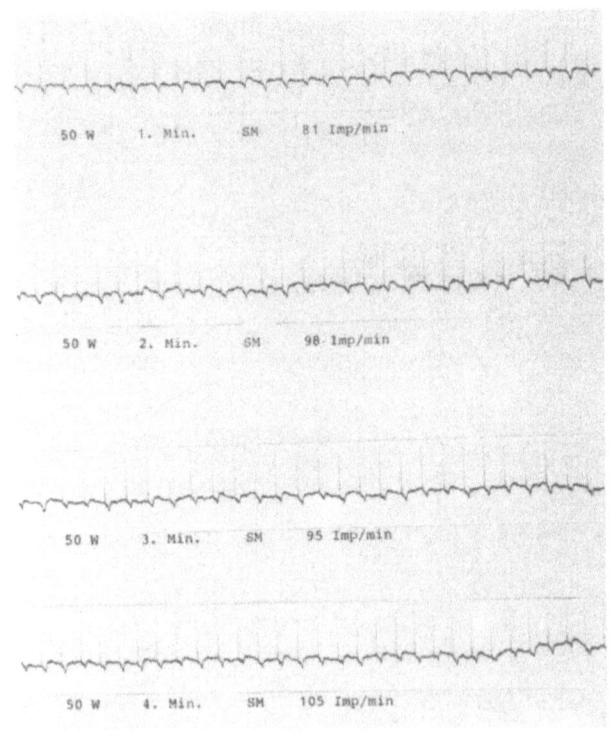

[+] Division of Thoracic and Cardiovascular Surgery (Head: Prof. Dr. Satter) and [*] Division of Nuclear Medicine (Head: Prof. Dr. Hör), University of Frankfurt/Main, West Germany

Respiration dependent pacemakers are based on the correlation between breathing frequency and heart rate. The concept of respiration dependent pacemakers was developed by Funke (1975), Ionescu (1980) and Rossi et al. (1983).

In the Division of Thoracic and Cardiovascular Surgery, University of Frankfurt/Main, respiration dependent pacemakers were implanted in 9 patients, average age 62.9 ± 8.5

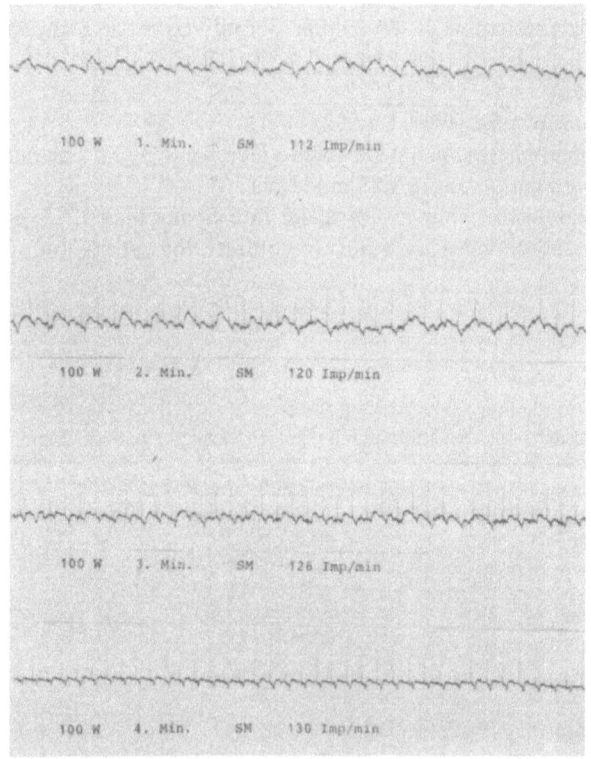

Fig. 2. Increase in heart rate during exercise (100 W) in a patient with a respiration dependent pacemaker.

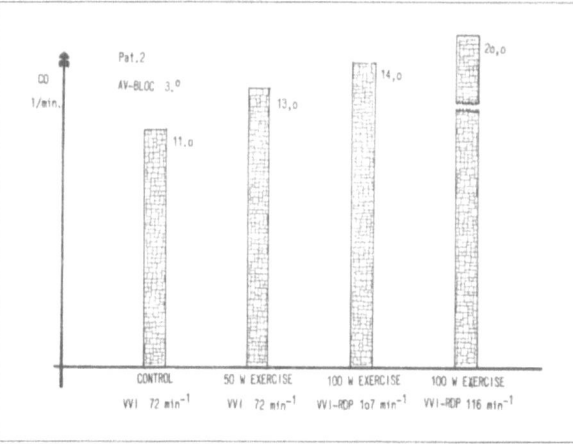

Fig. 3. Increase in cardiac output with a respiration dependent pacemaker during increasing exercise.

years (Mean ± SD). This system consists of the pacemaker, the auxiliary lead and the pacing lead. The auxiliary lead is easily inserted subcutaneously under local anaesthesia. The following parameters are programmable in these pacemakers:

(1) respiration dependency (On – Off); (2) relationship between respiratory rate and heart rate (8 settings); (3) respiratory sensitivity levels (8 settings); and (4) minimum heart rates.

During the follow-up examination 4–8 weeks after implantation all patients were examined by an exercise ECG and a determination of the cardiac output was made using radionuclide ventriculography.

The following results were obtained:

– heart rate always increases during exercise (Figs. 1 and 2)
– patients with respiration dependent pacemakers were able to increase their cardiac output by approximately 15–35% in relation to the VVI mode (Fig. 3);
– In older patients with myocardial insufficiency a ventricular rate greater than 120 bpm does not result in a further increase in cardiac output. In contrast, the cardiac output may fall again.

References

Funke HD (1975) Ein Herzschrittmacher mit belastungsabhängiger Frequenzregulation. Biomed Tech 20: 225
Ionescu VL (1980) An "on demand pacemaker" responsive to respiration rate. PACE 3: 375
Rossi P, Plicchi G, Canducci GC et al (1983) Respiratory rate as a determinant of optimal pacing rate. PACE 6: 326

Authors' address:
Dr. F. Beyersdorf
Abteilung für Thorax-, Herz- und Gefäßchirurgie
Zentrum der Chirurgie
Klinikum der J. W. Goethe-Universität
Theodor-Stern-Kai 7
D-6000 Frankfurt/M. 70
West Germany

Results with the SO_2-Controlled Pacemaker

E. Alt, A. Wirtzfeld, and R. Heinze

Summary: Currently available physiological pacing systems do not fully restore rate regulation, especially with respect to little or no atrial response to activity. Other biological parameters, detected by sensors, may provide the physiological responsiveness necessary for rate-regulating pacemakers. An optical sensor using mixed venous oxygen saturation may be the ideal parameter for such a pacing system. At present, further research is necessary to elaborate a suitable algorithm for optimal rate control.

As described elsewhere, a variety of biological parameters have been proposed and are suitable for a rate-responsive pacing system.

For different reasons, we believe that mixed venous oxygen saturation, measured as HbO_2 saturation, represents a very good physiological parameter for pacing regulation. Unlike the pH value or, to some extent, the blood temperature, the body has no marked O_2 pools, and venous O_2 saturation is exclusively determined by the cardiac output and the peripheral O_2 demand. By raising oxygen consumption any increase in physical activity results in an increment of the O_2 transporting capacity, which is accomplished by two mechanisms:
- an increase in cardiac output, and
- an enhancement of oxygen extraction from arterial blood.

This latter change leads to an increase in arteriovenous oxygen difference which is a consequence of a drop in mixed venous oxygen saturation as arterial saturation remains unchanged. With raised oxygen consumption the mixed venous HbO_2 saturation falls promptly and quickly reaches a new plateau.

The extent of the drop in HbO_2 saturation depends on the level of exercise as well as on cardiac performance and thus on cardiac output (Fig. 1).

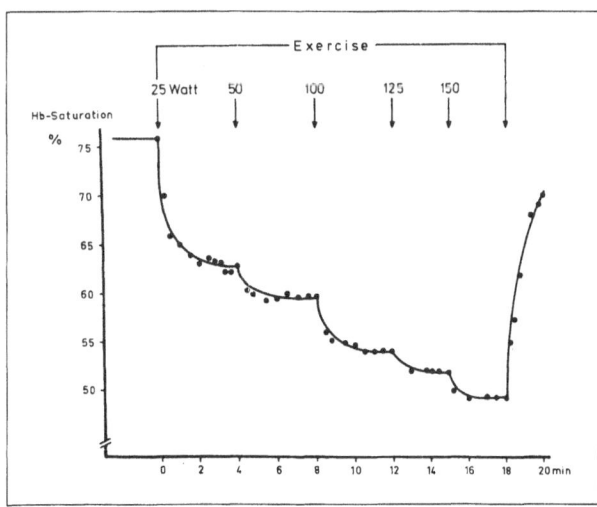

Fig. 1. Mixed venous oxygen saturation (SO_2) in a healthy volunteer during increasing physical work. 1 to 2 minutes after the beginning a new plateau is attained with a distinct relation between the level of exercise and the fall in SO_2. There is a rapid increase in SO_2 after the test is finished.

Figure 2 shows the different hemodynamic results and the respective mixed venous oxygen saturation (SO_2). The data were measured on 10 pacemaker patients at rest and during two exercise tests with 25 and 50 watts, each performed either with a rate VVI 70 or with atrial triggered VDD pacing. One can see that during VVI ventricular stimulation the cardiac output (CO) rises only slightly compared with the increase during VDD stimulation. Compensatorily the equal oxygen uptake by physical work is brought about by enhanced oxygen extraction from the blood, according to the formula oxygen uptake (VO_2) = cardiac output (CO) x arteriovenous oxygen difference ($AVDO_2$).

Fig. 2. SO_2 and cardiac output (CO) at rest and during exercise with 25, 50 and 75 watts. Ventricular stimulation with a rate of 70 (VVI 70) results in a smaller increase in CO, and thus in enhanced oxygen extraction and reduced SO_2 at a given level of exercise, whereas a VDD stimulation causes reduced oxygen extraction due to the enhanced CO.

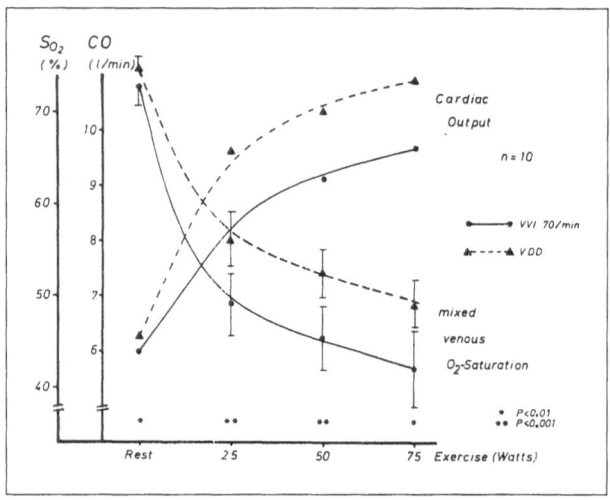

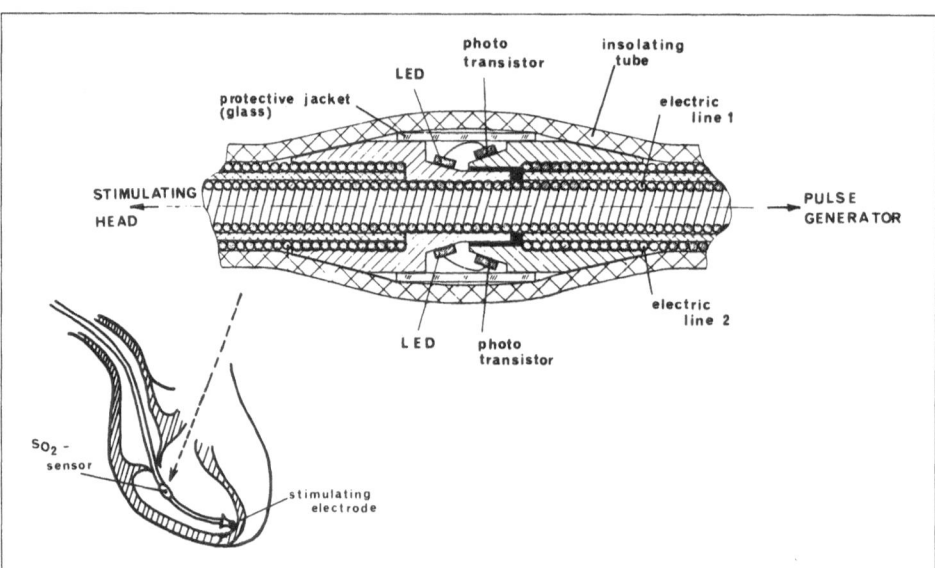

Fig. 3. Cross-section of the sensor. One can see the light emitting diode (LED) and the phototransistor that measures the reflected light. Two elements are shown, situated around the longitudinal axis of the lead.

136

As arterial oxygen saturation remains unchanged the mixed venous oxygen saturation renders the $AVDO_2$.

Following the concept of HbO_2-dependent rate responsive pacing we have developed an optoelectronical sensor, which is incorporated within the pacing lead, so that oxygen saturation in the right ventricle can be monitored by the means of the principle of hemoreflectorimetry. Monochromatic red light of a wave length of 660 nm is emitted by a LED, reflected by the red blood cells, received by a phototransistor, and thus the oxygen saturation of the erythrocytes is calculated (Fig. 3). The voltage of the phototransistor lies around 2.5 volts and is dependent on the saturation of the mixed venous blood. Fibrin coatings and thrombi, which were sometimes detected at the optical sensor during long-time studies in sheep, cause a downward displacement of the curve, but do not alter its characteristic.

When used in vivo the HbO_2 signal shows characteristic fluctuations with each cardiac cycle. These are probably caused by real changes of the signal due to the blood flow as well as by artefacts of the sensor. These artefacts are due to different reflexion characteristics at rest and during blood flow. However, a stable signal can be obtained when the measurement of the SO_2 is triggered by an intracardiac ECG signal (Fig. 4). Our experience so far has shown that with the oxygen sensor working in the triggered mode, a re-

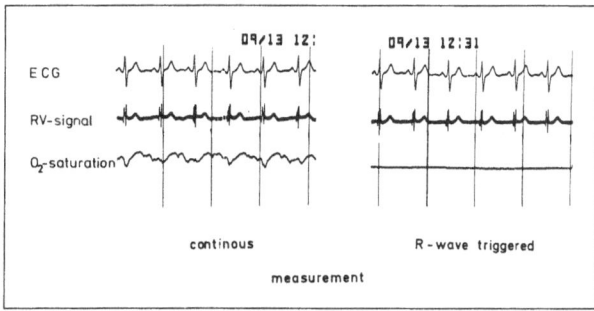

Fig. 4. Fluctuation of SO_2 with each cardiac cycle (Fig. 4a). Fig. 4b shows the same measurement when triggered by the R-wave.

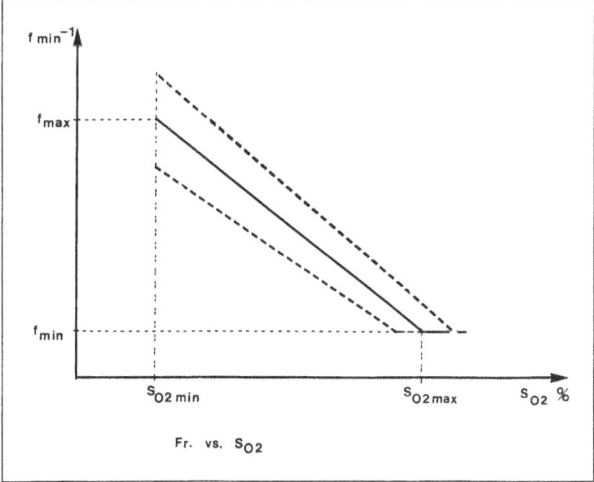

Fig. 5. Description of a feasible characteristic curve of pacing rate in relation to SO_2. High SO_2 correlates with a low pacing rate and vice versa. Within its limits the pacemaker changes its rate automatically and paces with the optimal rate according to the oxygen saturation.

liable reproduction of SO_2 can be obtained. The resolution capacity of the system lies at less than half a percent oxygen saturation. Due to the physiological role of mixed venous oxygen saturation, a physiological rate control is made possible, as a change in HbO_2 saturation depends only on the cardiac output and on the peripheral oxygen demand, and the oxygen saturation responds quickly to a change in physical activity.

The idea of this concept is a fully automatic physiological pacemaker, which at any given moment paces at the lowest possible rate achieving the highest venous oxygen saturation (Fig. 5). While the upper and lower limits of the oxygen saturation and the pacing rate are fixed, the pacemaker will always pace at the optimal rate, irrespective of the patient's rate-to-output curve or state of activity. The principle of SO_2 regulation may be used for any type of pacemaker including AAI and DDD units.

Thus a real physiological stimulation would be possible, especially in patients who cannot raise their heart rate sufficiently during physical activity.

Authors' address:
E. Alt, M.D.
I. Medizinische Klinik rechts der Isar
Technische Universität
Ismaninger Straße 22
8000 München 80
West Germany

Preliminary Clinical Results with a New Software-Controlled DDD Pacemaker

W. Hemmer, A. Markewitz, W. Funccius, and B. M. Kemkes

Summary: A software-controlled pacemaker is a pulse generator whose functions are all controlled by an integrated microprocessor. This paper deals with the clinical experience we gained with the implantation of the new Cosmos DDD device in 10 patients. It is the first pacemaker that contains a memory for diagnostic data which records patients' ECG events for months. Therefore, in addition to a great number of therapeutic advantages, it significantly facilitates function tests and the selection of long-term programming parameters for DDD-pacing.

Introduction

The term "software-controlled pacemakers" characterizes a new generation of pulse generators which incorporate a complete microprocessor to control the pacing system. Its functional capacities are fixed by the software fed into the external programmer; they can be changed by simply exchanging the software module. An adaptation of the implanted pacemaker to future developments in technology will thus be possible without any surgery being necessary.

Description of the implanted system

Our first experiences with this new generation of DDD-pacemakers were gained with the Cosmos, model 283-01[1]) (1). This multiprogrammable DDD device basically uses the semi-committed pacing mode (2).

In Table 1 the basic programmable parameters are listed. Their range comes up to what can be expected of a modern DDD device (3).

Furthermore, programming of the following adjustments is provided within a wide range:
– atrial refractory extension after PVC
– fallback response
– blanking period (special code must be used)
– non-physiological AV interval (special code).

All programmed values can be interrogated with the help of the external computer. Additionally, telemetry data referring to pacing rate and pacing energy, lead impedance, and state of the battery can be transmitted (Fig. 1).

During function tests external threshold measurements can be performed safely and quickly by temporarily (3 to 4 cycles) changing the parameters. At the moment only the Cosmos system incorporates a computer algorithm which automatically terminates endless-loop tachycardias (4).

Another new development is a memory which records diagnostic data of the patient's ECG. The computer's capacity provides a continuous recording for 5.5. months (100% pacing, rate 70 ppm, Table 2).

---

[1]) Intermedics Inc., P.O. Box 617, Freeport, Texas 77541, USA.

139

Table 1. Basic parameters of the Cosmos device.

Parameter	Range	Increments
Mode	DDD/VDD/DVI/DVI(C) DOO/VVI/VVT/VOO AAI/AAT/AOO/OOO	
Pacing rate	30–120 ppm	1 ppm
Maximum rate (DDD/VDD)	94–180 ppm	2 ppm
Fallback rate (DDD/VDD)	94–180 ppm	2 ppm
Pulse width (Atrium and ventricle)	0.03–1.5 msec	0.01 msec
Pulse amplitude (Atrium and ventricle)	2.7/5.4/8.1 V	
Sensitivity Atrium Ventricle	0.4–2.8 mV 1.0–7.0 mV	0.4 mV 1.0 mV
Refractory period Atrium (including AV delay)	220–570 msec	5 msec
Ventricle (VDD/DDD)	170–320 msec	5 msec
AV delay (DDD/VDD/DVI)	50–300 msec	5 msec
Hysteresis (AAI/VVI)	30–120 ppm	1 ppm

Fig. 1. Computer print-out; top: programmed parameters, bottom: measured values.

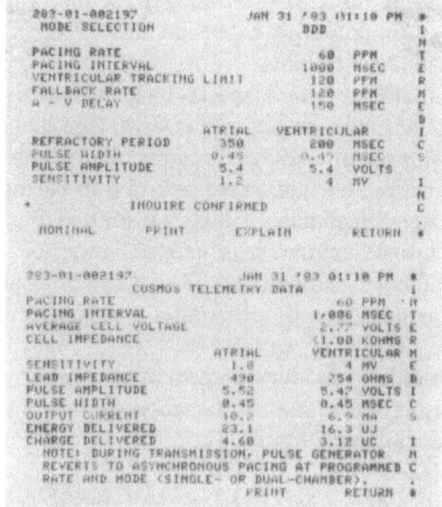

Table 2. Diagnostic data of the Cosmos device.

Number of times ventricular tracking limit reached	(Capacity 255)
Number of premature ventricular events	(Cap. 16.777.215)
Atrial sense events followed by a ventricular sense event	(Cap. 16.777.215)
Atrial sense events followed by a ventricular pace event	(Cap. 16.777.215)
Atrial pace event followed by a ventricular sense event	(Cap. 16.777.215)
Atrial pace event followed by a ventricular pace event	(Cap. 16.777.215)
Percent paced – atrium	(0–100%)
Percent paced – ventricle	(0–100%)
Number of signal peaks counted during last sense event	(Capacity 15)

Table 3. Patients' clinical data.

Number	10
Sex	6 × ♂ 4 × ♀
Age	58 ± 11 years (42–77 yrs)
Diagnosis	3 × Sinus node disease 5 × AV-block II° or III° 2 × Binodal disease

Table 4. Measurements during implantation.

Threshold – atrium (1 msec)	0.6 ± 0.2 V
Threshold – ventricle (1 msec)	0.5 ± 0.1 V
P-wave amplitude	2.8 ± 0.8 mV
P-wave slew rate	0.6 ± 0.4 V/sec
R-wave amplitude	8 ± 3 mV
Retrograde conduction	2 × present 220 or 380 msec

Clinical application

Between October and December 1983 ten patients were provided with a Cosmos pace-maker at the Department of Cardiac Surgery, University of Munich (Table 3). Underlying arrhythmias were sinus nodal and/or AV nodal diseases. The implanted leads were manufactured by Osypka[2]: screw-in leads in the atrium (Osypka VY61C) and tined electrodes in the ventricle (Osypka SF61D). Both leads were introduced via the cephalic (8 patients) or the subclavian vein (2 patients). Table 4 gives the values measured during implantation.

---

[2] Dr. Ing. P. Osypka GmbH, Basler Str. 109, 7889 Grenzach, FRG.

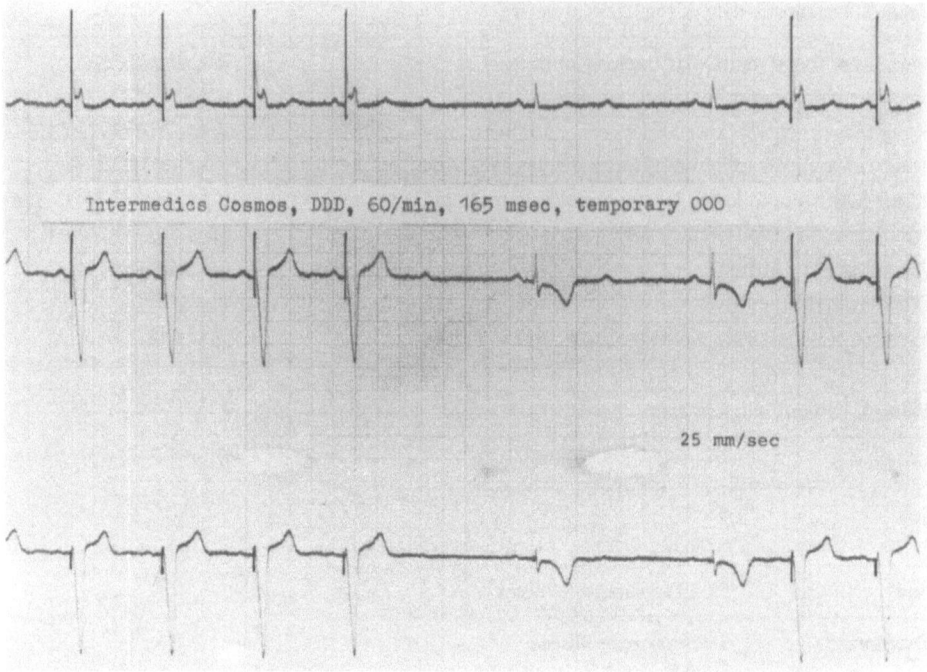

Fig. 2. Temporary switch-off of the pacemaker, the intrinsic rhythm shows a II° heart block.

Nine of the ten patients could be examined after an observation period of 20 patient-months (5). During the follow-up procedures we gained our first experience with the functional capacities of the pulse generator (6). The following examples will explain some significant aspects.

At the beginning of an examination quick information about the patient's intrinsic rhythm is obtained by switching the pacemaker off temporarily (Fig. 2). The 000-mode remains in effect as long as the programming head is held in place on the pacemaker. If an asystole should possibly result it can thus be managed safely. The determination of pacing thresholds can be performed in a short time and without any risk of a longer asystole by temporarily and gradually reducing pulse amplitude and pulse duration (Figs. 3a, b). To test the sensing thresholds sensitivity can be varied in the same way. Furthermore the device can mark sensed events at the surface ECG (Fig. 4). These markers also facilitate the diagnosis of pacemaker-induced and pacemaker-mediated tachycardias (7).

Figure 5 shows the automatic termination of an endless-loop tachycardia by a specific algorithm of the pacemaker. The tachycardia has previously been provoked by reducing the atrial pulse duration and programming a short atrial refractory period. Termination of the tachycardia is managed by omitting the 15th ventricular pacing event.

Until recently long-term programming of DDD-pacemakers could only be done with the aid of anamnesis and ECG-results. To judge rate adaptation under stress ergometry was necessary and sometimes it was possible to gain additional information by a Holter-ECG (8, 9). The diagnostic memory of the Cosmos device provides information that is a great help in selecting the individually most advantageous long-term programming. Tables 5

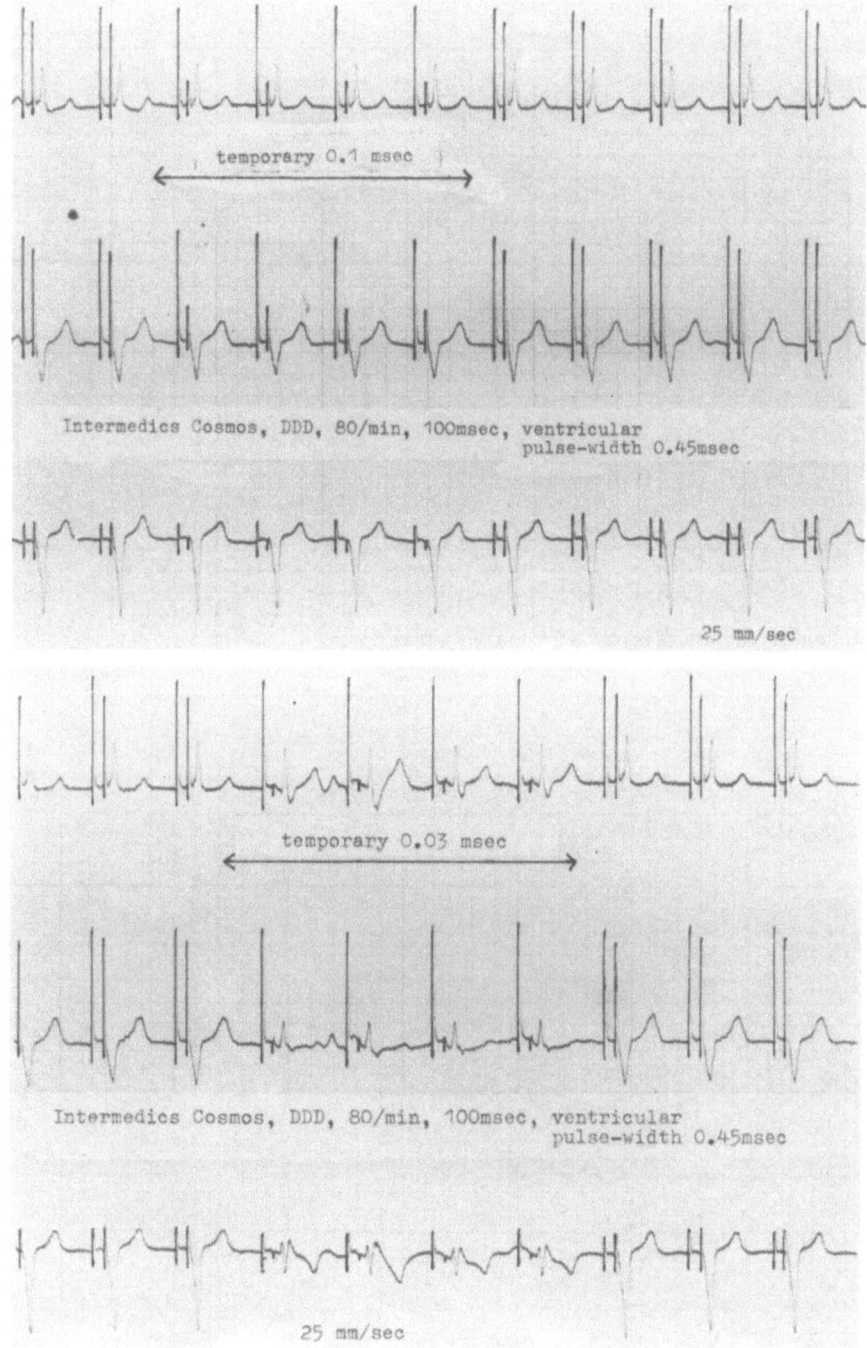

Fig. 3. External ventricular threshold measurement by temporarily reducing pulse duration; a) capture; b) no capture.

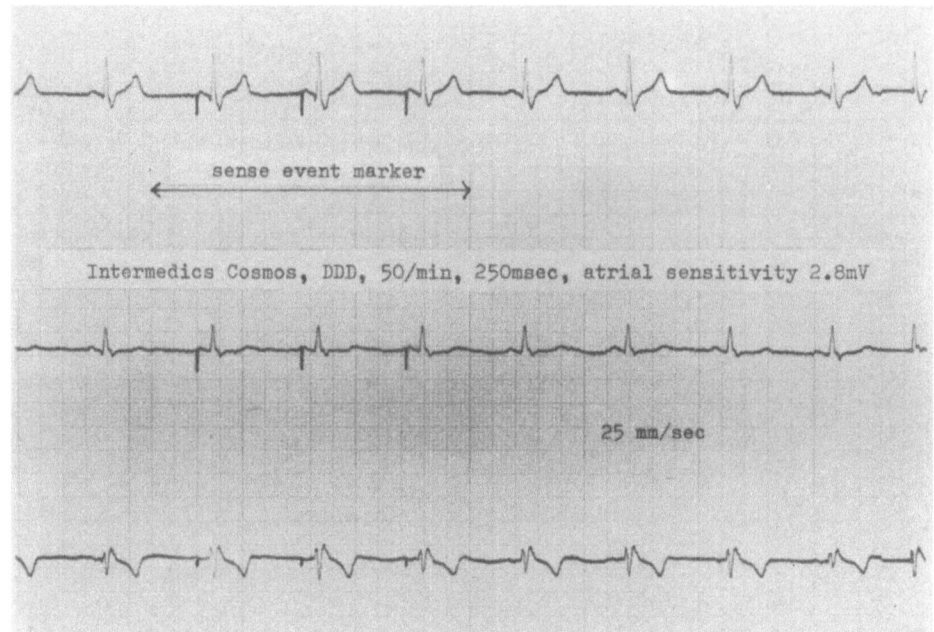

Fig. 4. Markers confirming correct detection of P-waves.

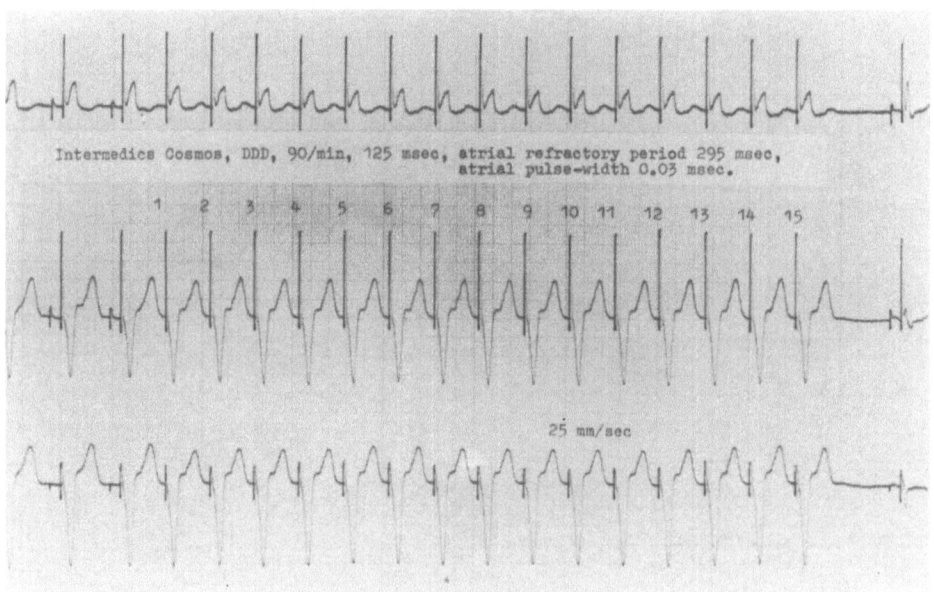

Fig. 5. Automatic termination of an endless-loop tachycardia.

Table 5. Diagnostic data of a patient with AV-block II°, 2 months after implantation, DDD 60–150/min, 175 msec.

Percent paced – atrium	23%
Percent paced – ventricle	100%
Number of times ventricular tracking limit reached	0
Number of premature ventricular events	491

and 6 give examples of two patients with different arrhythmias. The most important parameters are demonstrated. They provide useful additional information for the programming of basic rate, ventricular tracking limit, and AV interval. Furthermore, statements about the patients' intrinsic rhythm and pacemaker-mediated tachycardias are possible. The large number of premature ventricular events in Table 6 indicates an antiarrhythmic therapy whose effectiveness may easily be controlled with the diagnostic memory.

Table 6. Diagnostic data of a patient with sick sinus syndrome, 1 month after implantation, DDD 60–100/min, 175 msec.

Percent paced – atrium	73%
Percent paced – ventricle	84%
Number of times ventricular tracking limit reached	more than 255
Number of premature ventricular events	341.011

Table 7. Long-term programmings.

Mode		9 × DDD
Pacing rate		9 × 50–60 ppm
Maximum rate		5 × 140–150 ppm
		4 × 100–120 ppm
AV delay		8 × 165–175 msec
		1 × 250 msec
Pulse amplitude:	atrium	6 × 2.7 V
		3 × 5.4 V
	ventricle	3 × 2.7 V
		6 × 5.4 V
Pulse width:	atrium	9 × 0.3–0.5 msec
	ventricle	9 × 0.3–0.45 msec
Sensitivity:	atrium	9 × 1.2–1.6 mV
	ventricle	9 × 3–4 mV
Refractory period:	atrium	6 × 365–430 msec
		3 × 450–565 msec
	ventricle	9 × 200 msec

Table 7 summarizes the long-term programmings which were finally selected for the patients. DDD mode was maintained in all devices. Arrhythmias could be avoided by adequate programming. With standard programming pectoral muscle stimulation had occurred in four patients, but vanished when output was reduced to within the safety margin. In two cases a detection of muscle potentials was produced after programming the maximum atrial sensitivity of 0.4 mV (10).

It was striking that in almost all cases an atrioventricular crosstalk occurred when pulse amplitude or duration were increased, sometimes only slightly above the standard values (Fig. 6). In this context a programming of the blanking period without knowing the special code would be desirable. The nominal duration of 17.7 msec seems to be slightly short in some cases.

Fig. 6. Atrioventricular crosstalk: when atrial pulse duration is increased to 0.7 msec the ventricular electrode detects the atrial event and stimulates after the non-physiological AV interval (semi-committed mode).

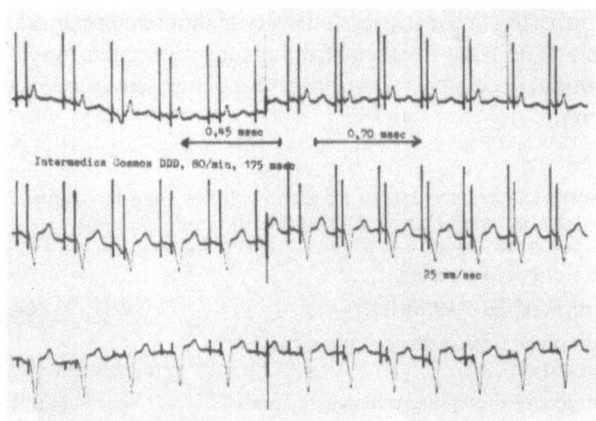

Conclusions

In spite of the bewildering complexity of this new generation of computer-controlled pacemakers – the Cosmos is currently the most versatile model – these systems offer a significant aid in the management of physiological pacing (11). The handling of the external programmer can be learnt in a short period of time. Reprogramming of individual parameters can be done quickly and easily. The diagnostic data represent a great aid when determining the best choice of long-term programmed parameters.

References

1. Cosmos ™-Model 283-01, Physician's Manual. Intermedics Inc, Freeport, Texas
2. Calfee RV (1983) Dual-Chamber Committed Mode Pacing. PACE 6: 387
3. Astrinsky E, Furman S (1983) Output Programmable Pulse Generator Adjustment: Pulse Duration or Amplitude. In: Steinbach K et al (eds) Cardiac Pacing. Steinkopff Verlag, Darmstadt p 281
4. Furman S, Fisher JD (1982) Endless-Loop Tachycardia in an AV-Universal (DDD) Pacemaker. PACE 5: 486

5. Rydén L, Kristensson B-E, Kruse J (1983) Dual Chamber Pacemakers-Follow Up. In: Steinbach K et al (eds) Cardiac Pacing. Steinkopff Verlag, Darmstadt, 469
6. Hemmer W, Beyer J, Kreuzer E, Weinhold Ch, Luther M (1983) EKG-Beurteilung und Nachsorge von Zweikammer-Schrittmachersystemen. Herz/Kreislauf 15: 598
7. Barold SS, Falkoff MD, Ong LS, Heinle RA (1983) Arrhythmias Caused by Dual-Chambered Pacing. In: Steinbach K et al (eds) Cardiac Pacing. Steinkopff Verlag, Darmstadt, p 505
8. Beyer J, Hemmer W (eds) (1983) Physiologische Stimulation mit Herzschrittmachern. Georg Thieme Verlag, Stuttgart
9. Hauser RG (1983) The Electrocardiography of AV Universal DDD Pacemakers. PACE 6: 399
10. Van Gelder LM, El Gamal MJH (1983) Influence of Myopotentials on Implanted DDD-M Pacemakers. In: Steinbach K et al (eds) Cardiac Pacing. Steinkopff Verlag, Darmstadt, p 555
11. Zipes DP (ed) (1981) Current Clinical Applications of Dual-Chamber Pacing. Proceedings of a symposium in Dallas, Texas, 1981

Authors' address:
W. Hemmer, M.D.
Städt. Krankenhaus München-Neuperlach
I. Chirurgische Abteilung
Oskar-Maria-Graf-Ring 51
8000 München 83
West Germany

DDI Mode: a New Stimulation Mode in the Therapy of Pacesetting Disorders

A. Markewitz, W. Hemmer, W. Funccius, and B. M. Kemkes

Summary: The indication for the large group of patients with an isolated pacesetting disorder, such as sick sinus syndrome, to implant a pacemaker device is the necessity to restore a sufficient basic rate. Because AV conduction is maintained P-wave controlled ventricular stimulation is of secondary importance. On the other hand pacemaker-mediated tachycardias by intermediate atrial fibrillation or supraventricular tachycardias are likely to occur in patients with sick sinus syndrome.

The DDI mode protects against this complication, retaining dual chamber detection and stimulation. The fact that P-wave controlled ventricular stimulation is not possible during physical activity is not a disadvantage. Therefore the DDI mode should be considered as a new physiological stimulation mode for patients with an isolated pacesetting disorder.

Fifty per cent of the patients suffering from rhythm disorders who underwent permanent pacemaker implantation in our hospital had isolated sinus node dysfunction (Fig. 1).

The indication for cardiac pacing in patients with severe deterioration of sinus node function is the restoration of a sufficient basic rate by stimulation. During exercise the rate of these patients depends on the remaining capabilities of the sinus node: sinus rate either increases or remains unchanged. In any case, however, P-wave synchronous ventricular pacing is of less importance in this patient group.

On the other hand there is one typical complication related to the fact that brady/tachycardia syndrome is a part of the basic disease: pacemaker mediated tachycardia. Figure 2 shows a normal ECG immediately after implantation of a dual chamber pacemaker device in a patient with sinus node dysfunction. Some days later another ECG recording shows a pacemaker mediated tachycardia due to intermittent atrial fibrillation (Fig. 3).

Unfortunately these patients tend to develop recurrent atrial fibrillation after successful cardioversion.

Fig. 1. Indications for cardiac pacing at the Department of Cardiac Surgery, University of Munich.

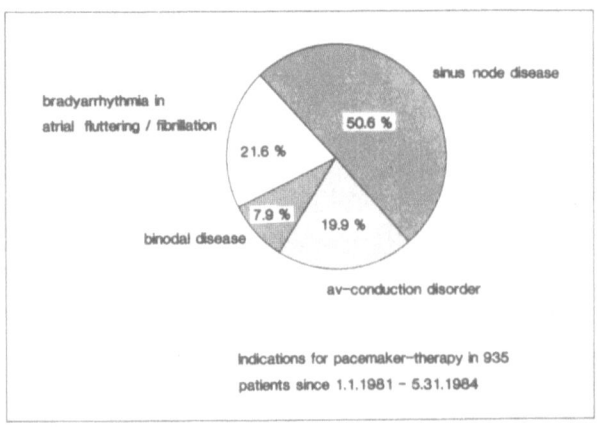

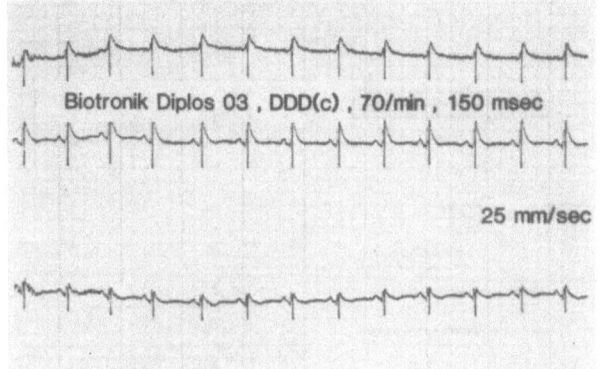

Fig. 2. Normal ECG findings after implantation of a dual chamber pacemaker device.

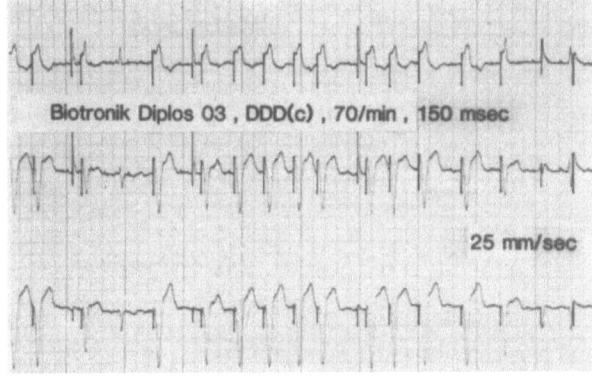

Fig. 3. Pacemaker mediated tachycardia due to atrial fibrillation.

Because of this complication the decision to implant a dual chamber pulse generator has been fairly rare. Since 1983 the DDI mode has offered a new alternative to pace patients with sinus node dysfunction in a dual chamber stimulation mode.

The patients are safely protected against pacemaker mediated tachycardias while dual chamber stimulation and detection is retained. The DDI mode, at present only programmable in a one pulse generator (Pacesetter* AFP 283), is characterized by 4 different ECG findings (Fig 4); native rhythm above the minimum programmed rate will inhibit the pacer (not shown in Fig. 4). In the case of a decreasing sinus rate an atrial stimulus is delivered after the atrial escape interval. A ventricular output pulse is discharged after the programmed interval unless a native QRS complex occurs. A native P-wave occurring before the atrial escape interval has been reached cannot initiate the AV interval counter. In this case the ventricular output pulse is delivered at the end of the pacing interval which comprises atrial escape interval and AV delay.

The consequence is obvious (Fig. 5): fast, P-wave synchronous, ventricular pacing is impossible. That means that neither a pacemaker mediated nor a pacemaker induced tachycardia can be started in this stimulation mode.

---

* Pacesetter Systems Inc., Sylmar, California, USA.

Fig. 4. Basic ECG configurations in the DDI mode.

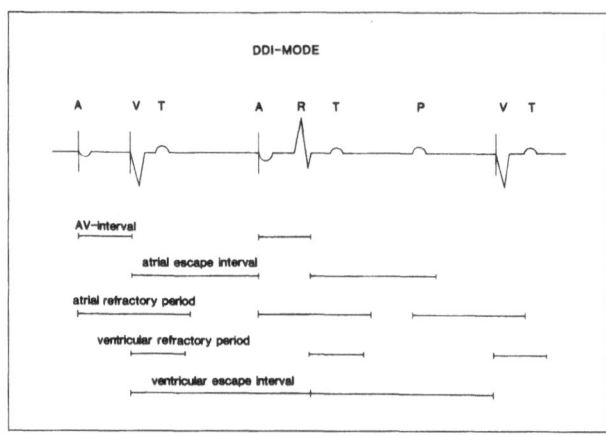

Fig. 5. Difference between DDD and DDI mode.

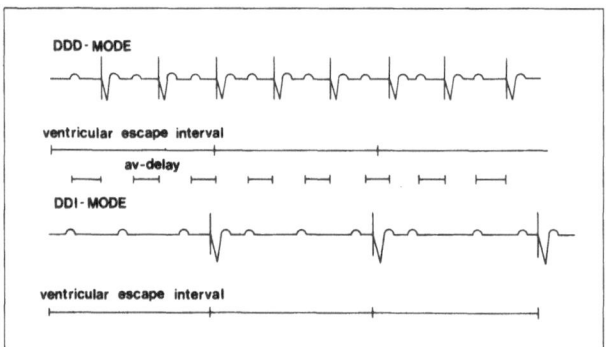

Fig. 6. Difference between DVI and DDI mode.

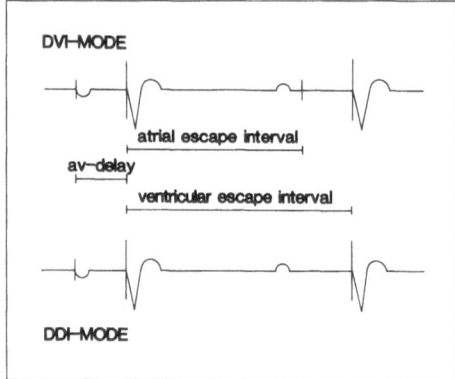

Up to now the most reasonable way to face the problem of a pacemaker mediated tachycardia due to intermittent atrial flutter/fibrillation in patients with sick sinus syndrome has been the DVI mode. This pacing mode, however, is disadvantageous as atrial detection is not possible. Thus an atrial stimulation may occur during the vulnerable period of a native atrial action and induce atrial fibrillation. This complication is impossible in the DDI mode as one can see in Fig. 6.

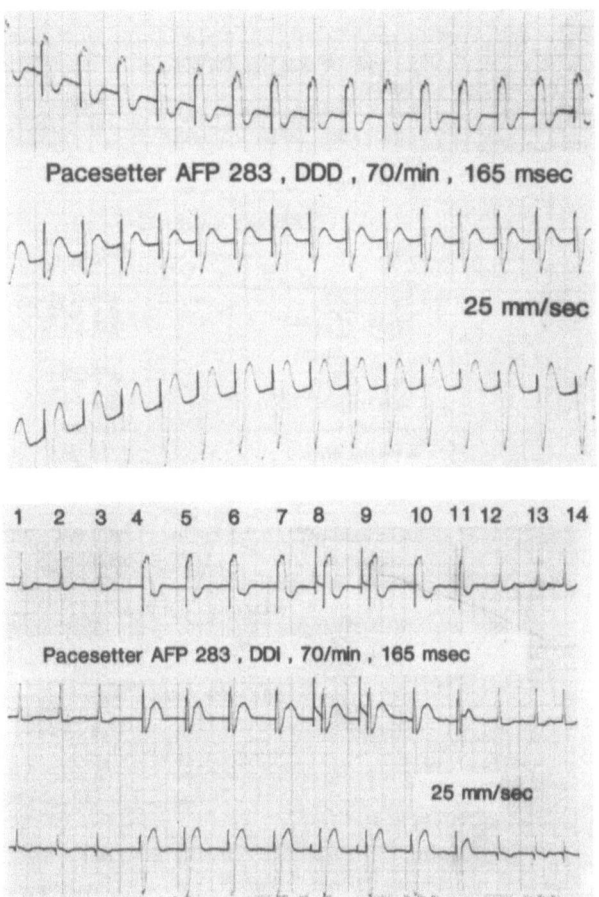

Pacesetter AFP 283 , DDD , 70/min , 165 msec

25 mm/sec

1 2 3 4 5 6 7 8 9 10 11 12 13 14

Pacesetter AFP 283 , DDI , 70/min , 165 msec

25 mm/sec

Fig. 7. Pacemaker mediated tachycardia due to atrial fluttering.

Fig. 8. Same patient as in Fig. 7 after programming to DDI mode.

The advantages of the DDI mode can be underlined with a clinical example: Figure 7 shows the ECG of a patient who developed atrial flutter after implantation of a dual chamber pacemaker. The result is a fast P-wave synchronous ventricular stimulation; in other words, a pacemaker mediated tachycardia.

After programming DDI mode (Fig. 8) this complication disappears. Flutter waves are partly detected (actions 4–7 and 10) and partly not detected (actions 8 and 9 with ineffective atrial pacing). After atrial pacing the ventricular output pulse is delivered after the programmed AV delay (actions 8 and 9).

After detection of a P-wave the ventricle is paced after reaching the end of the pacing interval independent of native atrial actions (actions 4–7 and 10). Actions 1–3, 12, and 13 show AV sequential inhibition, action 11 is a fusion beat.

Figure 9 shows a DDI program: this stimulation mode allows programming of the highest atrial sensitivity settings to guarantee atrial detection particularly when sinus rhythm is restored. In addition the patient is safely protected against fast P-wave synchronous ventricular stimulation.

Fig. 9. Example of a DDI program.

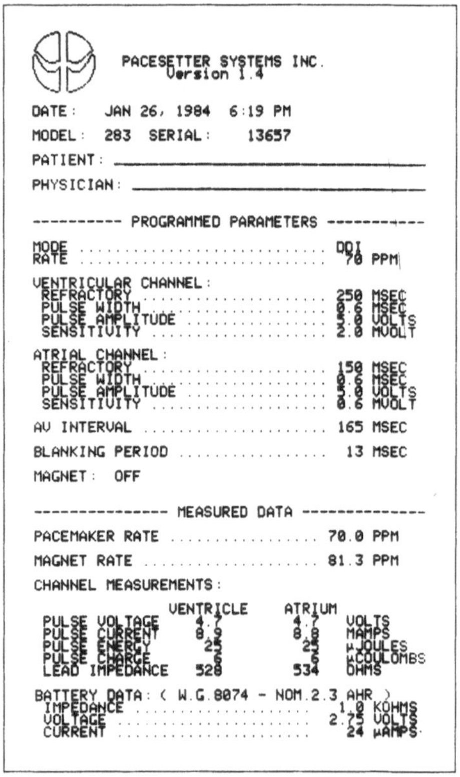

PACESETTER SYSTEMS INC.
Version 1.4

DATE: JAN 26, 1984 6:19 PM
MODEL: 283 SERIAL: 13657
PATIENT: ________________
PHYSICIAN: ________________

---------- PROGRAMMED PARAMETERS ----------

MODE .... DDI
RATE .... 70 PPM

VENTRICULAR CHANNEL:
REFRACTORY .... 250 MSEC
PULSE WIDTH .... 0.6 MSEC
PULSE AMPLITUDE .... 5.0 VOLTS
SENSITIVITY .... 2.0 MVOLT

ATRIAL CHANNEL:
REFRACTORY .... 150 MSEC
PULSE WIDTH .... 0.6 MSEC
PULSE AMPLITUDE .... 5.0 VOLTS
SENSITIVITY .... 0.6 MVOLT

AV INTERVAL .... 165 MSEC
BLANKING PERIOD .... 13 MSEC
MAGNET: OFF

--------------- MEASURED DATA ---------------

PACEMAKER RATE .... 70.0 PPM
MAGNET RATE .... 81.3 PPM

CHANNEL MEASUREMENTS:

	VENTRICLE	ATRIUM	
PULSE VOLTAGE	4.7	4.7	VOLTS
PULSE CURRENT	8.9	8.8	MAMPS
PULSE ENERGY	25	25	μJOULES
PULSE CHARGE	6	6	μCOULOMBS
LEAD IMPEDANCE	528	534	OHMS

BATTERY DATA: (W.G.8074 - NOM.2.3 AHR)
IMPEDANCE .... 1.0 KOHMS
VOLTAGE .... 2.75 VOLTS
CURRENT .... 24 μAMPS

In conclusion: patients with an isolated sinus node dysfunction benefit from the DDI mode for two reasons:

1. Basic atrial and ventricular stimulation rate is also guaranteed in the case of impairing AV conduction after pacemaker implantation.
2. Pacemaker-mediated tachycardia due to intermittent atrial flutter/fibrillation, a major complication in this patient group, is impossible.

Therefore the DDI mode must be considered as an alternative stimulation mode for patients suffering from sinus node dysfunction.

Authors' address:
A. Markewitz, M.D.
Herzchirurgische Klinik
Ludwig-Maximilians-Universität München
Marchioninistraße 70
8000 München 70
West Germany

A New Generation of Dual Chamber Pacemakers with Automatic in-built Rhythm Recognition Capabilities

B. Candelon, F. H. M. Wittkampf, and J. C. Jacobs

Summary: Actual generation of dual chamber cardiac pacemaker reacts to atrial and ventricular arrhythmia according to respective refractory period settings.
Recognition and identification of atrial arrhythmia enables the pulse generator to prevent inducing arrhythmia in the ventricle and to preserve and extend physiological rate adaptation for normal sinus rate. Recognition and identification of ventricular arrhythmia can be used to trigger special pacing modes to reduce the occurrence of these arrhythmias.

An algorithm for the analysis and recognition of atrial and ventricular rhythm patterns can be used in dual chamber pacemakers to determine the optimal pacing response in both chambers.

Such a recognition capability can be used to provide improved physiological adaptation of the ventricular pacing rate in the case of exercise-induced high atrial rates, and to prevent the artificial conduction of atrial arrhythmias to the ventricle. In addition, special pacing modes can be used to adapt the pacemaker response to certain types of arrhythmia.

Finally, the storage and subsequent retrieval, from the pacemaker memory, of information about the occurrence and frequency of the different rhythm patterns can provide an efficient tool for diagnosis and pacemaker programming.

Physiological and unphysiological atrial rates

In dual chamber pacemakers the discrimination between physiological and unphysiological atrial rates is usually determined by means of a single rate level called the "upper rate limit" or the "1 : 1 tracking limit". This very simple differentiation at an arbitrary level is often insufficient since an exercise-induced high atrial rate can exceed the rate of a tachycardia. A more sophisticated method should be used in order to ensure better discrimination. One of the possible solutions consists of the beat to beat monitoring of the atrial rate, which allows for an accurate analysis of the onset of any rate acceleration. The discrimination between an atrial tachycardia (sudden rate increase) and an exercise-induced high atrial rate (smooth rate increase) is then much more accurate, and the pacemaker can adapt the ventricular pacing response accordingly:

1. In the case of an atrial tachycardia, the pacemaker can limit the ventricular pacing rate in such a way that, while A-V synchrony is maintained, the ventricular pacing rate never exceeds an unphysiological value. Recognition of the atrial arrhythmia allows the pacemaker to avoid transmitting it to the ventricle, or to have an unphysiological high ventricular pacing rate. This type of response can be seen in Figure 1, where

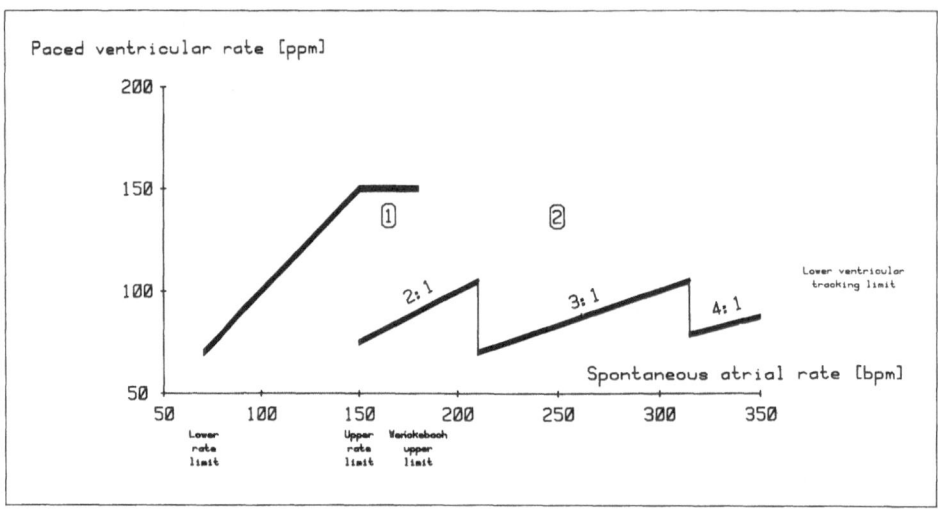

Fig. 1. Automatic ventricular response for different atrial rates. Zone 1. Extension of ventricular response (Wenckebach mode) to exercise-induced high atrial rates, or block response to atrial arrhythmias. Zone 2. Protection against high ventricular pacing rate in atrial tachycardia, achieved by automatic lowering of the maximum ventricular pacing rate.

the ventricular rate is the result of pacemaker-induced block of 2 : 1, 3 : 1 or 4 : 1 etc. In the case of such an atrial arrhythmia, limitation of the ventricular rate to a value around 100 ppm prevents the transmission of the arrhythmia to the ventricle.

2. In the case of an exercise-induced high atrial rate that exceeds the programmed upper rate limit the pacemaker can automatically extend the programmed upper sensing limit, and by so doing, allow the pacemaker to provide a physiological ventricular response and at the same time maintain A-V synchrony (1). Since the artificial A-V conduction is in the Wenckebach mode, the ventricular rate can be kept at the preset maximum ventricular pacing rate.

In Figure 1, zone I, the ventricular pacing response of the pacemaker is shown. In the case of a physiological rate increase, automatic Wenckebach is set instead of the block response. It is interesting to note that, in the system described in Figure 1, the Wenckebach response is at atrial rates above the programmed upper rate limit, thus extending the capabilities of physiological response of the pacemaker to exercise without introducing limitations due to a short atrial refractory periods. This is because the automatic extension is only effective when a physiological rate increase is detected.

Prevention of pacemaker-induced arrhythmias

Pacemaker-induced arrhythmias can easily be prevented if the pacemaker is able to recognise them and their causes. Of these arrhythmias, the pacemaker mediated tachycardia (PMT) is the most common. The causes of such artificial arrhythmias have been described extensively in the literature (2).

A major step towards the prevention of such arrhythmias is provided by an automatic Wenckebach response, as described above. This contributes to the prevention of pacemaker induced arrhythmias since it is the Wenckebach mode of ventricular response that is one of the main causes of PMTs. A second aspect is correct programming of the post ventricular atrial refractory period (PVARP). To determine the optimal PVARP one should first check for the existence of retrograde conduction and determine the associated V-A conduction time. This can be done directly by temporarily reprogramming the pacemaker to the VAO mode. In this mode the pacemaker paces asynchronously in the ventricle, simultaneously senses the atrial activity, and times the P-wave relative to the ventricular stimulus. A stimulus-P interval that remains constant from beat to beat is an indication of the presence of retrograde conduction (Figure 2).

In addition to the interval analysis capability, automatic prevention should be performed whenever a possible cause of PMT can be automatically recognised by the pacemaker. This is the case with ventricular premature beats which are either spontaneous (ventricular ectopic beats) or which are triggered by atrial oversensing. Sensing of retrograde conduction can then be prevented by automatic lengthening of PVARP.

A spontaneous ventricular premature contraction can be identified by the pacemaker since it is a ventricular event not preceded by a spontaneous or paced atrial event. In such a case the pacemaker can automatically prolong the PVARP.

In the case of atrial oversensing which triggers an artificial PVC, automatic prolongation of the PVARP can be achieved by incorporating a rate responsive A-V delay in the pacemaker. Since the total atrial refractory period is constant, premature oversensing in the atrium will automatically cause the A-V delay to shorten, and thus lengthen the PVARP.

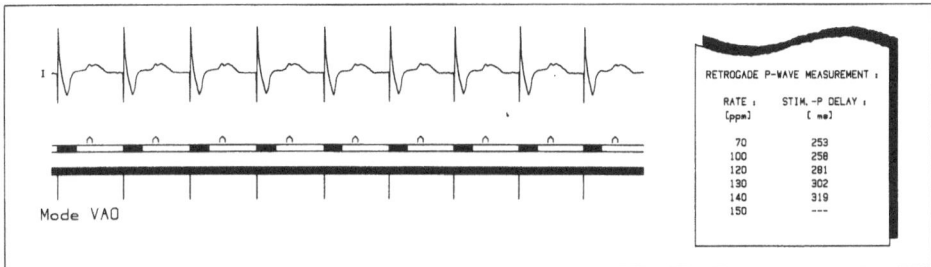

Fig. 2. Non-invasive analysis of retrograde conduction by means of VAO pacing mode and monitoring of V-A interval.

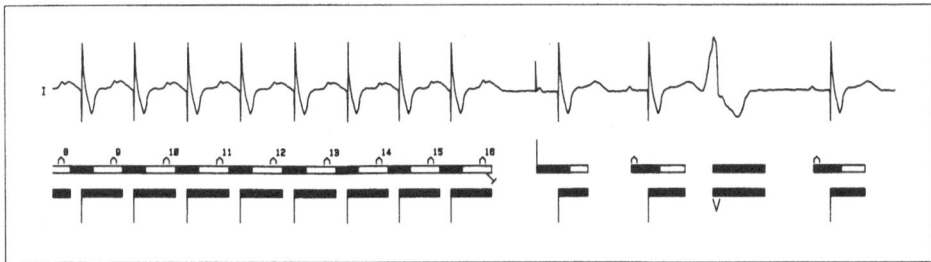

Fig. 3. Automatic recognition and termination of a pacemaker-mediated tachycardia by monitoring V-A conduction time and skipping A-V conduction.

In addition this feature would also provide the obvious physiological advantage of having a pacemaker that, at higher rates, automatically shortens the A-V delay in the same way as a normal heart.

In spite of the inclusion of a prevention algorithm and of various protection mechanisms, it should be realised that a PMT can still occur. It is therefore important that the pacemaker itself is able to recognise that it is helping to maintain an arrhythmia and is capable of interrupting it. This can be done by programming the pacemaker to automatically monitor the V-A conduction time whenever it is pacing at the ventricular upper rate limit. If a constant value is found the pacemaker can diagnose a PMT and interrupt it by skipping the A-V conduction for one cycle (Figure 3).

Automatic prevention of triggered ventricular arrhythmias

Since one of the main purposes of a DDD pacemaker is to restore A-V synchrony, any beat to beat variations in the atrial rate (within the programmed 1 : 1 conduction zone) will be transmitted to the ventricle. This means that irregular atrial rates induced by such arrhythmias as premature atrial contractions, S-A block or the bradycardia-tachycardia syndrome will result in an irregular ventricular pacing rate. Such irregularities can be prevented by making use of such pacing modes as "rate smoothing" (6) or the "flywheel" mode (4). Such special modes act as regulators of the ventricular pacing rate by only allowing beat to beat variations that are within a given time interval (7), thus preventing any sudden decrease in ventricular rate. In this way, arrhythmias such as the bradycardia-tachycardia syndrome or intermittent SA block are not passed to the ventricle.

Such modes can also be used to prevent arrhythmias. The rate smoothing mode can help to prevent sudden rate increases in case of PACs. However, A-V synchrony may be lost because the ventricular stimulus is no longer allowed to directly follow the sensed atrial event. The flywheel mode will react to a PVC or a PAC by first increasing the atrial pacing rate and then slowly decreasing it. The method of overdriving the arrhythmia suppresses further premature beats (8).

In order to be able allow a physician to check the functioning of the control algorithm, the pacemaker should also have a built-in Holter, in which information can be stored about the various spontaneous rhythm patterns. The analysis of such information can then, if necessary, be used to adjust the programmable parameters of the pacemaker. The storage of information about the duration of the various rhythm patterns, such as exercise-induced high atrial rates and atrial tachycardias, can provide valuable information about the programming of the upper rate limit, and can be an aid to the diagnosis of frequent atrial arrhythmias, which may be either true atrial arrhythmias or due to oversensing (e.g. myopotentials) by the atrial channel. PAC and PVC counters can also be a good tool for the evaluation of antiarrhythmia treatment (drug therapy or a special pacing mode). Such features in a dual chamber pacemaker will help the physician to concentrate more on the medical aspects of DDD pacing than on the complicated technical aspects sometimes linked to the use of DDD pacemakers.

Acknowledgement

The authors would like to thank Ron Whiteley for his help in preparing this manuscript.

References

1. Furman S (1983) Retreat from Wenckebach. PACE 7: 1, p 1
2. Harthorne JW, Eisenhauer AC, Steinhaus DM (1983) Pacemaker mediated tachycardias – an unresolved problem. PACE 7:6, 1140–1147
3. Physicians manual, Intermedics Cosmos model 283–01
4. User's manual, Vitatron Quintech DDD model 931
5. Van Gelder LM, El Gamal R, Baker R, Sanders RS (1983) Tachycardia termination algorithm – a valuable feature for interruption of pacemaker mediated tachycardias. PACE 7:2, 283–287
6. Physicians manual, Cardiac Pacemakers Inc, Delta DDD
7. Sermasi S, Marzaloni M, Rusconi L, Antioli GW (1984) RBM Vol 6: p 207
8. Winter UJ, Behrenbeck DW, Brill Th, Höher M, Hombach V, Hilger HH (1984) First clinical assessment of the hemodynamic and anti-ectopic effects of long-term dynamic overdrive pacing in implanted VVI pacemakers. In: Progress in Clinical Pacing; Proceedings edited by Santini M, Pistolese M, Alliegro A, Rome, p 813–818

Authors' address:
Mr. Bernard Candelon
Product Manager
Vitatron Medical B.V.
Kanaalweg 24
P.O. Box 76
NL-6950 AB Dieren
The Netherlands

Left Ventricular Function During VVI and DVI Pacing at Different Rates as Assessed by M-Mode and Two-Dimensional Echocardiography, Gated Single Photon Emission Computerized Tomography (GASPECT) and Thermodilution

B. Maisch[1], G. Ertl[1], C. Eilles[2], W. Gerhards[2], J. Knoblauch[1], and K. Kochsiek[1]

Summary: The influence of heart rate and pacing mode (ventricular pacing (VVI) versus atrial synchronous pacing (DVI)) on left ventricular volumes, cardiac index (CI) and ejection fraction (EF) was analyzed with M-mode and two-dimensional echocardiography, gated single photon emission computerized tomography (GASPECT) and compared to stroke volume indices (SVI) and CI obtained by simultaneous thermodilution measurements.

When compared to thermodilution the CI obtained by GASPECT ($r = 0.78$) gave better correlations than 2-D-echocardiography ($r = 0.57$). Similarly SVI assessed by GASPECT ($r = 0.69$) correlated more closely with the SVI from thermodilution than did SVI by M-mode ($r = 0.46$) or 2-D-echocardiography ($r = 0.61$). The percent changes in left ventricular volumes by 2-D-echocardiography during an increase in heart rate by either DVI or VVI stimulation are comparable to those previously reported: due to a disproportional decrease of left ventricular end-diastolic (LVEDVI) and end-systolic volume indices (LVESVI) stroke volume index decreases when heart rate is accelerated by pacing. The hemodynamic profit of atrial synchronous pacing at baseline frequency is demonstrated by a 14% increase of CI and is even higher (20 to 30%) at 120 beats per min. This persisting hemodynamic profit at high rates through DVI pacing is of clinical importance when rate adaptive VVI pacing is compared to fully physiological atrial synchronous pacing.

If the chronic hemodynamic benefit of pacing at different modes and rates is to be objectified repeated non-invasive measurements are mandatory in elderly patients for whom invasive methods are inadequate. M-mode and two-dimensional echocardiography (1–7) and radionuclide ventriculography (8) have been used to approximate left ventricular hemodynamics (11). In patients with ventricular pacemakers (VVI pacing), however, the use of M-mode echocardiography is limited since abnormal septal motion is present in the majority of cases (9). Abnormal septal motion results in the underestimation of the end-systolic diameters, and thus calculated stroke volume indices or cardiac indices derived from this parameter my also be wrong. Two-D-echocardiography has the problem of finding a clear endocardial echo, of tangential cuts, and of undistorted display of the apical portion of the left ventricle (1–4). When compared to cineangiography volumes are underestimated (1, 3, 5). Conventional radionuclide ventriculography may be superior to echocardiography in the determination of an ejection fraction index (10), but the ejection fraction itself is known to be unreliable as the representative parameter of left ventricular function. On the other hand the determination of left ventricular volumes by

University Hospital of Internal Medicine (1), and the Department of Nuclear Medicine (2), Würzburg, Germany.

radionuclide ventriculography is by indirect means only (10). Gated single photon emission computed tomography (GASPECT) applied to radionuclide ventriculography offers several advantages over conventional radionuclide ventriculography in the determination of absolute ventricular volumes (10, 11). The present study compares the reliability of M-mode und 2-D-echocardiography, of conventional and GASPECT radionuclide ventriculography with thermodilution cardiac output measurements to determine parameters useful to define left ventricular function in patients with pacemakers. The DVI and VVI pacing modes were compared in their influence on left ventricular function parameters at different heart rates.

Methods

Patients

Eight patients (6 female, 2 male) with DDD pacemakers (5 Versatrax II, 1 Symbios (Medtronic), 2 AFP (Pacesetter)), 10 patients (6 male, 4 female) with VVI devices (4 Spectrax SXT (Medtronic), 3 Optima MP (Telectronics), 2 Pacesetter 221, and 1 Vitatron C) were investigated. Mean age was 67 ± 9 years. Permanent DDD devices were implanted because of 2nd or 3rd degree AV-block in 6 and sinus bradycardia (< 40 bpm) in 2 cases. Indications for VVI pacemakers were sick sinus syndrome in 7 and pathological bradycardia with atrial fibrillation in 3 cases.

Study protocol

On days 5 to 10 after the implantation of a permanent pacemaker right heart cardiac output was measured with a Swan-Ganz thermodilution catheter. Simultaneous M-mode and 2-D-echocardiography was performed. GASPECT was carried out one day later or on the same afternoon at the same pacing rates. End-systolic and end-diastolic volume indices were determined as previously described (10, 11). End-diastolic and end-systole were defined by ECG gating.
The AV delay (DVI mode) was set to 160 ms (12).

Echocardiography

The study included only those patients in whom volume indices could be assessed by at least 80% of the endocardial surface in the RAO aequivalent or four chamber view with an electronic sector scanner (84°, 2,25 MHz transducer, Varian 3400 DPDM, Diasonic). TM echocardiograms were printed out immediately, 2-D-echocardiograms were recorded on videotape during end-exspiration. End-systolic and end-diastolic volumes were calculated using the rotating single-plane ellipsoid formula ($V = \dfrac{8A^2}{3\,T\,L}$, where V is the volume, A the area, L the length). End-diastolic was defined as peak of the R-wave, end-systole was set by ECG gating at the end of the T-wave. Volumes from M-Mode echocardiograms were calculated using the Teichholz formula.

Gaspect

ECG gated single photon emission computerized tomography (GASPECT) for cardiac bloodpool imaging was carried out with the gamma camera GE 400 Autotune ZS, which was rotated 180 degrees and made 32 single projections. The system was guided by a PDP 11–34 computer with a floating-point processor after the injection of 25 mCi 99 m Technetium-human serum albumin (Henning, Berlin) or radioactively labelled red blood cells. A 64 × 64/16 bit matrix was used for imaging, and new software, described previously (10, 11), was developed for data processing and reconstruction of images. Volumes were assessed by averaging the tomographic data for a period of 20 minutes. Pixel units were then transformed to ml using a factor of 0.091, which was predetermined in in vitro phantom studies and in comparison with left ventricular angiography (10, 11). Ejections fractions attained by GASPECT correlated well with the EF as measured by conventional radioventriculography (11).

A comparison of all 4 methods used for the assessment of SVI and CI was possible in 12 of 18 patients only due to unsatisfactory registration of the endocardial surface in 5 patients for 2-D-echocardiography and lack of satisfactory GASPECT in 2 patients (overlap of 1 patient).

Results

Comparison of thermodilution, M-mode, 2-D-echocardiography and GASPECT for the assessment of stroke volume and cardiac indices

When compared to thermodilution the cardiac indices of GASPECT (r = 0.78) and two-dimensional echocardiography (r = 0.57) gave the best correlations. The correlation between both echocardiography methods was slightly better. No satisfactory correlations were found for the CI, when GASPECT was correlated with either H-mode or 2-D-echocardiography (r = 0.40 and 0.32, respectively).

Fig. 1a. Regression analysis of the cardiac index (CI) as assessed by thermodilution and GASPECT.

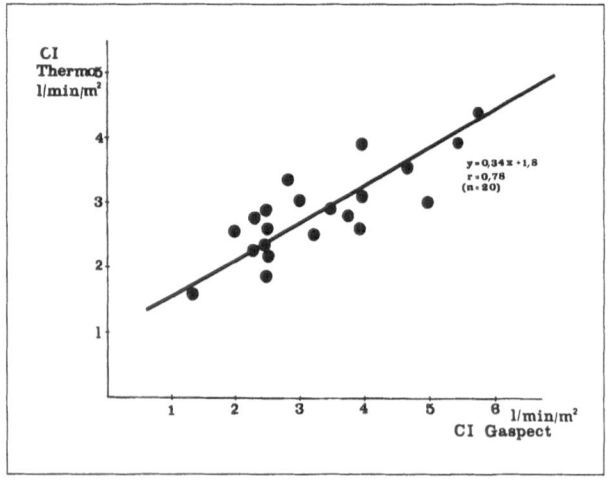

160

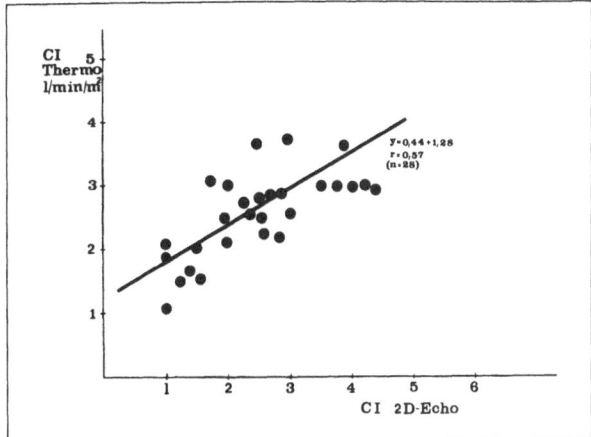

Fig. 1b. Regression analysis of the cardiac index (CI) as assessed by thermodilution and 2-D-echocardiography.

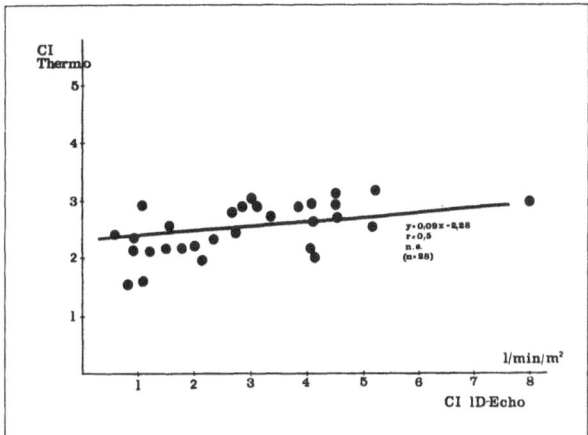

Fig. 1c. Regression analysis as assessed by thermodilution of the cardiac index (CI) and M-mode (1-D-)echocardiography. M-mode echocardiography is not suitable for the assessment of cardiac function in a heterogenous group of patients, some of whom have abnormal septal motion.

The line of regression in the comparison of the cardiac indices measured by thermodilution and GASPECT can be seen in Fig. 1a. Fig. 1b shows regression analysis between thermodilution and 2-D-echocardiography, while Fig. 1c demonstrates assessments by thermodilution and M-mode echocardiography.

When compared to thermodilution both 2-D-echocardiography and GASPECT overestimated the cardiac index in range of > 3 $1/min/m^2$, and underestimated it by < 1.5 $1/min/m^2$ as can be derived from the coefficients of the regression equations.

Correlations of the stroke volume index calculated from thermodilution are shown in Table 1.

161

Table 1. Comparison of thermodilution to echocardiography and GASPECT (r values).

	M-mode	2-D-Echo	GASPECT
Cardiac index	0.54	0.57	0.78
Stroke volume	0.46	0.61	0.69

Table 2. Regression analysis of left ventricular volume indices.

	2-D-Echo	M-mode
LVEDVI		
GASPECT	0.76	0.39
2-D-Echo	–	0.47
LVESVI		
GASPECT	0.43	0.35
2-D-Echo	–	0.22
Ejection Fraction		
GASPECT	0.58	0.42
2-D-Echo	–	0.37

Comparison of volume indices and ejection fractions assessed by 2-D, M-mode echocardiography and GASPECT

Left ventricular end-diastolic volumes assessed by 2-D and M-mode echocardiography were comparable, with 64 and 65 ml/m² respectively, whereas GASPECT yielded a volume 5 to 6 ml greater by over all analysis. This also holds for the data derived from different pacing modes and frequencies (Figs. 2a, 3).

Left ventricular end-systolic volume is also overestimated by GASPECT or underestimated by echocardiography (Fig. 2b).

Ejection fraction was consequently overestimated by both of the echocardiographic methods, particularly in M-mode echocardiograhy due to the relatively larger stroke volume indices.

The correlation between the 3 noninvasive techniques for left ventricular end-diastolic volume indices gave satisfactory r values only when GASPECT was compared to 2-D-echocardiography (r = 0.76). Correlations of the end-systolic parameters were less impressive with r = 0.43 when the LVESVI of GASPECT was compared to 2-D-echocardiography. Correlations of the ejection fraction between all 3 noninvasive methods also gave poor correlation coefficients, the best being 0.58 when GASPECT was compared to 2-D-echocardiography.

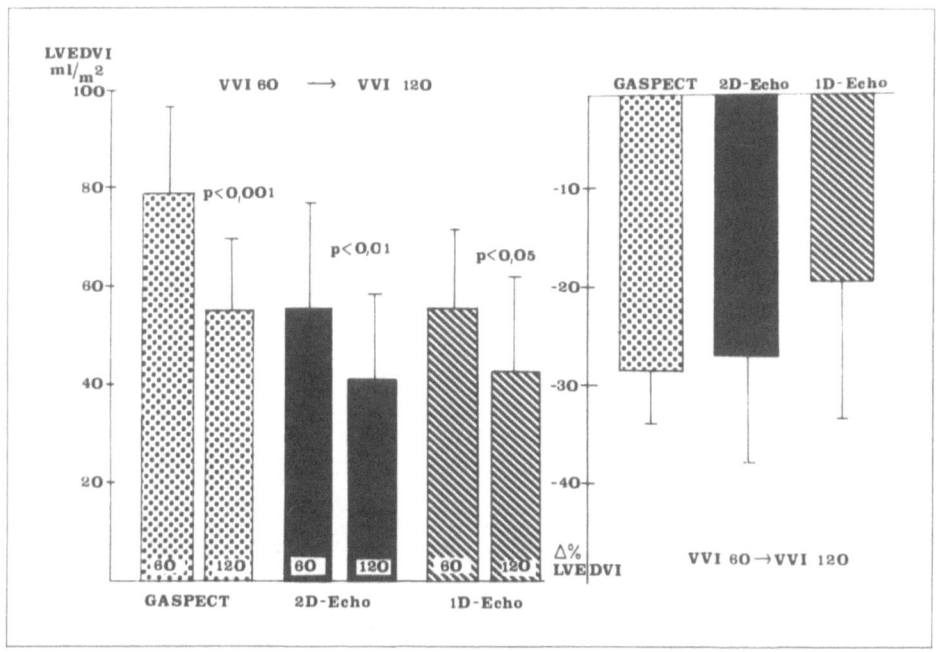

Fig. 2a. The decrease of LVEDVI (left ventricular end-diastolic volume index) in VVI pacing during an increase in rate from 60 to 120 bpm could be assessed with all 3 methods employed.

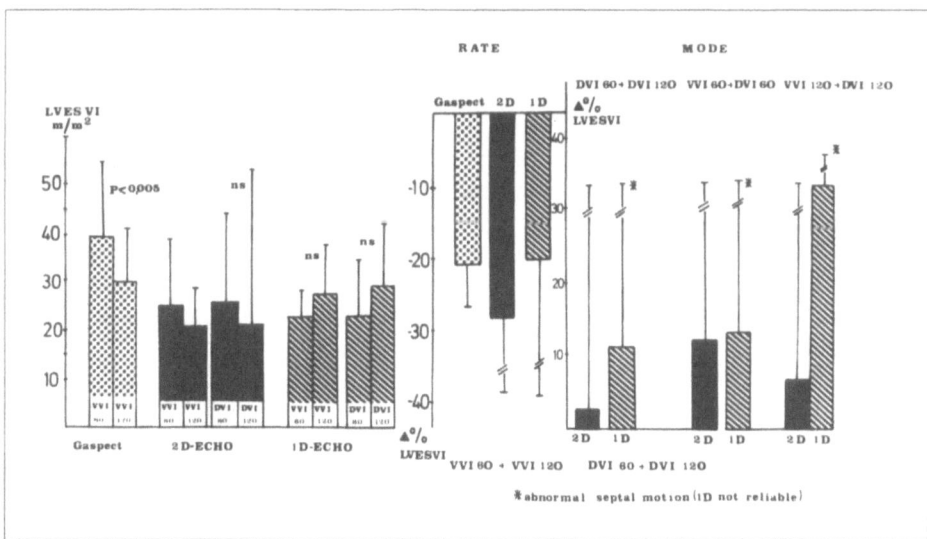

Fig. 2b. A decrease in the LVESVI (left ventricular end-systolic volume index) could be monitored by all methods independent of the pacing mode when rate was increased from 60 to 120 bpm. Differences obtained by M-mode echocardiography were not significant, however.

163

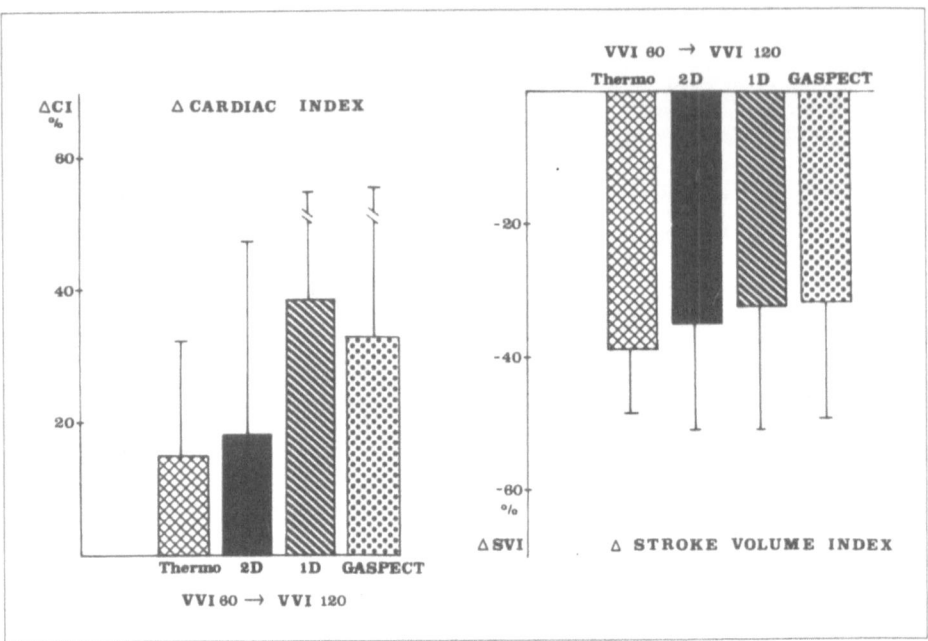

Fig. 2c. The rate dependent increase in cardiac index (CI in %) was overestimated by all noninvasive methods when compared to thermodilution. Stroke volume index was underestimated accordingly.

Hemodynamic parameters during changes of heart rate in VVI pacing

An increase in heart rate from VVI 60 bpm to VVI 120 bpm resulted in a moderate improvement of cardiac index by absolute values (Fig. 2c). The increase was significant when measured by either of the techniques. Correspondingly the rate-dependent percent decrease in stroke volume index was less prominent in M-mode echocardiography and GASPECT. All 4 techniques provided evidence for the same direction of change (increase of CI and decrease of SVI) both by analysis of all and of individual data. The percent increase in CI when the VVI pacing rate was changed from 60 to 120 showed considerable quantitative differences depending on the techniques used. The smallest percent increases for the cardiac index and consequently more prominent alterations of the SVI were found by thermodilution measurements. M-mode echocardiography and GASPECT overestimated the percent increase of CI considerably (15.5% by thermodilution as compared to 34.7% by GASPECT or 39.6% by M-mode echocardiography), whereas 2-D-echocardiography gave similar results.

LVEDVI decreased (Fig. 2a), when the rate was increased from VVI 60 to VVI 120 bpm by 27.6% (2-D-echocardiography) or 29.4% (GASPECT), whereas M-mode echocardiography showed a less prominent alteration, possibly due to the patients with aneurysms (n = 2).

LVESVI changed between –27.4% (2-D-echocardiography) and –20% (M-mode echocardiography), depending on the technique used when the heart rate was increased (Fig. 2b).

164

Ejection fraction was reduced significantly as assessed by GASPECT and 2-D-echo-cardiography from 52.6 or 57.3 to 48.3 or 46.7, respectively ($p < 0.05$ each), when the stimulation rate was changed from VVI 60 to VVI 120 bpm. Four of the 8 patients had reduced EF at VVI 60.

Hemodynamics during changes in heart rate by DVI pacing

A rise of heart rate from 60 bpm to 120 bpm during DVI pacing resulted in an increase in cardiac index (Fig. 2d). This result was consistent irrespective of the method used to determine cardiac index.

Irrespective of the method used, LVEDVI decreased with the increase in heart rate while LVESVI remained basically unchanged.

Heart rate correlated changes of EF were not statistically significant during pacing in the DVI mode.

Four patients who initially had a normal EF ($> 55\%$) did not decrease EF at higher rates.

Hemodynamic profit of atrial synchronous pacing (DVI mode)

Although correlations of hemodynamic parameters by the different techniques show considerable divergence in absolute numbers the hemodynamic profit during DVI when

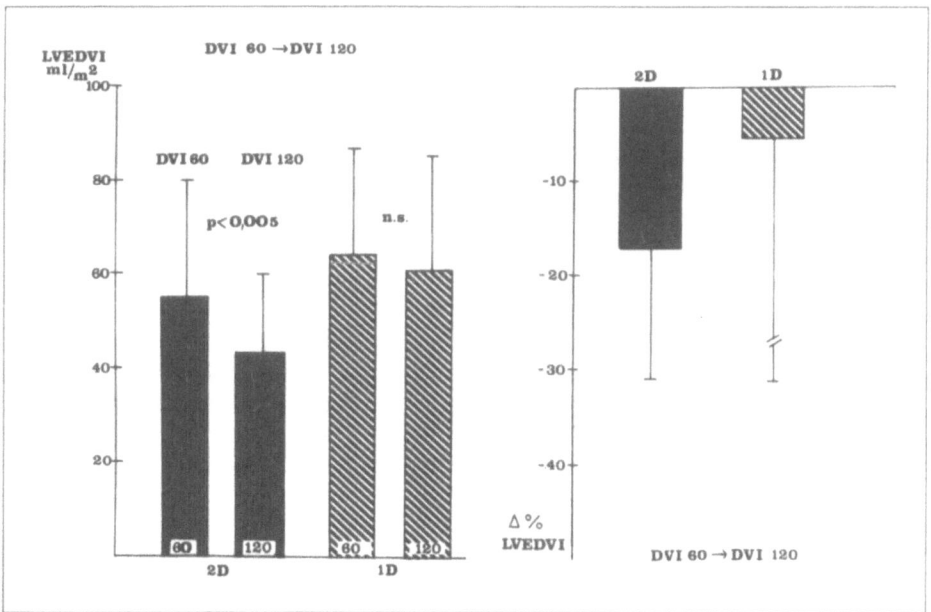

Fig. 2d. In DVI pacing a rate dependent increase of the cardiac index (CI) could be measured by all methods employed. There was some overestimation by both echocardiographic methods when compared to thermodilution.

165

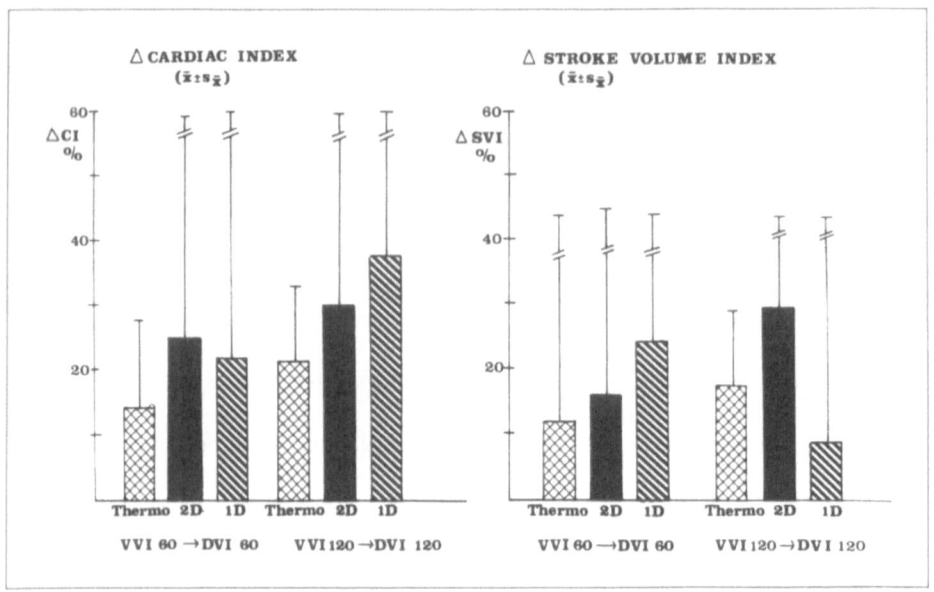

Fig. 3. Mode dependent changes (% increase when changing from VVI to DVI pacing) could be demonstrated by all methods. The percent increase of cardiac index and stroke volume index was lowest by thermodilution measurements, so echocardiography may overestimate the increase to a certain degree.

compared to VVI pacing is obvious. The hemodynamic improvement could be assessed by at least 2 of the 4 methods, most of the time by all 4 methods employed.

Cardiac index rose by 14% at 60 bpm and 21% at 120 bpm when the mode was switched from VVI to DDI when thermodilution was taken as reference method (Fig. 3). M-mode and 2-D-echocardiography revealed an even higher profit of DVI pacing mode (Fig. 3).

As to be expected mean stroke volume index (Fig. 3) increased by a similar amount when the DVI mode was established. This was by 13.1% at 60 bpm and by 17% at 120 bpm, With thermodilution and somewhat more when measured by 2-D and M-mode echocardiography.

LVEDVI at DVI mode was not significantly different from LVEDVI mode at 60 bpm. At 120 bpm LVEDVI increased when VVI was switched to DVI marginally (n.s.) as measured by 2-D-echocardiography (+10.7%) and 40% ($p < 0.01$) when assessed by 1-D-echocardiography.

Significant differences of LVESVI at VVI vs. DVI mode were not found.

Discussion

One of the purposes of these investigations was to compare noninvasive techniques such as M-mode and two-dimensional echocardiography and GASPECT with thermodilution

166

and to find out if reproducible data for follow-up studies can be assessed in patients at 65 to 80 years of age, in whom invasive techniques cannot be used routinely.

GASPECT correlated best with thermodilution as far as cardiac index and stroke volume index are concerned. This is probably due to the averaging of data by GASPECT for 20 to 30 minutes and the difficult echo-anatomy of elderly people with emphysema who do not have an optimal echocardiographic window.

Furthermore divergent results may depend on the model for the rotation ellipsoid, or even more prominently on the volume determinations with the Teichholz formula, the precise application of which demands the exclusion of segmental wall motion abnormalities. This prerequisite was not fulfilled in a quarter of our patients due to coronary artery disease. GASPECT on the other hand is hampered by the large amount of time necessary to obtain data of one volume at a time for one frequency and one mode only (10, 11).

In accordance with others (1, 15–19) LVEDVI, LVESVI and SVI decrease when heart rates is increased. Ejection fraction remains constant over a large range frequencies during VVI stimulation or is slightly decreased, as described by others (20). During DVI stimulation a rate dependent slight decrease of the ejection fraction also takes place, indicating that the reduction of EF observed by VVI stimulation is not only caused by the missing atrial systole.

Atrial systole in return causes an increase of cardiac index at 14% of baseline frequency stimulation in the VVI mode, an effect which is even more prominent at a rate of 120 bpm. This hemodynamic improvement of DVI stimulation is comparable to data from Hung et al. (21), Karlöf (22), Kappenberger et al. (23), and Kruse et al. (24). It can easily be calculated from cardiac indices that during bifocal stimulation the stroke volume index increased at baseline frequency (60 bpm) by 12 to 16% and even more so at 120 bpm by 17 to 29%, depending on the method employed for its assessment. This remaining and even more prominent effect of an increase of CI during DVI stimulation at higher frequencies does not confirm the data from Creplet et al. (25) but is in accordance with Hung et al. (21). These data may therefore be of clinical importance when rate adaptive VVI pacing is compared to atrial synchronous pacing, since there is still controversy on the relative importance of atrial systole at higher frequencies (26, 27). It should be noted in this context, however, that the left ventricular filling pressure during different pacing frequencies at rest is not subjected to significant alterations, whereas during exercise it can rise considerably, thus diminishing the relative importance of the atrial kick at higher rates.

References

1. DeMaria AN, Neumann A, Schubart PJ, Lee G, Mason DT (1979) Systematic correlation of cardiac chamber size and ventricular performance determined with echocardiography and alterations in heart rate in normal persons. Am J Cardiol 43: 1–9
2. Erbel R, Krebs W, Schweizer P, Richter HA, Meyer J, Effert S (1982) Comparison of single plane and biplane volume determination by two dimensional echocardiography: asymmetric model hearts. Eur Heart J 3: 469–480
3. Erbel R, Schweizer P, Lambertz H, Henn G, Meyer J, Krebs W, Effert S (1983) Echoventriculography – a simultaneous analysis of two-dimensional echocardiography and cineventriculography. Circulation 67: 205–215

4. Grube E, Richter R, Otten H, Janson R, Lackner K, Simon HJ (1979) Darstellung linksventriku-lärer Kontraktionsanomalien mit der zweidimensionalen Sektor-Echokardiographie. Dtsch Med Wschr 104: 703–707
5. Schiller NB, Acquatella H, Ports TA, Drew D, Goerke J, Ringertz H, Silverman NH, Brundage B, Botvinick EH, Boswell R, Carlsson EP, Parmley WW (1979) Left ventricular volume from paired biplane two-dimensional cardiography. Circulation 60: 547–555
6. Touche T, Prasquier R, Merillon JP, Barthelemy M, Hanoun HC, Verden P, Gourgon R (1980) Mesure des volumes ventriculaires gauches par echocardiographie bidimensionelle a partir d'une coupe apicale. Arch Mal Coeur 73: 691–700
7. Kan G, Visser CA, Lie KI, Durrer D (1981) Left ventricular volumes and ejection fraction by single plane two dimensional apex echocardiography. Eur Heart J 2: 339–343
8. Starling MR, Crawfort MH, Sorenson SG, Levi B, Richards KL, O'Rourke RA (1981) Comparative accuracy of apical biplane cross-sectional echocardiography and gated equilibrium radionu-clide angiography for estimating left ventricular size and performance. Circulation 63: 1975–1984
9. Maisch B, Kochsiek K (1983) Underestimation of stroke volume (SVI) and cardiac index (CI) by TM-echocardiography during ventricular pacing. In: Steinbach K, Glogar D, Laszkovics A, Scheibelhofer W, Weber H (eds) Cardiac Pacing. Proceedings of the VIIth World Symposium in Cardiac Pacing. Steinkopff Verlag, Darmstadt pp 193–197
10. Eilles C, Gerhards W, Reiners C, Börner W (1983) EKG-getriggerte Emissions-Computertomo-graphie der Herzbinnenräume. Methoden und klinische Ergebnisse. Nuklearmed 5: 275–283
11. Eilles C, Strauss P, Gerhards W, Reiners C, Börner W (1982) Klinische Wertigkeit der EKG-getriggerten Single-Photon-Emissionscomputertomographie (GASPECT) des Herzbinnenraums. In: Höfer R, Bergmann H (eds) Radioaktive Isotope in Klinik und Forschung. 15/2. Egermann Vienna, pp 675–683
12. Dicola VC, Stewart WJ, Harthorne JW, Weymann AE (1983) Doppler ultrasound measurement of cardiac output in patients with physiologic dual chamber pacemakers. In: Steinbach K, Glo-gar D, Laszkovics A, Scheibelhofer W, Weber H (eds) Cardiac Pacing. Steinkopff Verlag, Darmstadt, pp 231–239
13. Erbel R (1983) Funktionsanalyse des linken Ventrikels mittels zweidimensionaler Echokardio-graphie. Steinkopff Verlag, Darmstadt, 24–50
14. Curtis JJ, Walls JT, Boley TM, Madigan NP, Flaker GC, Reid JC (1983) Influence of atrio-ventricular contraction interval on hemodynamics In: Steinbach K, Glogar D, Laszkovics A, Scheibelhofer W, Weber H (eds) Cardiac Pacing. Steinkopff Verlag, Darmstadt, pp 175–179
15. Teichholz LE, Kreulen T, Hermann MV, Gorlin R (1976) Problems in echocardiographic vol-ume determination: Echocardiographic – angiographic correlation in the presence or absence of asynergy. Am J Cardiol 37: 7–11
16. Hirshleifer J, Crawford M, O'Rourke RA, Karliner JS (1975) Influence of acute alterations in heart rate and systematic arterial pressure on echocardiographic measures of left ventricular per-formance in normal human subjects. Circulation 52: 835–841
17. Thadani U, Lewis RJ, West RO, Chiong MA, Parker JO (1979) Clinical, hemodynamic and metabolic responses during pacing in the supine and sitting postures in patients with angina pectoris. Am J Cardiol 44: 249–256
18. McLaughlin PR, Kleimann JH, Martin RP, Doherty PW, Reitz B, Stinson EB, Daughters GT, Ingels NB, Alderman EL (1978) The effect of exercise and atrial pacing on left ventricular vol-ume and contractility in patients with innervated and denervated hearts. Circulation 58: 476–483
19. Erbel R, Schweizer P, Krebs W, Langen H-J, Meyer J, Effert S (1984) Effects of heart rate changes on left ventricular volume and ejection fraction: A 2-dimensional echocardiographic study. Am J Cardiol 53: 590–597
20. Ricci DR, Orlick AE, Alderman EL, Ingles NB, Daughters GT, Stinson EB (1979) Influence of heart rate in left ventricular ejection fraction in human beings. Am J Cardiol 44: 447–451
21. Hung J, Kelly DT, Hutton BF, Uther JB, Baird DK (1981) Influence of heart rate and atrial transport on left ventricular volume and function: relation to hemodynamic changes by su-praventricular arrhythmia. Am J Cardiol 48: 632–638
22. Karlöf I (1975) Haemodynamic effect of atrial triggered versus fixed rate pacing at rest and dur-ing exercise in complete heart block. Acta Med Scand 197: 195–206

23. Kappenberger L, Gloor HO, Babotai I, Steinbrunn W, Turina M (1982) Hemodynamic effects of atrial synchronization in acute and long-term ventricular pacing. PACE 5: 639–645
24. Kruse I, Arnman K, Conradson TB, Ryden L (1982) A comparison of the acute and long-term hemodynamic effects of ventricular inhibited and atrial synchronous ventricular inhibited pacing. Circulation 65: 846–855
25. Creplet J, Sarieaux A, Bohyn P, Achkar F, Sacre J, Adda JL, Azancot I, DeMey D (1983) Study of the left ventricular performance during sequential and ventricular pacing by quantitative two dimensional echocardiography. In: Steinbach K, Glogar D, Laszokovics A, Scheibelhöfer W, Weber H (eds) Cardiac Pacing. Steinkopff Verlag, Darmstadt, pp 199–204
26. Fananapazir L, Bennet DH, Monks P (1983) Atrial synchronized pacing: Contribution of the chronotropic response to improved exercise performance. PACE 6: 601–608
27. Pehrsson SK, Aström H (1983) Left ventricular pump function after long-term treatment with ventricular pacing compared to atrial synchronous pacing. In: Steinbach K, Glogar D, Laszkovics A, Scheibelhofer W, Weber H (eds) Cardiac Pacing. Steinkopff Verlag, Darmstadt, pp 187–192

Authors' address:
Professor Dr. Bernhard Maisch
Medizinische Universitätsklinik
Josef-Schneider-Straße 2
D-8700 Würzburg
West Germany

New Aspects on the Pathogenesis of Ischemia-Induced Ventricular Arrhythmias

Hj. Hirche and F. M. McDonald

Summary: The temporal distribution of ventricular arrhythmias occurring early in the course of myocardial ischaemia is briefly described, and some of the possible causal factors are discussed. These factors include the development of injury currents and ischaemia-induced transmembrane ion shifts, stretching of myocardial fibres, local and systemic catecholamine release, and the disturbances of fatty acid metabolism found in the ischaemic myocardium. The experimental evidence available to date suggests that no single factor alone is responsible for these arrhythmias, but rather that it is a multifactorial process depending on the interaction of several pathophysiologic changes.

With the exception of cardiogenic shock, severe ventricular arrhythmias are the most serious complication of disturbances of the coronary circulation. Following acute, complete occlusion of a coronary artery, ventricular arrhythmias usually occur within specific defined time intervals. More than 50% of patients dying from acute myocardial infarction develop severe ventricular arrhythmias, and in some cases ventricular fibrillation, within 30 to 60 min of the onset of symptoms.

Figure 1 shows the number of ventricular extrasystoles per minute following acute ligation of the left anterior descending coronary artery about one half to two thirds of the way from its origin in 49 anaesthetised pigs (1). Eight animals developed ventricular fibrillation during the 1a-phase of arrhythmias, i.e. in the first 10 min following coronary artery occlusion. Nine animals had very few arrhythmias in the 1a-phase, but developed ventricular fibrillation (VF) in the 1b-phase (15 to 25 min after the onset of ischaemia). In 21 pigs, a typical 1a and 1b-phase was observed, and these animals also fibrillated in the 1b-phase of arrhythmias. A further 11 animals showed ventricular arrhythmias in the 1a- and 1b-phases, which were in some cases delayed, but did not develop VF within the first 60 min of myocardial ischaemia. The top right-hand part of Fig. 1 shows the cumulative survival with respect to time following occlusion for these animals.

The causal mechanisms producing these early ischaemia-induced arrhythmias remain for the most part unclear. The electrical inhomogeneity which results from myocardial ischaemia may be most marked in the border zone, i.e. between ischaemic and normally-perfused myocardium, and there is considerable experimental evidence for the possible development of both re-entry circuits and focal automaticity. The conditions required for the development of a re-entry circuit are unidirectional block and a reduction in conduction velocity. As shown in Fig. 2, the normal impulse, which is blocked antegradely at C can, if conduction is sufficiently delayed, depolarise branch C retrogradely and thus initiate the re-entry circuit if B is no longer refractory. The induction of macro re-entry circuits, with diameters of several millimetres and more, and of micro re-entry circuits, with diameters of only a few millimetres or less, have been investigated in experimental studies using ECG-mapping techniques (2).

The induction of focal automaticity may be particularly dependent on the following factors:

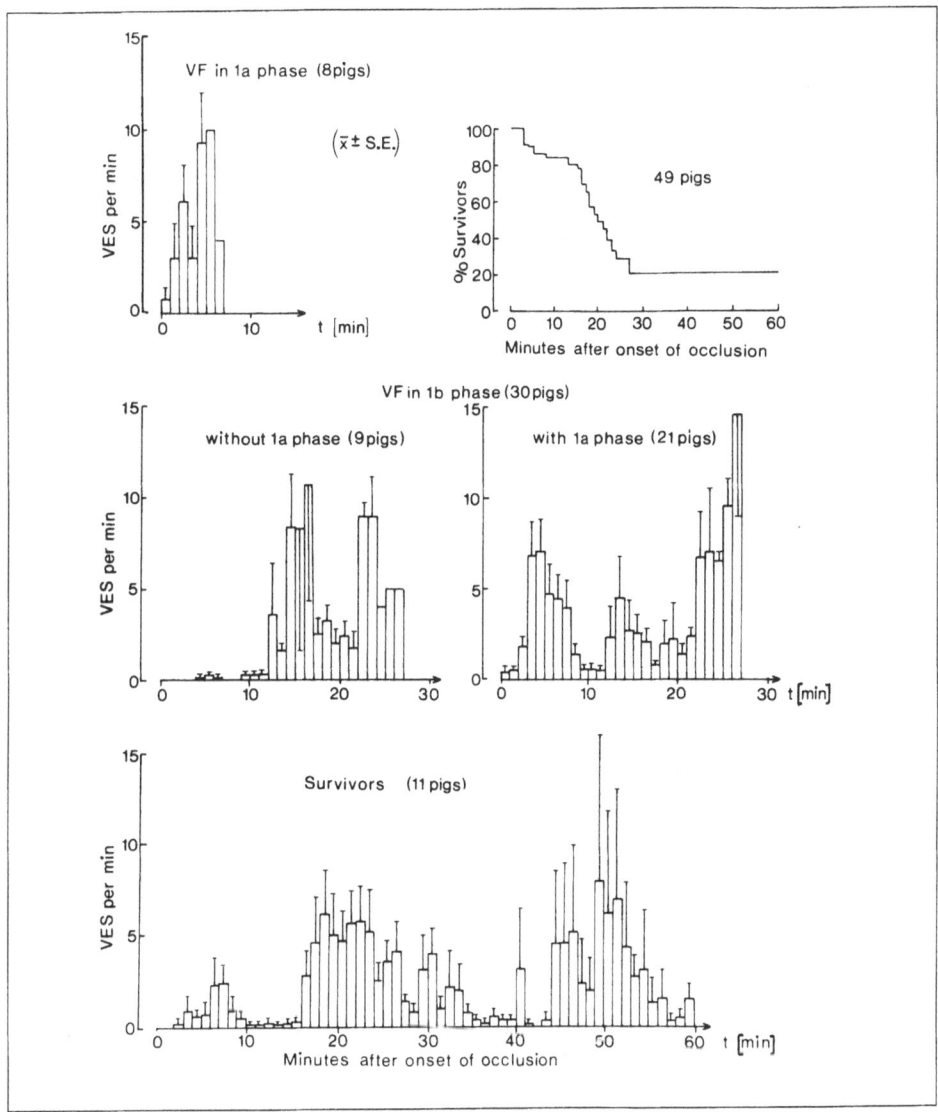

Fig. 1. Frequency of occurrence of ventricular extrasystoles (VES) and cumulative mortality curve due to ventricular fibrillation (VF) following coronary artery ligation in anaesthetised pigs.

1. the so-called injury currents between ischaemic and non-ischaemic myocardium (3);
2. the extreme stretching of myocardial fibres which have lost their tone as a result of the energy deficit in the ischaemic myocardium;
3. the local and systemic release of catecholamines resulting from myocardial ischaemia;
4. the changes in membrane function resulting from disturbances in fatty acid metabolism in the ischaemic myocardium.

There is at present experimental evidence supporting each of these causal factors.

Janse et al. (3) place particular emphasis on the importance of injury currents for ar-

Fig. 2. Diagrammatic representation of the development of reentry circuits. For further explanation see text (from (7)).

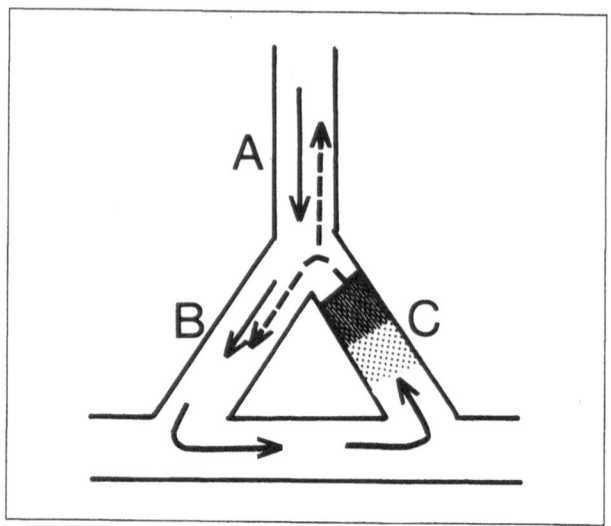

rhythmogenesis. The upper part of Fig. 3 shows an intracellularly recorded action potential from an isolated dog heart, and the lower part the DC-electrogram, both before and 5 min after LAD occlusion, with the normal and ischaemic recordings being projected on top of each other. As shown diagrammatically in the right-hand part of Fig. 3, ischaemia results in both intra- and extracellular potential differences, which form the basis of the currents of injury, and these potential differences vary during the heart cycle. At the point in time marked by the dotted line, for example, there will be flow of direct current intracellularly from the ischaemic area through the border zone into the non-ischaemic myocardium, which will depolarise the normal myocardial cells.

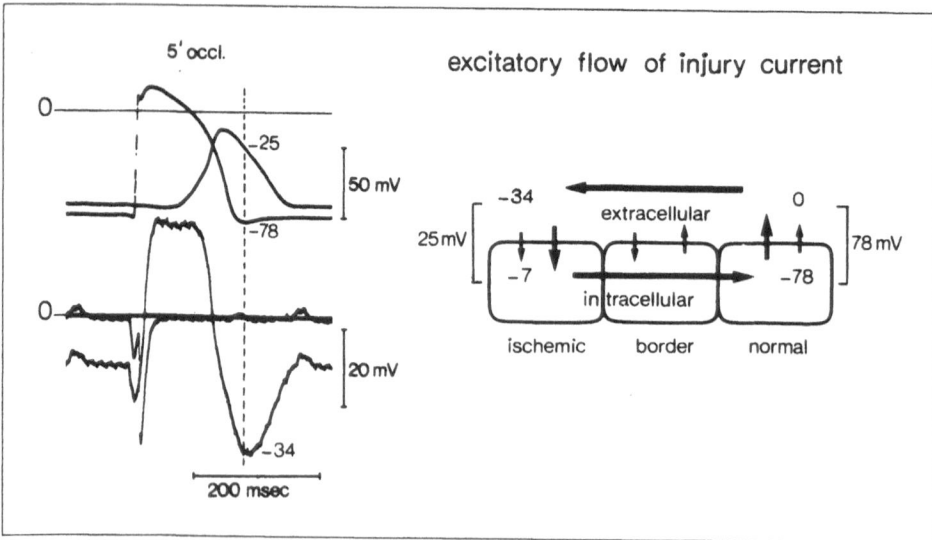

Fig. 3. Diagrammatic representation of the development of injury currents. For further explanation see text (from 3).

172

Winter et al. (4) attempted to imitate these injury currents by epicardial application of weak direct currents to pig hearts in situ. When the cathode and anode were placed only a few millimetres apart on the epicardial surface, direct current application produced similar electrocardiographic changes to myocardial ischaemia, including ventricular extrasystoles, tachycardia and fibrillation. The probability of inducing arrhythmias and ventricular late potentials in this model was not only dependent on the current strength but also on the position of the electrodes on the epicardium. Arrhythmias could be induced with the weakest currents when the electrodes were positioned in the paraseptal region. When the electrodes were positioned in the lateral or anterobasal regions, considerably higher current strengths were required for the induction of arrhythmias, but stimulation in these areas resulted more often in the recording of ventricular late potentials. It seems likely that Purkinje fibres play a considerable role in the development of these arrhythmias, as histological studies showed that the paraseptal region of the pig heart contains the most Purkinje fibres, whereas the lateral and anterobasal regions of the left ventricle contained very few Purkinje fibres. A similar role of Purkinje fibres in the induction of arrhythmias during acute myocardial ischaemia may also be present if injury currents are indeed the major causal factor.

The cause of ischaemia-induced myocardial electrical inhomogeneity is the transmembrane movement of ions which results in changes in the extra- to intracellular ion gradients (see Fig. 4). Na^+ and Ca^{2+} move into the cells, K^+ and H^+ move out into the extracellular space. As a result of the increase in intracellular osmotic pressure, there is also a movement of water into the cells (1, 5). this results in an intracellular oedema and shrinkage of the extracellular space, and this redistribution of water results in further changes of the transmembrane ion gradients. Experimental measurements using ion-selective electrodes have investigated the extent and time-course of the changes in ion activity in the extracellular space (1, 5, 6,). The most extensively investigated changes to date are those of the extracellular potassium concentration in the ischaemic myocardium (5, 6, 8–11).

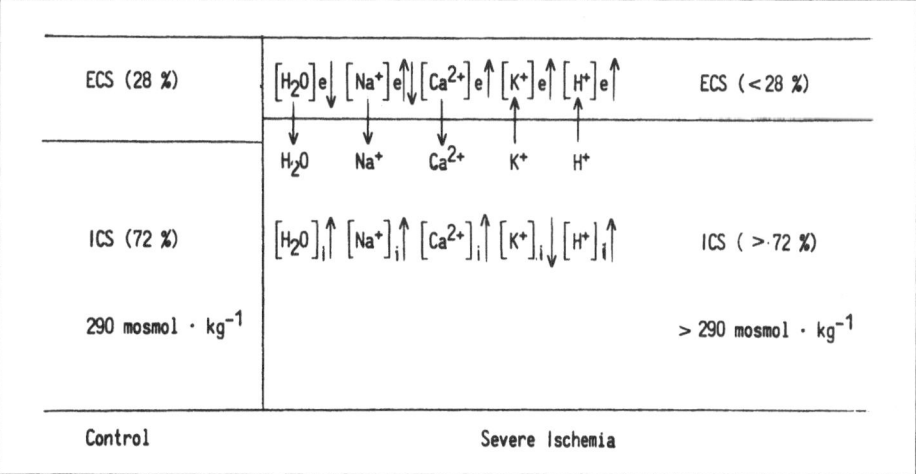

Fig. 4. Changes in the distribution of ions and water across the myocardial cell membrane during acute ischaemia (from (7)).

Following acute ligation of the LAD about half way from its origin, the epicardial extra-cellular potassium concentration ($[K^+]e$) begins to increase within 15 s of the onset of ischaemia. The maximum rate of rise of about 3 mmol/l/min is reached after 2 to 3 min (Fig. 5). After 4 to 5 min of ischaemia, the $[K^+]e$ in the centre of the ischaemic myocardium has reached values of about 14 mmol/l. This is followed by a transient reduction in $[K^+]e$ and a further, though slower, continuous rise beginning about 10 min after coro-

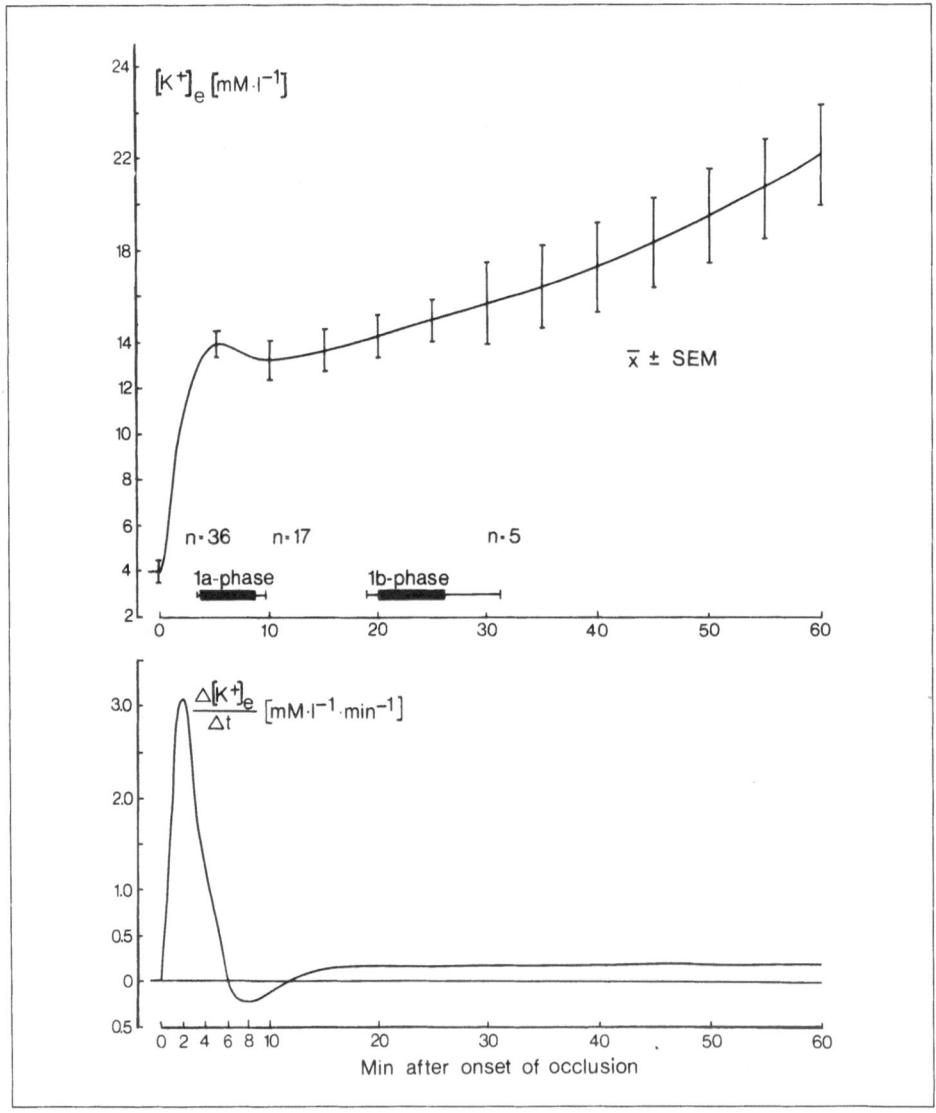

Fig. 5. Changes in epicardial extracellular potassium ion concentration and rate of change of potassium concentration measured in the centre of the ischaemic myocardium in anaesthetised pigs (from (7)).

nary artery occlusion. The causes of this triphasic change in [K$^+$]e remain unclear. The initial rate of rise of [K$^+$]e is probably influenced by heart rate, contractility and temperature (11). The plateau phase may result from an increased activity of the Na$^+$/K$^+$-pump, which is still active in the early phase of myocardial ischaemia. The third phase, showing a slow, continuous increase in [K$^+$]e, occurs within the phase during which ischaemia-induced myocardial injury becomes irreversible (12). Despite the fact that pig hearts, due to their virtual absence of coronary collateral circulation, develop severe transmural ischaemia following coronary artery ligation, considerable inhomogeneities in the increases in extracellular potassium during ischaemia have been observed, both on the epicardium and in deeper layers of the myocardium (1, 9). These workers have shown the the increases in [K$^+$]e are most marked in the centre of the ischaemic area and in deeper myocardial layers compared to the border and surface layers.

Changes in the potassium equilibrium potential can be estimated from the changes in extracellular potassium concentration. The results of such calculations show that within 5 min of the onset of myocardial ischaemia, the potassium equilibrium potential and therefore the resting membrane potential can reach values of less than –60 mV, i.e. the changes in the potassium equilibrium potential alone are sufficient to cause considerable electrical inhomogeneity between the ischaemic and non-ischaemic myocardium.

A further factor which could induce focal automaticity is the mechanical stretching of myocardial and Purkinje fibres. It is known that the diastolic tone is reduced within a few seconds of the onset of coronary artery occlusion, and that systolic contractile activity ceases after about 20 s. Studies in our own laboratory have shown that after about 60 s of severe ischaemia, the ventricular myocardium shows only passive stretching during systole. Such stretching in isolated preparations is known to result in oscillations of the membrane potential, which can have arrhythmogenic effects. We have also observed that in pig hearts subjected to 5 min of ischaemia followed by 60 min of reperfusion, recovery of diastolic tone and contractility in the previously ischaemic myocardium is often incomplete.

Ischaemia-induced local or systemic release of catecholamines may also play an important role in the genesis of arrhythmias following coronary artery occlusion. Measurements of intraneuronal catecholamine-induced fluorescence and catecholamine tissue concentrations in myocardial samples obtained during coronary artery occlusion have shown a reduction in catecholamine content of the ischaemic myocardium, assessed both as a reduction in the number of fluorescing fibres and a fall in noradrenaline concentration, within 5 to 15 min after the onset of severe myocardial ischaemia (13). This implies that catecholamines are released very early in the course of myocardial ischaemia and may exhibit their well-known arrhythmogenic effects (14). This local catecholamine release in the ischaemic myocardium may have a particularly marked arrhythmogenic effect due to the heterogeneity of the release; for example, it has been suggested that asymmetric stimulation of the sympathetic nervous system, e.g. by increased stimulation of the left stellate ganglion concomitant with decreased stimulation of the right stellate ganglion, can induce cardiac arrhythmias (14).

The probable importance of catecholamine release for the development of ischaemia-induced arrhythmias in the clinical situation can be deduced from the therapeutic effectiveness of β-blocking drugs in this situation. Experimental studies have shown that blockade of both β and α_1-receptors is effective in reducing the number of arrhythmias occurring after coronary artery occlusion. Clinical studies have also shown the effectiveness of anti-adrenergic therapy in the secondary prevention of sudden cardiac death (see 14).

Disturbances of fatty acid metabolism in the ischaemic myocardium may also play a role in the development of ischaemia-induced arrhythmias, as fatty acid esters and phospholipids showing hydrophobic and hydrophilic behaviour, which are found in increased concentrations in the ischaemic myocardium, may have arrhythmogenic activity. There is experimental evidence that relatively small increases in the concentration of these substances, and in particular the lysophospholipids, can result in membrane surface dysfunction and consequent electrophysiological disturbances (15).

In conclusion, a considerable number of factors may be involved in the genesis of ventricular arrhythmias early in the course of myocardial ischaemia, and it seems most likely that the development of these arrhythmias is dependent on a combination of these changes rather than on any one factor acting alone.

References

1. Hirche Hj, Kebbel U, McDonald FM, Knopf H, Bischoff A, Barth A (1985) Measurement of non-homogeneous changes of extracellular K$^+$ concentration within the ischaemic myocardium. In: Kessler M, Simon W (eds) International Symposium on the Theory and Application of Ion-selective Electrodes in Physiology and Medicine. Springer-Verlag, Berlin Heidelberg New York, in press
2. van Capelle FJL, Janse MJ (1983) A computer model for evaluation of mechanisms of cardiac arrhythmias. In: Breithardt G, Loogen F (eds) New aspect in the medical treatment of tachyarrhythmias. Role of Amiodarone. Urban und Schwarzenberg, München Wien Baltimore
3. Janse MJ, Moréna H, Cinca J, Klèber AG, Downar E, van Capelle FJL, Durrer D (1978) Role of re-entry and currents of injury in early ischemic ventricular tachyarrhythmias: which properties should theoretically make a drug effective in the management of these arrhythmias? In: Sandoe E, Julian DG, Bell JW (eds) Management of ventricular tachycardia – role of mexiletine. Excerpta Medica, Amsterdam, Oxford pp 183–195
4. Winter UJ, Ebeling H, Kebbel U, Arnold G, Schmahl M, Hirche Hj (1983) Induction of ventricular arrhythmias and ventricular late potentials by epicardial direct current (DC) application in pig heart in situ: Importance of the stimulation position. Circulation 68 (Suppl III): 288
5. Hirche Hj, Friedrich R, Kebbel U, McDonald FM, Zylka V (1982) Early arrhythmias, myocardial extracellular potassium and pH. In: Parratt JR (ed) Early arrhythmias resulting from myocardial ischaemia, mechanisms and prevention by drugs. MacMillan Press, London, pp 113–124
6. Hirche Hj, Franz C, Bös L, Bissig R, Lang R, Schramm M (1980) Myocardial extracellular K$^+$ and H$^+$ increase and noradrenaline release as possible cause of early arrhythmias following acute coronary artery occlusion in pigs. J Mol Cell Cardiol 12: 579–593
7. Hirche Hj (1984) Physiologie und Pathophysiologie des Koronarkreislaufs. In: Hombach V (ed) Kardiologie, Grundlagen – Fortschritte – Klinische Erfahrungen, Bd 1, Die koronare Herzkrankheit. FK Schattauer Verlag, Stuttgart–New York pp 1–18
8. Friedrich R, Hirche Hj, Kebbel U, Zylka V, McDonald FM (1982) Changes of extracellular electrolytes during myocardial ischemia. In: Grote J, Witzleb E (eds) Durchblutungsregulation und Organstoffwechsel. F Steiner-Verlag, Wiesbaden p 8
9. Hill JL, Gettes LS (1980) Effect of acute coronary artery occlusion on local myocardial extracellular K$^+$ activity in swine. Circulation 61: 768–778
10. Wiegand V, Güggi M, Meesmann W, Kessler M, Greitschus F (1979) Extracellular potassium activity changes in the canine myocardium after acute coronary occlusion and the influence of β-blockade. Cardiovasc Res 13: 297–302
11. Weiss J, Shine KJ (1982) Extracellular K$^+$ accumulation during myocardial ischemia in isolated rabbit heart. Am J Physiol 242 (Heart Circ Physiol): H 619–H 628
12. Jennings RB, Ganote ChE, Reimer KA (1975) Ischemic tissue injury. Am J Pathol 81: 179–198

13. McDonald FM, Addicks K, Bischoff A, Hartono S, Hirche Hj, Knopf H, Myocardial catecholamine release following acute coronary artery occlusion in anaesthetised pigs. In: Abstracts of
the 5th CA Symposium, Göteborg, 1983; Supplement to Progress in Neuropsychopharmacology
and Biological Psychiatry, p 327.
14. Sharma AD, Corr PB (1983) Adrenergic factors in arrhythmogenesis in the ischemic and reper-
fused myocardium. Eur Heart J 4 (Suppl D): 79–90
15. Corr PB, Gross RW, Sobel BE (1984) Amphipathic metabolites and membrane dysfunction in
ischemic myocardium. Circ Res 55: 135–154

Authors' address:
Professor Hj. Hirche
Lehrstuhl für Angewandte Physiologie der
Universität zu Köln
Robert-Koch-Straße 39
5000 Köln 41
West Germany

Pre-Implantation Evaluation of Candidates for an Antitachycardia Pacemaker

V. Hombach, H.-W. Höpp, D. W. Behrenbeck, A. Osterspey, T. Eggeling, U. J. Winter, and H. H. Hilger

Summary: In patients with chronic recurrent attacks of supraventricular, and in rare cases of ventricular tachycardia, chronic antitachycardia pacing using implantable pacemakers with different termination modes may be an attractive alternative to chronic drug therapy, particularly in patients with drug refractoriness or serious side effects. Before implantation of an antitachycardia pacemaker various clinical and technical conditions have to be considered and tested, such as reproducibility of tachycardia termination, effective and safe termination mode, optimal lead position, conditioning of the tachycardia by antiarrhythmic drugs for safe electrical termination, and the possible deterioration of the tachycardia by the antitachycardia pacing mode itself.

Chronic antiarrhythmia pacing seems to be relatively safe at the atrial level in the case of regular supraventricular tachycardias, even with the most potentially dangerous mode of burst pacing. However, one should be very restrictive with the implantation of a burst or multiple extrastimulus delivering antitachycardia pacemaker at the ventricular level, because of the potential danger of inducing ventricular flutter or fibrillation, at least with pacing devices without the safety of back-up cardioversion or defibrillation.

Introduction

Regular sustained supraventricular and ventricular tachycardias are mainly encountered in patients with underlying heart disease, such as coronary heart disease, cardiomyopathy, and aortic valve disease, but may also be found in 3–5% of individuals without cardiac disease (1). In more than 80% of patients with symptomatic tachycardias medical management seems to be the therapy of choice. However, antiarrhythmic drugs may exert serious side effects like hypotension, negative inotropy, bradycardia, affections of lung or liver or the central nervous system with or without patient intolerance to the drug, or the patients may be non-compliant to drug therapy and thus, long-term drug management of tachycardias, either prophylactically or therapeutically, may be a great problem. Therefore in recent years alternative electrical or surgical methods for control of tachycardias have been developed (3–6). In supraventricular tachycardias (SVT) or tachyarrhythmias with increased ventricular rates non-surgical catheter ablation of the bundle of His may be appropriate (5), or regular sustained forms of SVT in the WPW syndrome may be abolished by electrical (catheter ablation) or surgical interruption of the accessory pathway (6). Ventricular tachycardias (VT) may be abolished surgically by endocardectomy or circumcision of the area of the focus (2, 3), or even by endocardial catheter ablation. However, in certain cases surgery may be inappropriate, unsafe or even ineffective, and long-term drug therapy may be ineffective, and termination of tachycardias by implanted antitachycardia pacemakers may then be be considered as a reasonable alternative therapeutic measure.

General considerations

In patients with suspected or documented SVT or VT different therapeutic strategies may be adopted (4): prevention of tachycardia, reduction of ventricular rate during continued tachycardia, maintenance of tachycardia when changes to normal rhythm are badly tolerated, termination of tachycardia, and permanent abolition of tachycardia. Only in rare cases can an antitachycardia pacemaker be used for prevention of tachycardia, e.g. dynamic overdrive pacing at the atrial or ventricular level; in the vast majority of patients with sustained SVT or VT these devices are used for termination of an already running tachycardia. Although in animal experiments at least 3 different pathophysiological mechanisms of tachycardia initiation have been described (abnormal impulse formation with either focal or triggered activity and abnormal impulse conduction within a re-entrant circuit), in man most short and long-term sustained tachycardias may be based on a re-entrant mechanism (Table 1), as applies for AV-nodal tachycardias, WPW tachycardias, and about 1/3 of cases with VT (another 1/3 of VT may be focal in origin, and in the remaining cases VT mechanism may be uncertain, 12). This assumption may be confirmed by the fact that these tachycardias can be started by critically coupled single or double extrastimuli and may also be terminated by the same extrastimulus technique or by burst pacing, though experimentally triggered activity-related tachycardias could also be terminated by the extrastimulus or burst technique (4, 7).

A re-entrant circuit of tachycardia implies the presence of a continuously circulating electrical activity along a certain anatomical pathway with a partially or fully excitable period that circulates ahead of the advancing wave front (4, 7, 8, 9). Depending on the

Table 1. Survey on the suggested or confirmed pathophysiological mechanisms of the initiation of various types of supraventricular and ventricular tachycardias. (Gadsby et al. 1980, Allessie et al. 1980, Scherlag et al. 1983, El-Sherif et al. 1977, Josephson et al. 1978.)

Type of tachycardia	Abnormal impulse formation				Abnormal impulse conduction	
	Focal activity		Triggered activity		Circus movement (re-entry)	
	Animal	Man	Animal	Man	Animal	Man
Atrial tachycardia	+	(+)	+	(+)	+	+
A-V nodal tachycardia	–	–	–	–	+	+
WPA-supraventricular tachycardia	–	–	–	–	+	+
Atrial flutter	–	–	–	–	+	+
Atrial fibrillation	?	–	?	–	+	+ (multiple wavelets)
Non-paroxysmal junctional tachycardia	+	+	–	–	–	–
Multifocal atrial tachycardia	+	+	?	?	–	–
Ventricular tachycardia	(+)	(+)	?	?	+	+

speed of the circulating wavefront and the distance of the stimulation site from the site of the re-entrant pathway, an extrastimulus has to be delivered at a critical time interval to reach the re-entrant pathway at its excitable period ahead of the wavefront and to depolarize that part of the re-entry circuit (termination zone). If the extrastimulus is delivered slightly earlier, it will invade the excitable tissue in the tachycardia circuit ahead of the circulating impulse, and may itself continue to circulate within the pathway or advance the tachycardia (reset zone). If the extrastimulus is delivered too late the stimulated wavefront will collide with the impulse emanating from the tachycardia circuit (collision zone), and the tachycardia remains unaffected. If the extrastimulus interval is further delayed it may fail to evoke a response within the tachycardia circuit due to tissue refractoriness resulting from re-entrant depolarisation (refractory zone). Since the tissue between the stimulation site and the tachycardia circuit must also be invaded by the extrastimulus

Table 2. Clinical assessment of patients considered for the implantation of an automatic antitachycardia pacemaker.

Clinical history	Tachycardia episodes
	Syncopes
	Resuscitations
Clinical examination	Signs of heart failure
	Signs of valve disease
	Mitral valve prolapse
Conventional 12 lead electrocardiogram	Ischemic ST segment changes
	Pathological Q waves
	LV aneurysm
	LV hypertrophy
	Ventricular pre-excitation
	Bundle branch block
Chest X-ray	Heart size
	Left heart failure
Echocardiogram	LV performance
	Valve function
	LV hypertrophy
	Mitral valve prolapse
Exercise test	Blood pressure response
	Heart rate response
	Ischemic ST-segment changes
	Induction of arrhythmias
Holter electrocardiogram	Heart rate level
	Attacks of tachycardias
	Atrial fibrillation in WPW syndrome
	Arrhythmia profile
	Ischemic ST-segment changes
Left ventricular and coronary angiography	LV global and regional function
	LV aneurysm
	Number and size of coronary artery stenoses
Electrophysiological study	Determination of type of tachycardia
	Optimal stimulation site for termination
	Optimal termination mode
	Deterioration of tachycardia on antitachycardia stimulation
	Reproducibility of tachycardia termination

to reach the excitable gap of the tachycardia, different types of single or double extrastimuli or more, or burst pacing techniques have been proposed for effective termination of
a tachycardia. In principle, three different modes of antitachycardia pacing have been
developed for termination of tachycardias: underdrive pacing, overdrive or burst pacing,
and extrastimulus pacing (4), and SVT and VT have been found to respond differently to
these pacing techniques in man (Table 2). In general, the overall success rate of antitachycardia pacing depends on the following criteria: size and location of the re-entry circuit,
distance from the pacing site to the site of tachycardia circuit, rate of the tachycardia,
time interval of the extrastimulus or extrastimuli relative to the tachycardia wave front,
and the number and energy of the stimuli delivered (4, 11, 12).

Each patient considered for an antitachycardia pacemaker therapy should initially be
investigated by clinical methods (Table 3), e.g. taking history, physical examination,
chest X-ray, 12-lead ECG, exercise ECG, Holter ECG, echocardiogram and sometimes
left ventricular and coronary angiography. By this means the relevance of underlying

Table 3. Response of various types of supraventricular and ventricular tachycardias to the termination by different antitachycardia pacing modes.

Type of tachycardia	Underdrive	Dual site sequential	Overdrive (burst)	Extrastimulus
Atrial fibrillation	–	–	(+)	–
Atrial flutter	–	–	+	–
Atrial tachycardia	(+)	–	+	–
AV-nodal tachycardia	(+)	+	+	+
WPW tachycardia	(+)	+	+	+
Ventricular tachycardia	(+)	–	+	(+)

Table 4. Pre-conditions for the implantation of an antitachycardia pacemaker.

1. Patient site:
   a. Recurrent paroxysmal tachycardia (not repetitive or incessant)
   b. Severe tachycardia-induced symptoms and signs (including those of heart failure)
   c. Failure of antiarrhythmic drug therapy (drugs ineffective, patient non-compliant,
      patient intolerance to drugs, serious side effects of antiarrhythmic drugs)
   d. Patient's ability to cooperate with pacemaker implantation

2. Tachycardia site:
   a. Reproducibility of tachycardia termination
   b. Safe and repeatable termination mode without deterioration of the tachycardia
   c. Optimal endocardial pacing site for chronic antitachycardia pacing

3. Pacemaker site:
   a. Stable fixation of the endocardial pacing electrode(s)
   b. Facility of reprogramming the pacemaker
   c. Facility of switching off the pacemaker in case of inappropriate function
   d. Facility of additional demand pacing for control of basic heart rate
   e. Convenient size of the pacemaker

heart disease, the exclusion of valvular heart disease, and the symptomatology and response of the circulatory system to the tachycardia can be assessed as well as concomitant supraventricular or ventricular arrhythmias, that may accompany tachycardias, e.g. short runs or bursts of supraventricular or ventricular premature beats. In addition, before the implantation of an antitachycardia pacemaker some prerequesites should be met, as outlined in Table 4. From the patients's site: the occurrence of drug refractory tachycardias (failure of therapy, patient non-compliance, serious side effects of antiarrhythmic drugs), cardiac failure induced by the tachycardia, surgically noncorrectable type of tachycardia, and cooperation of the patient to pacemaker implantation and follow-up. From the tachycardia site: reproducibility of tachycardia termination, no degeneration of the tachycardia, particularly with ventricular tachycardias (acceleration, ventricular flutter or fibrillation) on the antitachycardia pacing episode. From the pacemaker site: the ability of stable fixation of the pacing electrodes at endocardial sites with optimal termination of

Table 5. Modifying factors of tachycardia termination.

1. Reproducibility of tachycardia termination
    a. Diurnal variations (sympathetic tone)
    b. Day-to-day variations (sympathetic tone)
    c. Postural changes (sympathetic tone)
    d. Physical activity (sympathetic tone)
    e. Change of termination rate by cardioactive drugs

2. Optimum site of stimulation (definitive fixation of intracardiac electrode(s)
    a. Right atrium (appendage, lateral part)
    b. Right ventricle (apex, outflow tract)
    c. Coronary sinus (suboptimal for chronic electrode location)

3. Optimum and safe termination mode
    a. Underdrive mode
    b. Overdrive mode
    c. Extrastimuls mode

4. Deterioration of tachycardia by antitachycardia pacing
    a. Atrial fibrillation in patients with the WPW syndrome
    b. Acceleration of the tachycardia
    c. Induction of ventricular flutter or fibrillation

5. Deterioration of hemodynamics
    a. Response of LV performance and blood pressure to the tachycardia itself
    b. Additional fall in blood pressure by the antitachycardia pacing (particularly with ventricular burst pacing)

6. Conditioning of tachycardias to successful termination by antiarrhythmic drugs
    a. A-V conduction delay in supraventricular tachycardias incorporating the A-V node as part of the re-entry circuit (digitalis, beta-blockers, calcium channel blockers) or conduction delay within the accessory pathway (certain class I antiarrhythmics)
    b. Slowing down the rate of ventricular tachycardias (certain class I and class III antiarrhythmic drugs)

the tachycardia, facility of re-programming the antitachycardia pacemaker and switch-off of the antitachycardia pacing mode, demand or back-up pacing, and finally an acceptable size of the pulse generator.

Special considerations

Prior to the implantation of an antitachycardia pacemaker an extensive electrophysiological evaluation of the patient has to be performed to obtain sufficient information on the reproducibility of tachycardia termination, the optimal site of stimulation, the optimal termination mode, the facultative deterioration of the tachycardia on pacing or deterioration of hemodynamics during antitachycardia pacing, and lastly the facility of conditioning the tachycardia to antitachycardia pacing by administration of antiarrhythmic drugs (Table 5). For EPS multiple intracardiac electrodes have to be placed at special areas within the heart, e.g. within the right atrial appendage, the His bundle area, the right ventricular apex and/or right ventricular outflow tract (septum), and the coronary sinus (Figure 1). Reproducibility has to be tested during pacing with one of the different antitachycardia pacing modes (Table 6). It is a common clinical experience that the rate of the tachycardia as well as the initiation and termination zone of the tachycardia can be considerably altered by an elevated sympathetic or parasympathetic tone. Simple standing or physical activity may increase the tachycardia rate and shorten the termination zone, at least in SVT involving the AV-node as part of the re-entrant circuit, whereas antiarrhythmic drugs may slow down the tachycardia rate and prolong the termination zone (Figure 2). In a previous study we have found that ergometric exercise considerably changed the tachycardia or echo zones of SVT as compared to the conditions at rest, and the antiarrhythmic effect of beta-blockade on the initiation of SVT was partially antagonized

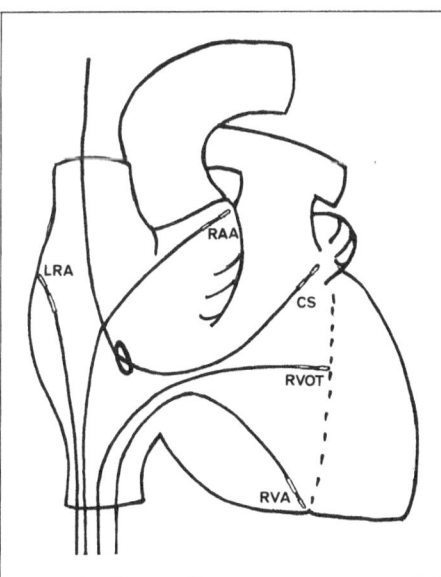

Fig. 1: Schematic representation of the stimulation sites commonly used for testing site and optimal termination mode in supraventricular or ventricular tachycardias. LRA: lateral right atrium, RAA: right atrial appendage, CS: coronary sinus, RVOT: right ventricular outflow tract, RVA: right ventricular apex.

Table 6. Modes for termination of supraventricular or ventricular tachycardias.

1. Underdrive mode:
   a. Simple fixed rate pacing
   b. Dual-demand pacing
   c. Marginal underdrive pacing

2. Overdrive mode:
   a. Single site pacing
   b. Dual site stimulation
   c. Continuous high rate pacing
   d. Paired stimulation
   e. Coupled stimulation
   f. Burst pacing
      1. fixed rate
      2. orthorhythmic
      3. Concertina
      4. autodecremental
   g. Entrainment with premature stimulation

3. Extrastimulus mode:
   a. Static adjustable coupling interval
   b. Short high frequency burst
   c. Scanning extrastimuli
      1. sequential scanning
      2. self-search stimulation
      3. centrifugal geometric scanning
      4. high pulse energy scanning

Fig. 2: Effect of postural changes and antiarrhythmic drugs on tachycardia cycle length and termination zone in supraventricular tachycardia (adapted from Camm and Ward (4)). CS_p: proximal coronary sinus, RVA: right ventricular apex, I: Einthoven lead I, PR: propranolol, FL: flecainide. Note that with increasing sympathetic tone tachycardia rates increase and the termination zone is shortened, whereas antiarrhythmic drugs like propranolol or flecainide slow down tachycardia rates and prolong the termination zone.

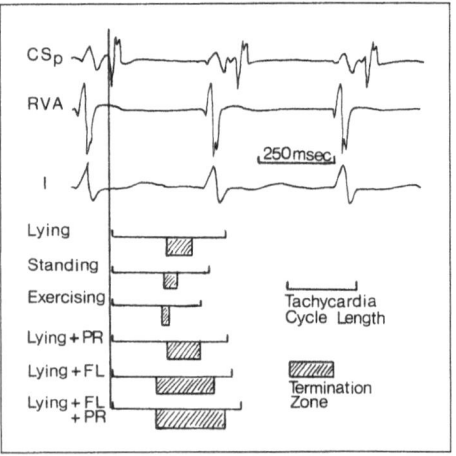

by submaximal ergometric exercise (13). Therefore it is essential to evaluate the influence of diurnal variations, of day to day variations, of positional changes, and of antiarrhythmic drugs on the termination characteristics of tachycardias, before considering a patient for implantation of an antitachycardia pacemaker.

184

A second important practical item to clarify is the search for an optimal electrode position for antitachycardia pacing. Several strategically favoured intracardiac areas have been proposed and regularly used for electrode placings, the right atrial appendage, sometimes the low lateral right atrium, the right ventricular apex, and the right ventricular outflow tract. For termination of SVT the right auricular location is the most convenient place for long-term electrode positioning, as is the right ventricular apex or sometimes the right ventricular outflow-tract for long-term antitachycardia pacing of VT. Because of a relatively high complication rate, placement of electrodes within the coronary sinus for long-term pacing cannot be recommended any longer (14, 15). Therefore, in clinical practice right auricular and right ventricular apical or outflow tract locations should be preferred for primary testing of any antiarrhythmic pacing mode, and only in the case of failure of antitachycardia pacing should other electrode locations be evaluated for chronic antitachycardia pacing. In addition, only one or two pacing modes should be tested for their efficacy in terminating the tachycardia, and this testing should be performed at a different time of day and different positional states (supine, upright, exercise). One should bear in mind that the three antitachycardia pacing modes of underdrive pacing, overdrive pacing and extrastimulus pacing may be differently efficacious in the various forms of SVT or VT. Thus, it has been reported that the success rates of underdrive and/or single extrastimulus pacing in SVT were significantly lower than the success rates of overdrive and/or double or triple extrastimulus antitachycardia pacing. Moreover, increasing the sympathetic tone decreased the chance of terminating SVT, and A-V nodal tachycardia with rates of more than 160 bpm almost invariably required at least double extrastimulus pacing for successful termination (18). In VT termination rates were also dependent on the mode of antitachycardia pacing (19). In general, overdrive pacing with rates of 40 stimuli/min faster than the the spontaneous VT rate revealed success rates of around 80% of VT episodes, whereas termination rates with single to triple extrastimuli were around 50% of VT episodes. In only 4% did ventricular overdrive pacing establish the VT rate – a rather low incidence of VT acceleration –, and external DC-cardioversion was required in 12 individuals in this study (19).

Atrial flutter may be reverted to sinus rhythm in about 45% of cases by atrial high rate overdrive pacing (4), and the reversion rates for atrial tachycardias may be in a similar range (Fig. 3). However, in a certain percentage of patients atrial overdrive pacing may induce atrial fibrillation with a reduction of ventricular rates. In our own studies we found relatively high conversion rates to sinus rhythm in various types of SVT (atrial tachycardia: 4/4 episodes, atrial flutter: 3/6 episodes, A-V nodal tachycardia: 2/2 episodes, WPW-SVT: 5/7 episodes), whereas in atrial fibrillation the conversion rates to sinus

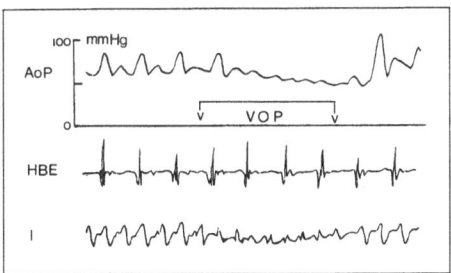

Fig. 3: Effect of ventricular tachycardia itself (left panel) and additional ventricular overdrive pacing (center) on arterial blood pressure (AoP). HBE: His bundle electrogram, I: Einthoven lead I, VOP: ventricular overdrive pacing (adapted from Camm and Ward (4)).

rhythm were significantly lower (3/16 episodes, 27). In A-V nodal tachycardias as well as in WPW-SVT relatively high termination rates have been reported with the extrastimulus technique, be it the self searching extrastimulus mode, the geometrical scanning or the sequential scanning mode (4, 23, 24, 25). In clinical practive one should test the overdrive mode and one or two of the extrastimulus modes for termination of the tachycardia, and then choose the implantable automatic antitachycardia pacemaker for definite implantation.

When testing the optimal termination mode one has to find out whether antitachycardia stimulation will deteriorate the tachycardia (acceleration of the tachycardia) or will induce new types of arrhythmias. It has been observed that atrial overdrive pacing for termination of WPW-SVT may precipitate atrial fibrillation, that will sometimes become precarious for the patients because of unusually high ventricular rates due to predominant A-V conduction via the accessory pathway. In patients with VT an acceleration of the tachycardia may be induced by both single or double extrastimulus and by overdrive pacing (4, 17). In addition, one has to test whether the stimulation protocol applied during the run of the tachycardia will further deteriorate the hemodynamic situation of the patient, e.g. systolic blood pressure during VT may fall to systolic values of 70–80 mm Hg, and overdrive pacing during the VT attack may further decrease systolic blood pressures to 50–60 mm Hg (4, see Figure 4).

If the reproducibility of tachycardia termination is poor in patients with SVT or VT with either method of antitachycardia pacing, one should evaluate the effect of antiarrhythmic

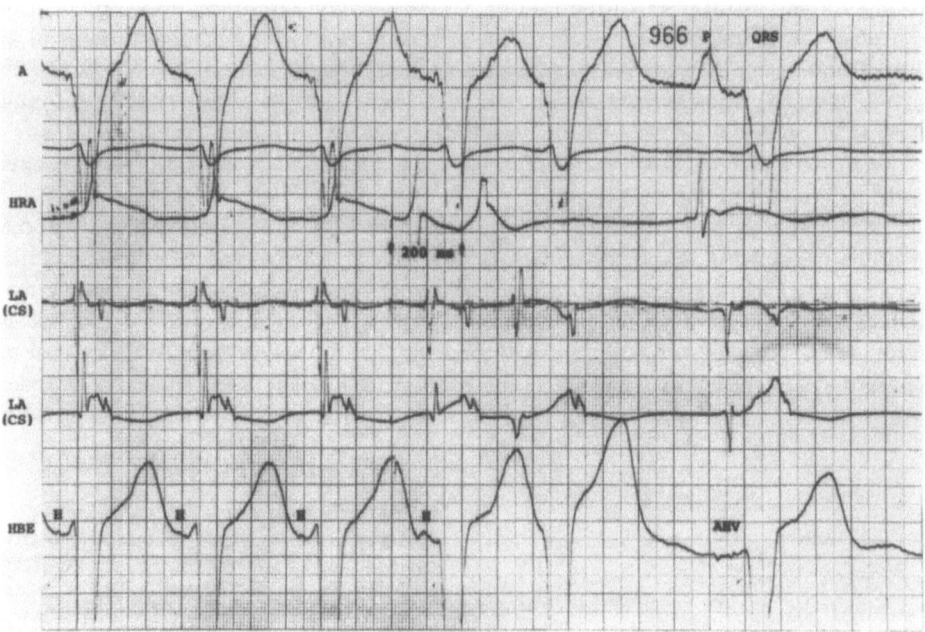

Fig. 4: Effective termination of a run of A-V nodal tachycardia in a 66 year old female by two critically coupled atrial extrastimuli. A: Lead A according to Trethewie (bipolar lead from manubrium to processus xiphoideus sterni), HRA: high right atrial ECG, LA(CS): left atrial ECG (from coronary sinus), HBE: His bundle ECG, A: low medial right atrial ECG, H: His bundle spike, V: ventricular depolarisation.

186

drugs for conditioning the tachycardia to the special pacing termination mode. SVT may be conditioned for chronic automatic pacing by digitalis, beta-blocking drugs or by some calcium-antagonistic substances (verapamil, gallopamil, diltiazem). In patients with VT antiarrhythmic drugs of classes I or III may be very effective in conditioning the tachycardia for most types of antitachycardia pacing. But again, the long-term efficacy of combined therapy (antiarrhythmic drugs plus antitachycardia pacing) has to be tested at different times and in different postural situations, in order to achieve a reproducible and safe long-term therapy regimen in these patients.

To give an idea of the percentage of patients who might be considered for the implantation of an antitachycardia pacemaker for VT termination, the results of our own study will be discussed briefly (Table 7). 154 patients with complex ventricular arrhythmias without or with syncopes were examined for ventricular vulnerability by programmed right ventricular stimulation (single or double extrastimuli at basic pacing rates of 100, 120, 140, 160 stimuli/min). In 111 of 154 patients a repetitive ventricular response equal or more than 3 consecutive ventricular echo beats could be elicited. Ventricular fibrillation was induced in 11/154 patients, and a sustained VT was observed in 13/154 patients following the diagnostic pacing protocol. Termination of sustained VT with a single or double extrastimulus was possible in only 1/13 cases, whereas ventricular overdrive pacing terminated the tachycardia in 9/13 cases. After stabilization by antiarrhythmic drugs (Table 8) only 3/13 patients with formerly inducible sustained VTs remained suitable for

Table 7. Termination of sustained ventricular tachycardias in 154 patients with CHD and complex VBPs.

	Number of patients	Percent
Diagnostic PVS	154	100%
RVR (more than 3 VEB)	111/154	72%
VF_{ib} induced	11/154	7%
VT_{sust} (more than 15 beats)	13/154	8%
$VT_{non\text{-}sust}$ induced	8/154	5%
Termination of VT_{sust} (single or double extrastimuli)	1/13	8%
Termination of VT_{sust} (burst stimulation)	9/13	69%

Table 8. Termination of sustained ventricular tachycardias: stabilization on antiarrhythmic drugs (AAD).

	Number of patients	Percent
Ventricular fibrillation	11/11	100%
Sustained VTs	10/13	77%
Non-sustained VTs	8/ 8	100%
Candidates for AT-PM (Cyber-Tach 60)	3/13	23%

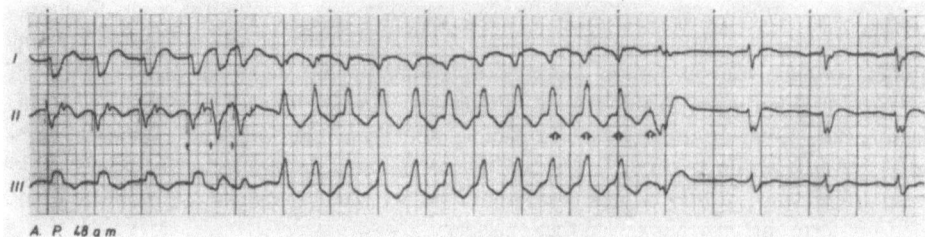

Fig. 5: Termination of an episode of ventricular tachycardia by a short burst of four ventricular stimuli (open arrows, right center). Small arrows (left panel): induction of the tachycardia by two ventricular extrastimuli.

chronic antitachycardia pacing, and in these patients an automatic antitachycardia burst pacemaker (Cyber-Tach 60) has been implanted (Fig. 5), the follow-up data of which have been reported elsewhere (30).

In conclusion, in patients with recurrent attacks of SVT or VT, chronic automatic antitachycardia pacing by an implantable pacemaker may be an attractive alternative to conventional therapy, particularly in patients who do not sufficiently respond to chronic oral antiarrhythmic therapy or who complain of side effects of these drugs and who are not candidates for antiarrhythmic surgery. Before implantation of such an antiarrhythmic pacing device various practical conditions and criteria have to evaluated, such as reproducibility of tachycardia termination, effective and safe termination mode, optimal lead position, conditioning of tachycardia termination by antiarrhythmic drugs, and possible deterioration of the tachycardia by the pacing procedure. Chronic antiarrhythmic pacing seems to be relatively safe at the atrial level in cases with SVT, even with the most dangerous form of overdrive burst pacing. However, one should be very restrictive in the application of burst or multiple extrastimulus pacing at the ventricular level in patients with sustained VT, because of the potential danger of inducing ventricular flutter or fibrillation, at least with pacemakers which do not provide the facilities of back-up endo-epicardial cardioversion-defibrillation (26, 27, 28) in case of degeneration of the ventricular tachycardia.

References

1. Bjerregard P. Prevalence and variability of cardiac arrhythmias in healthy subjects. In: Chamberlain DA, Kulbertus H, Mogensen L, Schlepper M (eds) Cardiac arrhythmias in the active population. Lindgren & Söner, Mölndal, pp 24–32
2. Fontaine G, Guiraudon G, Frank R, Cabrol C, Grosgogeat Y (1979) The surgical management of ventricular tachycardia. Herz 4: 276
3. Josephson ME, Harken AH (1983) Surgical therapy of arrhythmias. In: Rosen MR, Hoffman BF (eds) Cardiac Therapy. Martinus Nijhoff Publishers, Boston, The Hague, Dordrecht, Lancaster p 337
4. Camm J, Ward D (1983) Pacing for tachycardia control. Telectronics, Australia
5. Scheinman MM, Morady F, Hess DS, Gonzalez R (1982) Catheter-induced ablation of the atrioventricular junction to control refractory supraventricular arrhythmias. J Am Med Ass 248: 851
6. Gallagher JJ (1978) Surgical treatment for arrhythmias, current status und future directions. Am J Cardiol 41: 1035

7. Allessie MA, Bonke FIM (1980) Atrial arrhythmias: Basic concepts. In: Mandel WJ (ed) Cardiac Arrhythmias, their mechanisms, diagnosis and management. JB Lippincott Company, Philadelphia, p 145
8. Janse MJ. The acute phase of experimental myocardial ischemia, electrophysiology and mechanisms of arrhythmias. In: Hombach V, Hilger HH (eds) Holter Monitoring Technique. FK Schattauer-Verlag, Stuttgart, New York (in press)
9. El-Sherif N, Hope RR, Scherlag BJ, Lazzara R (1977) Re-entrant ventricular arrhythmias in the late myocardial infarction period. 2. Patterns of initiation and termination of re-entry. Circulation 55: 702
10. Scherlag BJ, Brachmann J, Harrison LA, Harrison L, Lazzara R. Mechanisms of chronic ventricular arrhythmias: The concept of latent ischemic damage. In: Hombach V, Hilger HH (eds) Holter Monitoring Technique. FK Schattauer-Verlag, Stuttgart, New York (in press)
11. Josephson ME, Seides SF (1979) Clinical Cardiac Electrophysiology, Techniques and Interpretation. Lea and Febiger, Philadelphia
12. Mason J (1984) Management of intractable ventricular tachycardia. Clinical Tutorial, NASPE Meeting, New York
13. Hombach V, Höpp HW, Braun V, Gil-Sanchez D, Deutsch H, Behrenbeck DW, Tauchert M, Hilger HH (1983) Relevance of physical activity to the antiarrhythmic effects of β-blockade on supraventricular tachycardias. Drug 25 (Suppl 2): 186
14. Messenger JD, Ellestad MH (1977) Coronary sinus pacing: indications and clinical problems. In: Hawthorne JW, Thalen HJT (eds) Cardiac Pacing. Martinus Nijhoff Publishers, The Hague, p 83
15. Joseph SP, White J (1979) Permanent atrial pacing, functional characteristics of coronary sinus and right atrial appendage electrodes. Proceedings of the VIth World Symposium on Cardiac Pacing, Pacesymp Montreal, Chapter 20-6
16. Ward DE, Camm AJ, Spurrell (1979) The response of regular re-entrant supraventricular tachycardia to right heart stimulation. PACE 2: 586
17. Rowland E, Curry PVL, Krikler DM (1979) The assessment of underdrive pacing in the early termination of re-entrant atrioventricular tachycardia. Proceedings of the VIth World Symposium on Cardiac Pacing, Pacesymp Montreal, Chapter 9-5
18. Wellens HJJ, Bär FW, Gorgels AP, Muncharaz JF (1978) Electrical management of arrhythmias with emphasis on the tachycardias. Am J Cardiol 41: 1025
19. Fisher JD, Mehra R, Furman S (1978) Termination of ventricular tachycardia with bursts of rapid ventricular pacing. Am J Cardiol 41: 94
20. Lister JW, Cohn LS, Bernstein WH, Samet P (1968) Treatment of supraventricular tachycardias by rapid atrial stimulation. Circulation 38: 1044
21. Zipes DP (1973) The contribution of artificial pacemaking to understanding the pathogenesis of arrhythmias. Am J Cardiol 28: 211
22. Vergara GS, Hildner FJ, Schoenfeld CB, Javier RP, Cohen LS, Samet P (1972) Conversion of supraventricular tachycardias with rapid atrial stimulation. Circulation 46: 788
23. Spurrell RAJ, Bexton R, Nathan A, Hellestrand K, Nappholz T, Camm AJ (1982) Implantable automatic scanning pacemaker for termination of supraventricular tachycardia. Am J Cardiol 49: 753
24. Nathan AW, Camm AJ, Bexton RS, Hellestrand K, Spurrell RAJ (1982) Initial experience with a fully implantable scanning extrastimulus pacemaker for tachycardia termination. Clin Cardiol 5: 22
25. Sowton E, Elmqvist H, Segerstad C (1981) Two years' clinical experience with a self-searching tachycardia pacemaker. Am J Cardiol 47: 476
26. Jackman W, Zipes DP (1982) Low energy synchronous cardioversion of ventricular tachycardia using a catheter electrode in a canine model of subacute myocardial infarction. Circulation 66: 187
27. Zipes DP, Jackman WM, Heger JJ, Chilson DA, Browne KF, Naccarelli GV, Rahilly GT, Prystowsky EN (1982) Clinical transvenous cardioversion of recurrent life-threatening ventricular tachyarrhythmias. Low energy synchronized cardioversion of ventricular tachycardia and termination of ventricular fibrillation in patients using a catheter electrode. Am Heart J 103: 789
28. Mirowski M, Reid PR, Watkins L, Weisfeldt ML, Mower MM (1981) Clinical treatment of life-threatening ventricular tachyarrhythmias with the automatic implantable defibrillator. Am Heart J 102: 265

29. Hombach V, Höpp HW, Braun V, Osterspey A, Behrenbeck DW, Hilger HH. Akute und chronische diagnostisch-therapeutische Elektrostimulation des Herzens bei supraventrikulären und ventrikulären Tachykardien. In: Weikl E (ed) Physiologische Stimulation des Herzens. Perimed-Verlag (in press)
30. Behrenbeck DW, Hombach V, Höpp HW, Braun V, Hilger HH (1983) Treatment of drug-resistant supraventricular and ventricular tachycardias with a new programmable antitachycardia pacemaker. In: Levy S, Gerard R (eds) Recent Advances in Cardiac Arrhythmias. John Libbey Company, London, p 430

Authors' adress:
Professor V. Hombach
Medizinische Universitäts-Klinik III
Josef-Stelzmann-Straße 8
5000 Köln 41
West Germany

Subthreshold Burst Pacing

E.-R. von Leitner and Th. Linderer

Summary: During electrophysiological studies in patients with recurrent ventricular tachycardia, we and others made the observation that critically timed extrastimuli within the refractory period may prolong ventricular refractoriness and thus lead to interruption of a tachycardia, even though the extrastimulus itself does not induce ventricular depolarization.

These observations made us think of the possibility of trying to interrupt runs of ventricular tachycardia by applying extrastimuli below the patient's stimulation threshold.

While single subthreshold stimuli in our experience were not able to terminate tachycardias in a significant number of VT episodes, the technique that we named subthreshold burst stimulation gave quite promising results.

Methods

We performed bipolar right ventricular pacing with 10 to 30 impulses at a rate of 800 per minute. The impulse width was 2.0 msec., the current strength was adapted to 10 to 20% below patients' individual stimulation threshold.

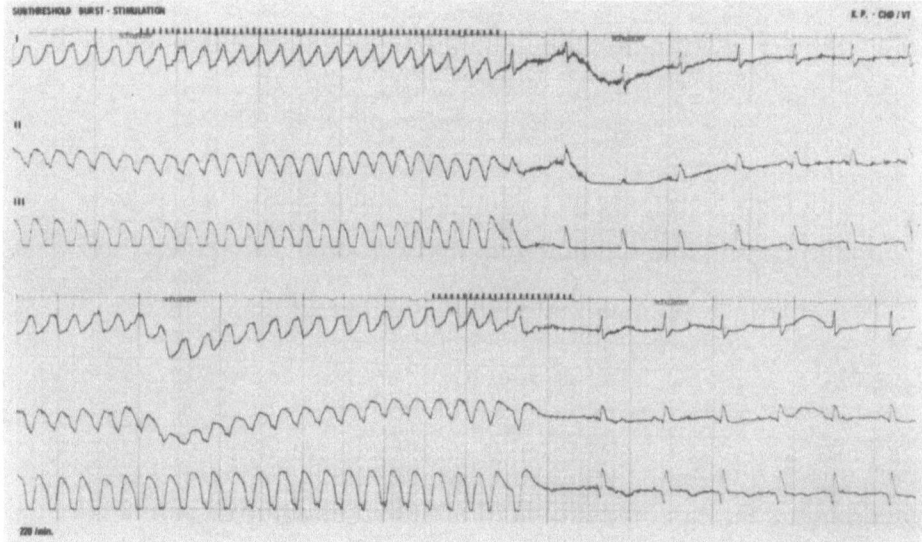

Fig. 1. Termination of two episodes of ventricular tachycardia in a patient with coronary heart disease and history of myocardial infarction and malignant ventricular tachyarrhythmias. Three limb leads are recorded. In the upper tracing, a long subthreshold burst is necessary to interrupt the ventricular tachycardia. The subthreshold stimuli are indicated by extra marks on the upper board of the tracing. At the time of interruption of the tachycardia, the tracing is disturbed by movement artifacts of the patient due to hemodynamic impairment as a consequence of this very rapid tachycardia.

In the bottom part, a short burst is sufficient to interrupt ventricular tachycardia. Although, after termination of the ventricular tachycardia, subthreshold burst pacing continues for a little while, no ventricular depolarization is induced.

191

So far 11 patients with coronary heart disease or dilative cardiomyopathy and recurrent ventricular tachycardia at rates of 120 to 240 per minute have been studied. In addition two patients with WPW-syndrome and circus movement tachycardia at rates of 160 and 220 per minute were studied.

Results

In seven of eleven patients with ventricular tachycardia subthreshold burst pacing was successful in reproducibly terminating the tachycardia. A representative example of tachycardia termination is shown in Figure 1. In all patients with successful subthreshold burst stimulation, the stimulation energy was kept constant. But instead of applying bursts we repeated the stimulation sequence which had been used before to induce ventricular tachycardia with higher amplitude of the stimuli. As can be seen in Figure 2, in most cases the subthreshold impulses did not introduce ventricular complexes. Some impulses, however, were propagated to the rest of the myocardium, although such a low

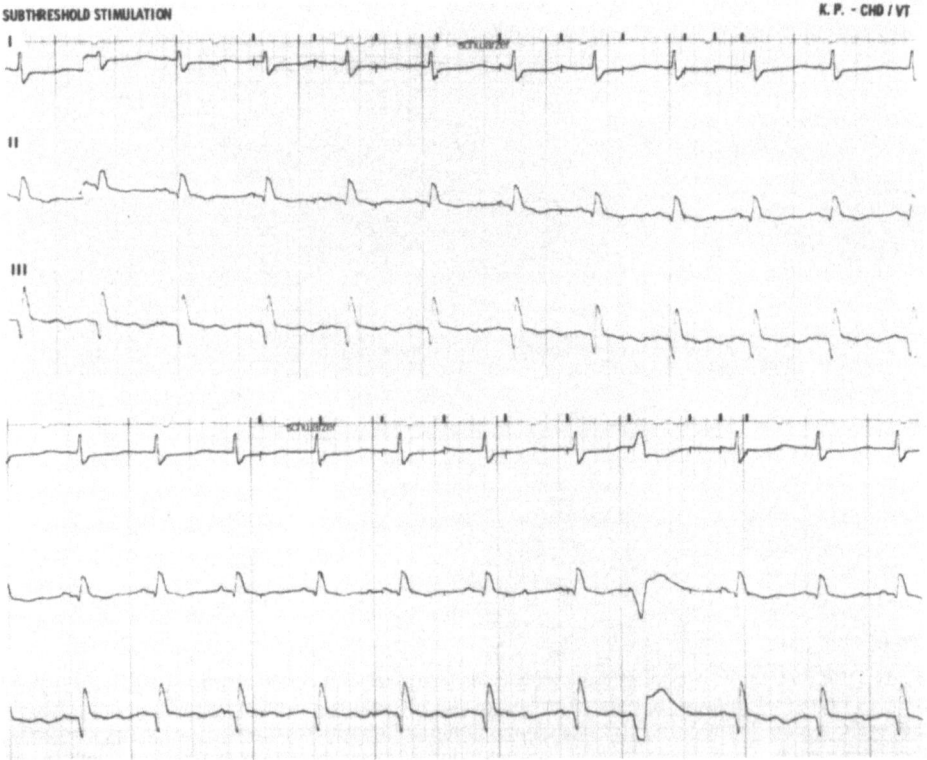

Fig. 2. In the same patient subthreshold stimulation energy was kept constant. But instead of applying bursts, we repeated the stimulation sequence which had been used before to induce ventricular tachycardia with higher amplitude of the stimuli. In most cases subthreshold impulses do not induce ventricular complexes. In the bottom part, however, it can be seen that propagation of the impulse to the rest of the myocardium sometimes does occur even when such low stimulation energy is used.

stimulation energy was used. Degeneration into more rapid tachycardia or into ventricular fibrillation was not observed.

In the patient with left-sided accessory pathway, circus movement tachycardia could be terminated by subthreshold burst stimulation from the coronary sinus, but it failed in another patient with right-sided accessory pathway, although several stimulation sites in the right atrium were used.

Conclusion

Subthreshold burst pacing may be a promising new technique for the treatment of patients with recurrent ventricular or supraventricular tachycardia, but a number of open questions remain to be answered by further systematic studies:

The precise mode of action will have to be determined, and the reliability of the method on a long-term basis remains to be shown. Furthermore, the importance of stimulation site, rate, and energy have to be evaluated. Finally, the risk of degeneration of ventricular tachycardia into more rapid forms or into ventricular fibrillation, although significantly smaller than with conventional anti-tachycardia pacing, will have to be studied by further investigations.

Authors' present address:
Priv.-Doz. E.-R. von Leitner
Städt. Krankenhaus Siloahr
II. Medizinische Klinik
Roesebeckstr. 15
3000 Hannover 91
West Germany

Tachycardia Recognition by Implantable Devices

A. J. Camm[+] and D. E. Ward[*]

Summary: Early tachycardia interruption pacemakers relied on the recognition of tachycardia by the patient and manual activation of the device. The first generation of automatic pacemakers utilized one or more specific heart rates to trigger the tachycardia conversion response. Such systems were vulnerable to activation by sinus tachycardia resulting from physical or emotional stress. In such situations the burst or competitive pacing which resulted was particularly likely to provoke unwanted and potentially dangerous arrhythmias. Second generation anti-tachycardia pacemakers utilize other criteria to distinguish pathological from physiological tachycardia. Amongst these additional criteria the rate of change of heart rate has been most widely applied. This has reduced the likelihood of false diagnosis of pathological tachycardia but there are still many situations in which the implanted device may be activated inappropriately. The most common setting for mistaken diagnosis is immediately following a pacemaker intervention when pathological tachycardia may be "reconfirmed" when only a post tachycardia fast sinus rate is present. Of the many tachycardia recognition criteria which have been proposed cardiac activation sequence, for example AV interval during tachycardia, is the most promising technique for the accurate diagnosis of specific pathological tachycardias.

Introduction

Accurate diagnosis of specific tachycardias is essential for the proper functioning of an automatic implantable tachycardia termination device. The first implantable pacemakers used to terminate tachycardia were conventional demand pacemakers temporarily converted to asynchronous or fixed rate pacing by the application of a magnet. The use of a magnet or another form of external device to trigger or drive an implanted pacemaker requires that the tachycardia is sufficiently symptomatic to be noticed by the patient. Provided that the patient is mature, intelligent and co-operative and is not disabled by the tachycardia, the patient's ability to recognise tachycardia can be used to activate a pacing response. On the other hand, if the tachycardia is either asymptomatic or severely symptomatic, or if a prompt and adaptive response to tachycardia is essential it is necessary for the implanted device to recognise the arrhythmia and respond accordingly. Automatic triggering of an antitachycardia response has other advantages and some disadvantages compared with the manual response (Table 1). A major advantage of manual triggering is the ability to restrict the use of the device by witholding the external component from the patient. In these circumstances the patient must attend hopsital for supervised termination of tachycardia. Another advantage is the ease of logging termination attempts.

Electrodes

Early pacemakers (e.g. Siemens P 43 and Biotronic Phylax) and some current systems (e.g. Vitatron DPG, Siemens 668, Telectronics Optima MP), which are designed to recog-

+ St. Bartholomew's Hospital, London, England.
* St. George's Hospital, London, England.

Table 1. Advantages of manual and automatic triggering of antitachycardia pacing.

Manual	Automatic
a) Accurate sensing not essential	a) No external device is required
b) Incidence of tachycardia and usage of the device is known	b) Arrhythmias are treated promptly
	c) Asymptomatic arrhythmias may be treated
b) The usage of the device can be restricted (e.g. to hospital or to physican)	d) Different arrhythmias may be distinguished and treated differently
	e) Pacing modalities which require sensing can be utilized
	f) Patient co-operation is not required
	g) May be used in patients with syncope or pre-syncope

nise tachycardia automatically, use the unipolar electrode disposition. However, such systems are easily deceived by myopotentials and electromagnetic interference. Therefore, most modern antitachycardia pacemakers (e.g. Intermedics Cybertach, Telectronics PASAR and Siemens P 46) utilize bipolar electrode systems. Bipolar pacing is, in theory, more hazardous than unipolar cathodal stimulation and the combination of bipolar sensing and unipolar pacing will soon be available in some conventional bradycardia support pacemakers (e.g. Intermedics 284-02, Cosmos) and this arrangement will no doubt be applied to tachycardia interruption pacing. There may also be considerable advantages from combined unipolar and bipolar sensing for respective recognition of timing and shape of electrograms. In addition, dual chamber, or dual channel, sensing will aid the differentiation of cardiac rhythms.

Recognition of tachycardia

a) Prodromal events

The majority of paroxysmal tachycardias are triggered by premature beats, sinus tachycardia or specific rhythms. In some cases detectable conduction block or delay is necessary to the initiation of the tachycardia. If these prodromal events are recognised tachycardia initiation may be prevented or immediately countered by an implantable device. For example, the AV conduction delay which follows any atrial premature beat and which may be necessary to initiate atrioventricular reentrant tachycardia may be prevented by automatic delivery of a ventricular stimulus shortly after sensing the atrial premature beat (1). Thus tachycardia initiation may be prevented. Alternatively, the pacemaker could stimulate the atrium shortly after the spontaneous atrial premature beat (2). Such an induced atrial depolarisation may preempt circus movement and prevent the initiation of tachycardia. Effective action following a prodromal event requires a pacemaker which may be programmed to respond specifically to certain trigger events.

b) Tachycardia

Tachycardia is usually recognised when the heart rate exceeds a preset trigger rate. In some automatic devices, e.g. Intermedics Cybertach 60, only two trigger rates were provided (3). In later generations such as Telectronics PASAR (4151) many programmable trigger rates were available to allow better separation between sinus tachycardia and pathological tachycardia (4). Although this development was an improvement it was not entirely satisfactory and a sudden rate change criterion was introduced in the Siemens P43 (Tachylog) (5) and later incorporated in several other commercial pacemakers, e.g. Medtronic Symbios. Although it is theoretically possible to distinguish the abrupt onset of pathological tachycardia from the more gradual acceleration of sinus rhythm this criterion is not always useful because pathological tachycardia may be provoked by sinus tachycardia or may be provoked by a train of gradually more closely coupled premature beats. Alternatively sinus arrhythmia or sudden sinus tachycardia in response to a change in posture, emotional stimulation or physical excitement may simulate the abrupt onset of pathological tachycardia. In the Intermedics 262-12 (Intertach) more programmable criteria have been introduced. In addition to heart rate and rate of change of heart rate, rate stability and duration at high rate are also incorporated into recognition algorithms. The requirement to detect a persistently rapid heart rate necessarily introduces a delay in the response of the pacemaker. Rate stability also involves sampling many tachycardia cycles and precludes present diagnosis and therapy. It is also uncertain that, in the physically active and autonomically intact individual, the cycle length of pacemaker terminatable tachycardia is any more regular than sinus tachycardia. It may, however, be a reasonable way to distinguish tachycardias responsive to pacemaker termination from atrial fibrillation. Nonetheless these new criteria are not tried and although they are welcome, their usefulness is not yet evident.

The sensors being developed for rate-responsive pacing may be applied inversely to distinguish between sinus (appropriate) tachycardia and pathological (inappropriate) tachycardia. Although response times are likely to be slow, pO_2, pH, pCO_2, central blood temperature, QT sensing, stroke volume (intracavitory impendance) and intramyocardial pressure are all possible parameters by which to judge tachycardia.

The most feasible method of distinguishing between tachycardias is the recognition of particular electrogram shapes or particular electrogram timing sequences. In this way, not only can sinus tachycardias be recognised but several varieties of pathological tachycardia may be differentiated. For example the ratio of atrial to ventricular complexes might be used to diagnose atrial tachycardia (more atrial events than ventricular events) and ventricular tachycardias (more ventricular than atrial signals). As yet no antitachycardia pacemaker utilizes this principle but the application of dual chamber (or dual site) sensing technology should lead to the early development of such a system.

c) Evoked response(s)

The presence of an evoked response indicates that tissue is not refractory and this information could be utilised to adjust the timing of a pacing stimulus in pacing algorithms of the 'hunting' or 'searching' type. Similarly the duration of the evoked response may reflect tissue refractoriness and predict the optimal timing of stimulation. During a contin-

196

ued burst of pacing an analysis of the evoked response may be used to evaluate fusion (and entrainment) or nonfused capture (and termination). Sensing of a local evoked response is still technically difficult but is increasingly feasible. It is also relatively easy to sense a response remote from the pacing electrode. It is therefore very likely that "evoked response" sensing technology will become an important aspect of antitachycardia pacing. It has been suggested that sinus tachycardia may be distinguished from pathological tachycardias by the ventricular response to an atrial premature stimulus. For example, during sinus rhythm the ventricular complex (QRS) may be advanced by an atrial premature stimulus. In junctional tachycardia this response is uncommon but advance of the QRS complex by atrial stimulation may sometimes occur. In ventricular tachycardia it is quite common, given appropriate timing, to capture the ventricles by atrial stimulation, even when 1 : 1 atrial conduction is present. It therefore seems unlikely that the ventricular response to atrial stimulation will reliably differentiate sinus from pathological tachycardia.

d) Rhythm after pacing

A pacing intervention may convert tachycardia to sinus rhythm, accelerate tachycardia, reset tachycardia or leave the tachycardia completely unaffected.
There has been virtually no consideration given to criteria for reconfirmation of the presence of tachycardia following a pacing intervention. Only the rate criterion has been applied and rate of change of rate is obviously inappropriate. Since relatively short-lived sinus tachycardia often emerges when pathological tachycardia has been successfully terminated and because termination may be immediately followed by a short burst of rapid ectopic activity it is clearly impossible to confirm tachycardia or diagnose sinus rhythm using simple rate criteria over one or two cycles. Similarly the compensatory pause which may follow a burst of pacing may confound prompt and accurate determination of the cardiac rhythm when pacing stops. Although some pacemaker algorithms (e.g. Siemens Tachylog) appear to use only the first two post-pacing intervals to determine the subsequent pacemaker response, it would be better if the first (as in the Telectronics 4151) or preferably the first two post-pacing intervals were ignored and the following two or more intervals were considered. The application of more sophisticated criteria for the recognition of both sinus rhythm and pathological tachycardia (e.g. activation sequences) will allow a more ready and reliable distinction between these rhythms.
Pacing during tachycardia may accelerate tachycardia or convert one tachycardia to another. Future antitachycardia pacemakers must be able to sense such events and distinguish them from simple continuation of tachycardia in order that the pacemaker may make the most appropriate response. The Intermedics 262-12 (Intertach) may be able to recognise two tachycardias and make specific responses to each.
The timing of post-pacing tachycardia complexes has been used to direct the subsequent pacing response. In the algorithm of the Siemens Tachylog (P 43 and P 46) reset of tachycardia (which implies tissue capture) is used to move pacemaker stimulation to a more premature point in the tachycardia cycle whereas non reset of continued tachycardia (which is thought to imply ineffective stimulation) moves stimulation away from the tachycardia complex. This principle has been used to implement the hunting method by which the tachycardia termination zone is rapidly searched out (5).

Conclusion

The technology required for the positive recognition of sinus tachycardia and regular pathological tachycardias is already available. However, the best criteria for the distinction between these rhythms have yet to be established. Combinations of bipolar sensing (rate and timing criteria) and unipolar sensing (morphology criteria) will probably emerge as the best methods of tachycardia detection and diagnosis by implanted devices.

References

1. Spurrell RAJ, Sowton E (1976) Pacing techniques in the management of supraventricular tachycardia. Part 2. J Electrocardiol 9: 89
2. Kuck K-H, Kunze K-P, Bleifeld W (1983) Electrophysiologic prevention of reentrant tachycardia intitiation. Circulation 68: III-312
3. Falkoff MD, Ong LS, Heinle RA, Barold SS (1981) Implantable multiprogrammable automatic burst antitachycardia pacemakers for refractory ventricular tachycardia. Pacing and Clin Electrophysiol 4: 44
4. Spurrell RAJ, Nathan AW, Bexton RS, Hellestrand KJ, Nappholz T, Camm AJ (1982) Implantable automatic scanning pacemaker for termination of supraventricular tachycardia. Am J Cardiol 49: 753
5. Sowton E (1983) Clinical results with an intelligent anti-tachycardia pacemaker. Circulation 68: III-312

Authors' address:
Professor A. J. Camm
Department of Cardiology
St Bartholomew's Hospital
West Smithfield
London EC1A 7BE, England

The Use of the Ventricular Paced Evoked Response in Antitachycardia Pacemaker Design

E. J. Perrins and A. F. Rickards

Summary: Recent advances in sensing technology allow the recording of the evoked response within 5 ms of an applied stimulus in the ventricle. The method is currently unsuitable for the atrium. The evoked T-wave can be sensed and the stimulus to peak T-wave interval measured (st-T). In antitachycardia pacemaker design incorporation of this feature may help in discrimination between pathological and physiological tachycardia, detection of capture or non-capture, prediction of ventricular refractory period and improvement in noise performance.

The relationship between evoked st-T and cycle length was studied during atrial pacing and isoprenaline infusion. Separation was seen for rates between 100 and 150 bpm. Loss of capture could be reliably detected even at very high ventricular rates. Fractionation of the evoked QRS complex was noted to occur close to the ventricular refractory period. The relationship between st-T interval at the driving cycle length and the ventricular refractory period was investigated using an extrastimulus method and a modification to the external evoked response pacemaker to allow it to be externally triggered by a programmed stimulator. A remarkably linear relationship was found which if substantiated during varying conditions (e.g. drugs and exercise) will allow continuous prediction of the ventricular refractory period from the evoked response alone. Sensing of both T-wave and QRS complexes using dual channel narrow bandwidth filters will significantly improve noise rejection characteristics.

Evoked response sensing will make a significant contribution to future designs of antitachycardia pacemakers.

Introduction

Until recently it has not been possible to record the endocardial signal which follows a ventricular stimulus due to the distortions introduced by polarisation effects and other after potentials at the lead/tissue interface. An implantable pacing system has now been developed however which can reliably sense within 5 ms of an applied stimulus (1). The signal following a pacing stimulus has been termed the "evoked response" and the characteristics of the evoked response have recently been reviewed (2). The pacing system allows detection of the evoked T-wave which follows the ventricular depolarisation. A T-wave sensing window is set following the QRS complex during which a peak detector senses the peak of the evoked T-wave (Fig. 1). The stimulus-peak T-wave interval can be accurately measured by the device (st-T). The changes in the st-T interval follow closely changes, in the QT interval and the relationship between shortening of the QT interval and exercise has been exploited in a rate responsive ventricular pacemaker (3). This paper will describe how this technology might be applied to the design of antitachycardia pacemakers. Currently it is not possible to reliably sense an atrial evoked response due to its very low amplitude, so that the considerations which follow are only applicable to tachycardia terminating systems in the ventricle.

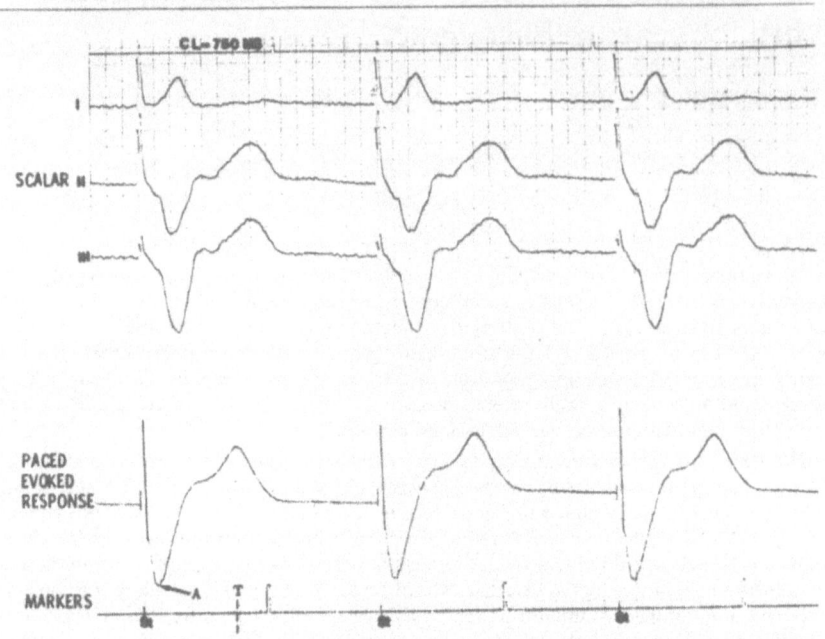

Fig. 1. Recording of the paced evoked response. The ventricular response is seen followed by the evoked T-wave. The peak of the evoked T-wave occurs earlier than the peak of the surface T-wave indicating the local nature of the evoked response. The T-wave peak detector has an adjustable window for T-wave sensing. The detector generates a marker pulse exactly 100 ms following the detected peak of the T-wave.

Current antitachycardia pacemakers have many deficiences, but four major areas of function might be enhanced by incorporating sensing of the evoked response. These are: discrimination between pathological and physiological tachycardia, detection of capture and non-capture during termination sequences, prediction of the ventricular refractory period and improvement in noise discrimination. These four areas will be discussed separately.

Detection of pathological tachycardia

Current detection algorithms rely on rate alone or in some designs on rate of change of rate. These systems are poor discriminators however, particularly during exercise. Wide complex tachycardia might be appreciated by sensing either the QRS duration or the QT interval of the spontaneous rhythm but at present the amplitude of the spontaneous T-wave (as opposed to the evoked T-wave following a pacing stimulus) is too small to be reliably sensed. Several authors have however documented that changes of the QT interval during exercise are dependent on both the intrinsic rate as well as the level of circulating catecholamines (4–6). It might be predicted therefore that the st-T interval of the evoked response might be longer during pathological tachycardia than during exercise at the same heart rate unless there is considerable sympathetic outflow consequent on the ef-

200

fects of the tachycadia on the patient. To test this hypothesis the following experiment was performed.

"Pathological" tachycardia was reproduced by atrial pacing between rates of 80 and 200 bpm with the patient supine and at rest. "Physiological" tachycardia was simulated by isoprenaline infusion. At each heart rate the ventricular pacemaker was driven just above the spontaneous rate (Fig. 2) and then the evoked response and st-T interval were record-

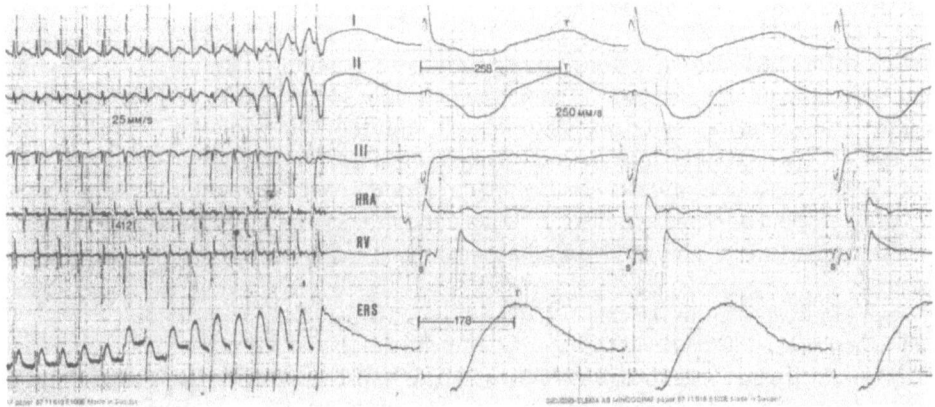

Fig. 2. Measurement of the evoked response during a tachycardia. The patient is being atrially paced at a cycle length of 412 ms. The ventricular pacing rate is increased until it just entrains the tachycardia. The recording speed is then increased to 250 mm/sec and the evoked response and st-T is measured.

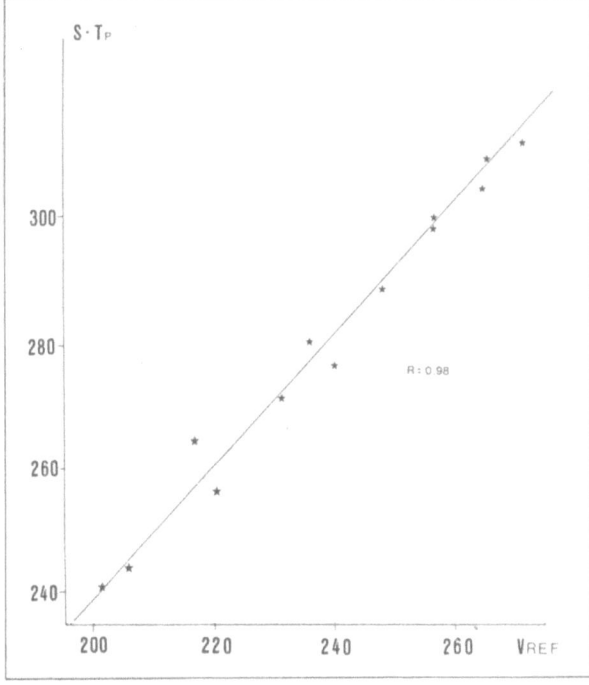

Fig. 3. Plot of evoked stimulus – peak T interval against cycle length during atrial pacing and spontaneous sinus tachycardia following isoprenaline administration. Separation of the two curves occurs at heart rates between 100 and 150 bpm with the evoked st-T interval being shorter during isoprenaline infusion. At high rates however the rate effect becomes dominant.

ed. The results are shown in Figure 3. It can be seen that there is separation of the st-T intervals at cycle lengths between 600 and 400 ms (100–150 bpm). It is the slower pathological tachycardias which are most difficult to detect by conventional means and it might therefore be possible to apply this principle. However it is likely that any reliable algorithm would have to be calibrated to the individual patient.

Detection of capture vs. non-capture

Many existing tachycardia terminating algorithms incorporate a searching or scanning method in order to find the correct termination zone for the tachycardia. This may cause pacing during refractory and detection of loss of capture would be useful to improve the efficiency of the algorithm. Detection of changes of tachycardia cycle length are not sufficient to detect loss of capture as it is possible to produce ventricular capture during a tachycardia without affecting cycle length. Detection of the evoked T-wave following a ventricular capture might however allow reliable detection of capture even during rapid cycle lengths.

In order to investigate this the external evoked response pacemaker was modified to allow external triggering of the device by a programmed stimulator. This was then used to assess the ventricular evoked response during programmed ventricular stimulation with a single extrastimulus and varying cycle lengths. The ventricular evoked response could be reliably detected until ventricular refractory was reached for basic cycle lengths up to 270 ms. A typical recording showing loss of capture is seen in Fig. 4. The complete absence of electrical activity on the evoked response channel within 125 ms of the applied stimulus will allow detection of failure to capture. As the ventricular extrastimuli became close to the ventricular refractory period widening and splintering (fractionation) of the evoked

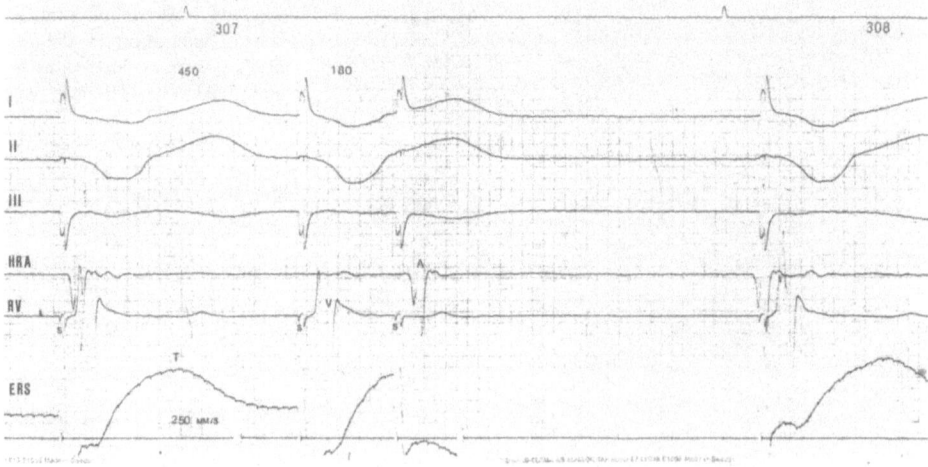

Fig. 4. Loss of ventricular capture. The ventricular cycle length is 450 ms. An extrastimulus is seen which apparently captures on the surface leads. However the cavity ventricular electrogram shows loss of capture. No evoked T-wave is detected and the evoked response has fallen to zero potential within 100 ms of the applied stimulus.

QRS complex was seen (Fig. 5). This phenomenon which has previously been described in the ventricular cavity electrogram may indicate non-uniformity of refractory period in the myocardial tissue close to the stimulating electrode. This fractionation of the evoked response might possibly be detected during attempted termination by the pacemaker and indicate imminent loss of capture. This might cause the pacemaker to change to a different mode of termination rather than continue to stimulate very close to refractor, thereby minimising the likelihood of triggering dangerous ventricular arrhythmias. This is particularly important when a ventricular lead is being used to terminate a supraventricular arrhythmia which might not be life-threatening in itself.

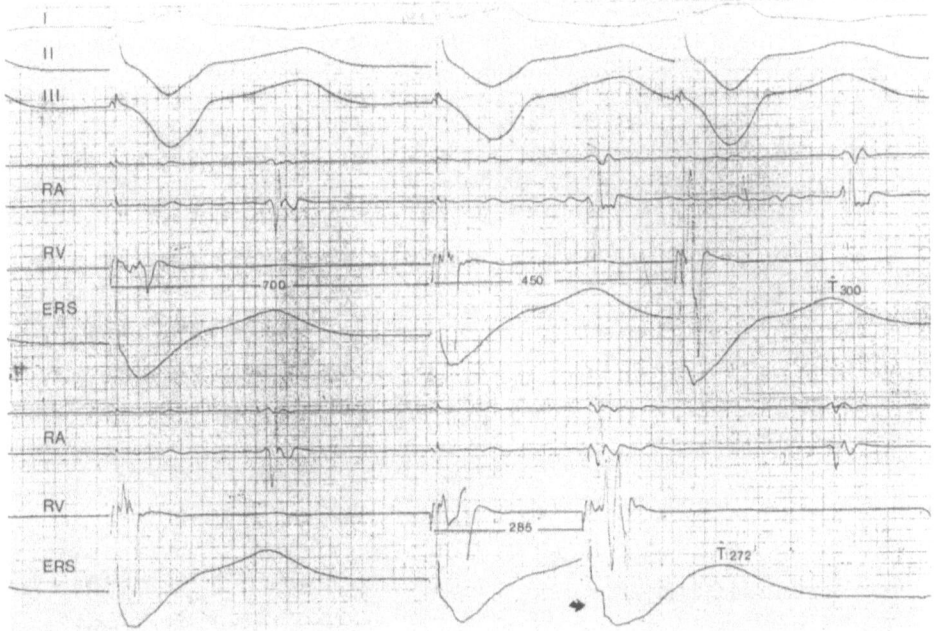

Fig. 5. Fragmentation of the evoked response with premature ventricular stimuli. The basic cycle length is 700 ms. The upper panel shows an extrastimulus with a 450 ms coupling interval. No significant widening or fragmentation of the evoked QRS is seen. The lower tracing shows an extrastimulus at 285 ms (5 ms above refractory). Marked widening and fragmentation of the evoked response is seen (arrow).

The prediction of ventricular refractory period during tachycardia

The ventricular refractory period (VRP) is dependent on many factors including heart rate, catecholamine drive, ischaemia and drugs. Accurate estimation of the VRP would allow more efficient termination as described above. Donaldson (7, 8) has recently shown that the time course of the ventricular evoked response closely follows that of the local monophasic action potential, not only during changes in rate but also during ischaemia and following some drugs. Hoffman (9) described a close relationship between re-fractory period and the 90% repolarisation time of the monophasic action potential. The relationship between the evoked response and the VRP was therefore investigated. Ven-tricular pacing at varying cycle lengths from 800 to 270 ms was performed and the st-T interval of the evoked response measured. The effective refractory period at each cycle length was then determined by the single ventricular extrastimulus method. The results are shown in Figure 6. A remarkably linear relationship was found between the basic ventricular cycle length (CL) and the ventricular refractory period for that base rate. (VRP = 0.943CL –22.1 ms, r = 0.98, p < 0.001.) Ventricular pacing at a rate just above the tachycardia rate would therefore allow close prediction of the ventricular refractory period merely by measuring the st-T interval of the evoked response. If this relationship is found to be consistent over a wide range of conditions (for example after one or more extrastimuli during a tachycardia) then complete avoidance of the "vulnerable" period may be possible and termination algorithms would be more efficient as they could be linked to the refractory period.

Fig. 6. Linear relationship be-tween the effective ventricular refractory period and the st-T interval of the evoked response at the basic pacing rate (see text).

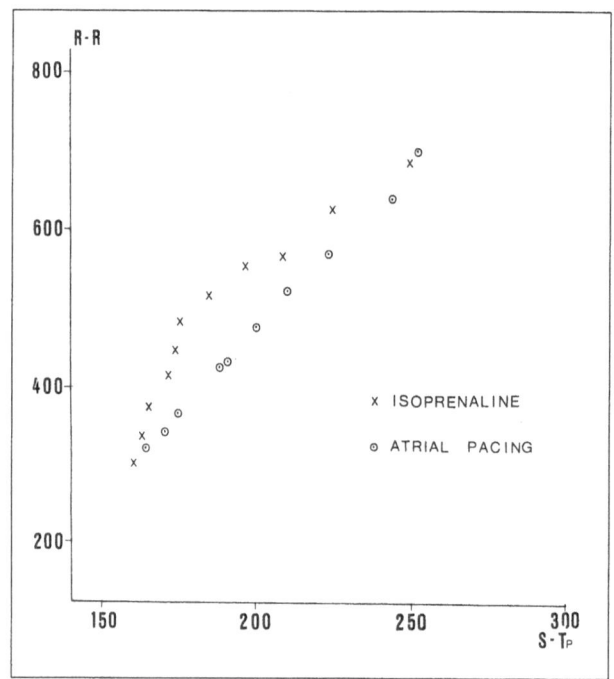

Noise performance

Noise may cause false triggering of the tachycardia detection circuit if it is interpreted by the pacemaker as high rate ventricular activity. Noise sensing might also cause false inhibition of the device, particularly if the unit has a low rate back-up mode to protect

204

against post termination bradycardia. Finally triggering of the pacemaker's noise detection circuitry may cause reversion to VOO pacing (depending upon the particular model). This may cause competitive pacing which may initiate a tachycardia. The frequency spectra of the T-wave is markedly different from the QRS complex as it is a low frequency event. It is possible therefore to construct separate filters (high pass and low pass respectively) to sense the QRS and T-waves. This will allow a significant increase in noise rejection as well as an increase in the sensitivity of the T-wave channel, particularly if noise does not trigger noise reversion mode unless sensed on both QRS and T-wave channels. Similarly false triggering of the QRS amplifier could be detected by the absence of an evoked response at the same QRS rate. Finally the noise reversion behaviour of the pacemaker could be altered to incorporate the "flywheel" principle whereby the noise reversion rate is always just above the last sensed R-R rate. This would minimise the chance of competitive pacing during noise reversion.

Conclusions

This paper has examined some of the possible applications of sensing the ventricular paced evoked response during tachycardia. The results are preliminary and at present based on only a few patients, however some important conclusions are possible.

The present sensing system is only applicable to a ventricular channel. Sensing of the evoked st-T may allow the discrimination between pathological and physiological tachycardia to be made but this will probably require individual patient calibration and will not always be reliable in situations of high catecholamine drive. The detection of ventricular capture is possible even during tachycardia and in addition fractionation of the evoked response might be sensed, indicating imminent loss of capture. Measurement of the evoked st-T interval may provide an accurate guide to the ventricular refractory period at that rate and will allow safer and more efficient termination sequences. Finally, refinement of the T-wave sensing mechanisms could allow significant improvements in noise rejection to be made. Evoked response sensing is likely to play a prominent role in the design of future antitachycardia pacing systems.

References

1. Rickards AF, Norman J (1981) Relation between QT interval and heart rate. New design of a physiologically adaptive cardiac pacemaker. Br Heart J 45: 56–61
2. Donaldson RM, Rickards AF (1983) The ventricular paced evoked response. Pace 6: 253–259
3. Rickards AF, Donaldson RM (1983) Rate responsive pacing. Clin Prog Pacing and Electrophysiol: 12–19
4. Rickards AF, Akhras F, Baron DW Effects of heart rate on Q-T interval (abstract). In: Meere C (ed) Proceedings of the VI World Symposium on Cardiac Pacing, Montreal, Chap 2: 7
5. Milne JR, Camm AJ, Ward DE, Spurrell RAJ (1980) Effect of intravenous propranolol on QT interval. A new method of assessment. Br Heart J 43: 1–6
6. Fananapazir L, Bennett DH, Faragher EB (1983) Contribution of heart rate to QT interval shortening during exercise. Eur Heart J 4: 265–271
7. Donaldson RM, Rickards AF (1982) Evaluation of drug induced changes in myocardial repolarisation using the paced evoked response. Br Heart J 48: 381–387

8. Donaldson RM, Hashat FS, Noble D, Taggart P (1982) The effect of ischaemia on the paced evoked response and monophasic action potentials in the dog. J Physiol 336: 65–66 P (abstract)
9. Hoffman BF, Cranefield PF, Lepeschkin E, Surawicz B, Herrlich HC (1959) Comparison of cardiac monophasic action potentials recorded by intracellular and suction electrodes. Am J Physiol 196: 1297–1301

Authors' address:
Dr. E. J. Perrins
Dept. of Medical Cardiology
The General Infirmary at Leeds
Great George Street
Leeds LSI 3EX
England

Detection and Discrimination of Supraventricular Tachycardia from Sinus Tachycardia of Overlapping Cycle Lengths

M. B. Sweeney and B. D. Pless

Summary: For more than 15 years, pulse generators (PG) have been implanted for the control of tachyarrhythmias. Patient-activated systems have not achieved wide acceptance due mainly to the need for direct patient participation. Automatic antitachycardia PGs have been limited by lack of flexibility of programmable parameters and the inability to discriminate pace-terminable (PT) tachycardias from sinus tachycardia and other non-PT rhythms.

The Intermedics InterTach, a microprocessor-based second generation automatic antitachycardia pulse generator utilizes four programmable detection criteria to discriminate PT tachycardias from sinus and other non-PT tachycardias. These criteria, high rate, sudden onset, rate stability and sustained high rate can be programmed to any nine configurations.

These detection criteria coupled with the PG's diagnostic counters and the capability to perform non-invasive programmed stimulation via the programmer afford the physician greater flexibility in selecting the most efficacious parameters for individual patients. This flexibility is needed to expand the potential patient population for implantation of automatic antitachycardia devices.

For over 15 years pulse generators have been implanted for the control of tachycardias. These devices have been either patient-activated or automatic. Patient-activated devices range from conventional pulse generators converted to fixed rate with the application of a magnet (1, 2) to sophisticated scanning generators delivering stimuli coupled to the patient's intrinsic rhythms via transmission to the implanted device from a hand-held transmitter (3, 4).

All types of patient-activated systems require direct participation by the patient in first detecting the arrhythmia and then activating the system. This participation may prove to be psychologically disturbing to the patient and will eliminate from consideration patients with frequent tachycardias and patients in whom the tachycardia induces syncope (5, 6). Due to this limitation, recent technology advances have been directed toward automatic antitachycardia devices which do not require patient interaction.

A significant limitation of current automatic antitachycardia devices is the inability of the device to correctly discriminate pace terminatable tachycardias from sinus tachycardia and other non-pace terminatable rhythms. This inability to differentiate rhythms has resulted in numerous reported incidences of false positives or inappropriate detection. Thus the physician is required to apply very stringent patient selection criteria which to this point has limited the patient population receiving antitachycardia devices for the control of supraventricular tachycardia.

Currently available automatic antitachycardia systems, such as the CyberTach 60, rely soley upon the sensing of high rate to identify supraventricular tachycardia. The tachycardia criterion consists of two programmable choices of high rate. If the intrinsic rate is

Fig. 1. CyberTach 60 – Sinus tachycardia at a rate greater than the high rate criterion (137 ppm) triggers atrial burst pacing, which continues until the sinus rate decreases below 137 ppm.

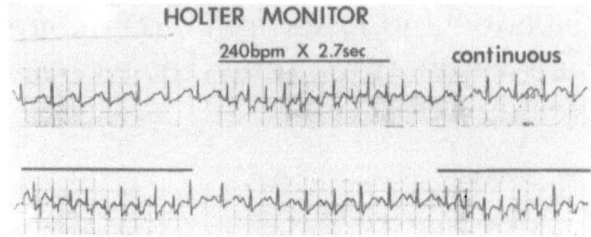

HOLTER MONITOR
240bpm X 2.7sec   continuous

consistently above the high rate criterion for seven intervals, a burst of pacing pulses is delivered at a preprogrammed cycle length and duration (7). Therefore, in sinus tachycardia due to physical exertion if the rate satisfies the programmed tachycardia criteria inappropriate burst pacing ensues (8) (see Figure 1).

With the advent of microprocessor-based pacing systems for the control of tachycardia, sophisticated algorithms can be utilized for rhythm identification. The microprocessor-based InterTach, a second generation antitachycardia pacemaker, in addition to a greatly expanded programmable high rate criterion, also features adtional criteria, sudden onset, rate stability and sustained high rate.

High rate criterion

Automatic antitachycardia pacemakers, using high rate as the sole criteria to identify pace-terminatable tachycardia have exhibited good sensitivity and problems in terms of specifity. An obvious area for improvement is increased flexibility in program selections of the high rate criteria. The InterTach offers greatly expanded parameters in high rate selection and in the number of intervals required above the high rate criterion to initiate therapeutic pacing.

The ability to "fine tune" the high rate criteria enables the physician with data gathered from electrophysiology studies, exercise testing and cumulative monitoring to select a high rate criterion above the maximal sinus rate and yet below the rate of the pace-terminatable tachycardia. While this is not always feasible, due to overlapping cycle lengths, increased programmability will certainly aid in eliminating inappropriate responses.

Another important feature is programmability of the number of intervals required before antitachycardia pacing is initiated. The wide range of choices (5–99 intervals), allows the physician to define sustained tachycardia with non-sustained episodes being ignored. This also helps to eliminate responses to sinus tachycardia with short excursions above high rate resulting from fright, sudden exertion, excitement or changes in posture.

Sudden onset criteria

The paroxysmal onset of reentrant supraventricular tachycardia has often been mentioned as a possible criterion to be used to differentiate it from sinus tachycardia with a more gradual rate acceleration (9). Therefore, when this criterion is coupled with a highly

208

flexible high rate criterion, tachycardias of overlapping cycle lengths can be differentiated.

Sudden onset criteria is the monitoring of the derivative (dR/dt) of the intrinsic rate. With microprocessor based pacing systems, the cycle lengths of intrinsic events can be stored in memory. When a measured interval satisfies the preprogrammed high rate criterion, the microprocessor measures the preceeding intervals to determine if the rate acceleration is gradual or paroxysmal in nature. The amount of rate change or delta is programmable from 120 msec–502 msec. The larger the delta value the more difficult for this criterion to be satisfied.

As an example (see Figure 2), with the pulse generator programmed to a high rate criterion of 150 ppm (400 msec), and the number of intervals above high rate criteria programmed to 10 and a sudden onset delta of 250 msec, an exercise induced sinus tachycardia is seen by the pulse generator. When the intrinsic rate reaches 150 ppm (400 msec), the microprocessor "looks back" to the interval immediately preceding the "high rate" to see if the rate change is greater than 250 msec. In this instance the sinus rate has gradually "ramped up" to 150 ppm and the preceding intervals do not, in fact, satisfy the sudden onset. The correct diagnosis of sinus tachycardia is made.

Using the example (see Figure 3) of A-V nodal supraventricular tachycardia with the pulse generator programmed to the same parameters as in the preceding example, during normal sinus rhythm, a premature atrial contraction with a cycle length of 360 msec to the preceding sinus P-wave initiates supraventricular tachycardia. The microprocessor "looks back" to the preceding interval which has a cycle length change greater than the

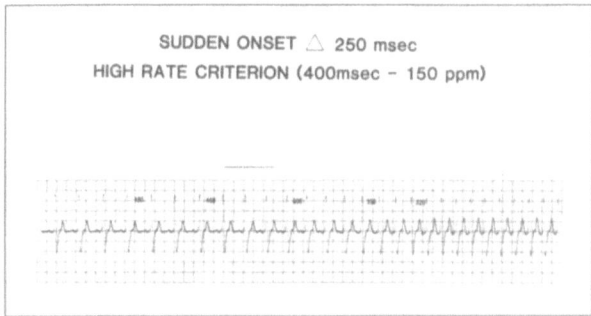

SUDDEN ONSET △ 250 msec
HIGH RATE CRITERION (400msec – 150 ppm)

Fig. 2. Using a simulated ECG, a rate greater than the high rate criterion (150 ppm–400 msec) is achieved. The interval change preceding high rate is not greater than the sudden onset delta of 250 msec. The diagnosis: non-paroxysmal onset tachycardia.

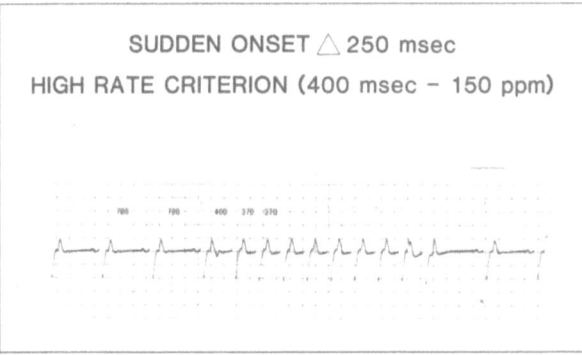

SUDDEN ONSET △ 250 msec
HIGH RATE CRITERION (400 msec – 150 ppm)

Fig. 3. Using a simulated ECG, a paroxysmal tachycardia is initiated by a single APD with a coupling interval of 400 msec. In this case, the sudden onset criterion is satisfied.

Fig. 4. Using a simulated ECG, during a "high rate" tachycardia, a pause of 630 msec is followed by a 370 msec interval which satisfies the high rate criterion (150 ppm–400 msec). This would result in an incorrect diagnosis of paroxysmal tachycardia. To avoid this, the microprocessor measures the intervals preceding the pauses which are above high rate. Therefore, the diagnosis: non-paroxysmal onset.

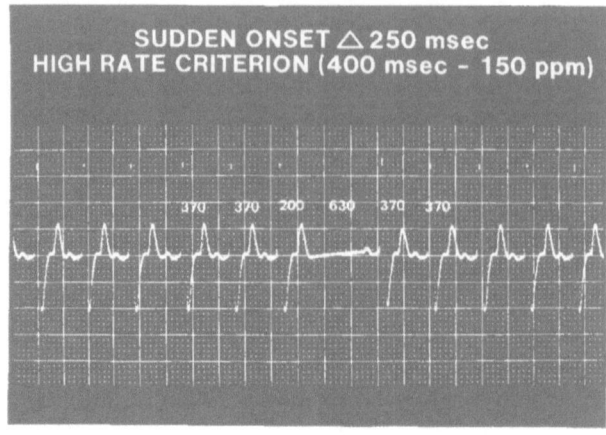

sudden onset delta of 250 msec and the diagnosis of paroxysmal onset tachycardia is made. If the tachycardia remains above the high rate for the required number of intervals which in this case is 10, antitachycardia pacing ensues.

Another example (see Figure 4) is one in which in the midst of a "high rate" sinus tachycardia, a premature contraction results in a compensatory pause with the interval following the pause again satisfying the high rate criterion. This high rate or short interval would result in the microprocessor "looking back" to the preceding interval, which, depending upon the length of the compensatory pause, could satisfy the sudden onset delta resulting in an incorrect diagnosis of paroxysmal tachycardia. For this reason the processor will sample the two preceding intervals which in this case are of "high rate" and therefore categorized as "short," the diagnosis – non-paroxysmal tachycardia.

Rate stability

Exercise induced reentrant pace terminatable tachycardia, sudden increases in sinus rate and other non-pace terminatable high rate rhythms with sudden onset such as atrial fibrillation pose problems with a system relying upon high rate and sudden onset as the only criteria for rhythm differentiation. For this reason, the InterTach incorporates additional detection criteria including rate stability.

Rate stability is the measured cycle length variation over a programmed number of intervals after the high rate criteria has been satisfied. The rate stability delta is programmable from 10 msec to 154 msec. In this case the smaller the delta the more difficult it is for this criterion to be satisfied.

The number of intervals in which the cycle lengths are compared is also programmable, from 8 to 250 intervals. Once the high rate criterion has been satisfied, the microprocessor will monitor cycle length variation for rate stability. If the rate stability criterion is met, antitachycardia pacing is initiated.

Rate stability can also be programmed in conjunction with sudden onset where both sudden onset and rate stability are required, or in the case of exercise induced supraventricular tachycardia or other tachycardias where sudden onset can be missed, the pacer can be programmed to sudden onset OR rate stability required. This combination of criteria will

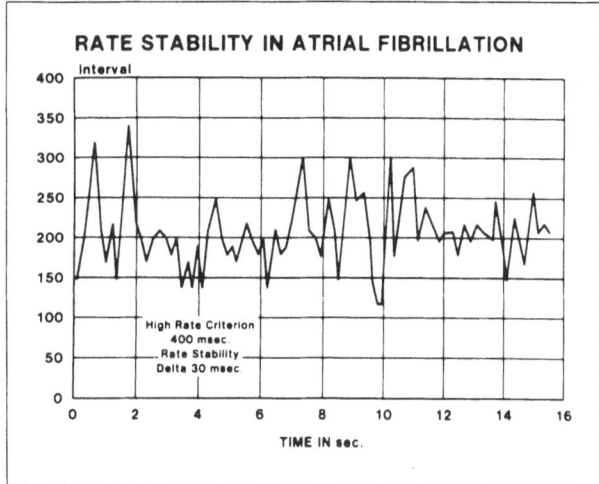

RATE STABILITY IN ATRIAL FIBRILLATION

Fig. 5. Cycle length variation in atrial fibrillation. Although the rate is continually above the high rate criterion (400 msec), the cycle length variation exceeds the rate stability delta of 30 msec.

prove helpful in distinguishing atrial fibrillation from other pace terminatable high rate rhythms (see Figure 5).

Sustained high rate

The final detection criterion available is sustained high rate which is used as a backup to sudden onset and rate stability and therefore cannot be programmed as a primary detection criterion.

The sustained high rate criterion is satisfied if the measured tachycardia rate is continually above the programmed high rate. The number of intervals above high rate is programmable from 6 to 250 intervals.

The InterTach can be programmed to any one of nine combinations of the detection criteria of high rate, sudden onset, rate stability and sustained high rate (see Table 1).

In the event that programmed antitachycardia response fails to terminate a tachycardia, the "restart control" feature offers additional flexibility. Based upon previous electrophysiologic studies to determine the effectiveness of pacing to terminate the tachycardia, these restart control criteria can be utilized to avoid repeated pacing of sinus tachycardia. These restart controls are 1) no restart, 2) restart if rate stability is reestablished, 3) restart

Table 1. The InterTach can be programmed to any one of the above combinations.

1. High Rate Only
2. High rate and sudden onset
3. High rate and rate stability
4. High rate and (sudden onset or sustained high rate)
5. High rate and (rate stability or sustained high rate)
6. High rate and (sudden onset and rate stability)
7. high rate and (sudden onset and rate stability or sustained high rate)
8. High rate and (sudden onset or rate stability)
9. High rate and (sudden onset or rate stability or sustained high rate)

if sustained high rate is reestablished, 4) restart if rate stability or sustained high rate is reestablished.

To help the physician in selecting the most effective detection and response parameters, the InterTach features "Diagnostic Counters" which monitor and store events including the number of times each of the four detection criteria has been satisfied. Additionally, non-invasive programmed stimulation with up to four critically timed extrastimuli for the induction of reentrant tachycardias can be performed via the programmer. This enables post-operative evaluation of changes in tachycardia cycle lengths and efficacy of programmed antitachycardia pacing responses.

As we look toward future generation antitachycardia devices with expanded microprocessor capabilities, more elaborate detection schemes have been suggested. These include the monitoring of A-V timing, activation sequences, waveform analysis (10) and the monitoring of other physiologic functions via sophisticated sensors to further improve the specifity of antitachycardia devices which becomes more critical in devices designed to terminate ventricular arrhythmias. These and other exciting concepts are made possible in future devices by the power and flexibility afforded by microprocessor technology which will enable more effective treatment of supraventricular and ventricular arrhythmias.

References

1. Ryan GF, Easly RM, Zaroff LJ, Goldstein S (1968) Paradoxical Use of a Demand Pacemaker in Treatment of Supraventricular Tachycardia Due to Wolfe-Parkinson-White Syndrome. Circulation 38: 1037–1043
2. Cooper TB, MacLean WAH, Waldo AC (1978) Overdrive Pacing for Supraventricular Tachycardia: A Device of Theoretical Implications and Therapeutic Techniques. PACE 1: 196–221
3. Scheibelhofer W, Probst P (1983) Treatment of Tachyarrhythmia by Implantable Devices: Patient Activated Pacemaker. In: Steinbach K et al (eds) Cardiac Pacing, Proceedings of the VIIth World Symposium on Cardiac Pacing, Vienna, 1983. Steinkopff Verlag, Darmstadt, pp 785–792
4. Camm J, Ward D. The Extrastimulus Mode for Tachycardia Termination. In: Pacing for Tachycardia Control, Chapter 6. Telectronics
5. Camm AJ, Spurrell RAJ (1983) Automatic Implantable Devices for Termination of Tachycardia. In: Steinbach K et al (eds) Cardiac Pacing, Proceedings of the VII World Symposium on Cardiac Pacing, Vienna, 1983. Steinkopff Verlag, Darmstadt, pp 793–801
6. Lister W (1978) A New Technology: Patient Triggered Pacemakers. Ann Intern Med 88: 120–121
7. Hardage ML, Sweeney MB. Automatic Tachycardia Terminating Burst Pacemakers. In The Third Decade on Cardiac Pacing
8. Lerman BB, Waxman HL, Buxton AE, Sweeney M, Josephson ME (1983) Tachyarrhythmias Associated with Programmable Automatic Atrial Antitachycardia Pacemakers. Am Heart J Vol 106, 5: 1029–1035
9. Fisher JD, Goldstein M, Ostrow E, Matos JA, Kim SG (1983) Maximal Rate of Tachycardia Development: Sinus Tachycardia with Sudden Exercise Versus Spontaneous Ventricular Tachycardia. PACE 6: 221–228
10. Furman S, Fisher JD, Pannizo F (1980) Computer Analysis of Signals During Detection of Tachycardia. Cardiostim 80. Mugica J SEPFI, Paris, p 11

Authors' address:
Michael Sweeney
Director of Electrophysiological Studies
Intermedics Inc.
P.O. Box 617
240 Tarpon Inn Village
Freeport, Texas 77541, USA

A Description of Reliable Pacemaker Holter Functions in the Future Antitachycardia Pacemaker

B. Candelon and F. H. M. Wittkampf

Summary: Treatment of tachyarrhythmias by means of permanent implantable cardiac pacemakers requires a means to evaluate efficiency and safety of the given treatment. In-built memory capabilities in the pacemaker can be used for such a purpose; first to optimise treatment by classification of optimal treatments per type of tachyarrhythmia and second by memorising the effect and consequences of every treatment to enable monitoring of dangerous sequences.

Introduction

The treatment of such arrhythmias as tachycardias requires an in-depth knowledge of both the arrhythmia itself and of the efficiency of the treatment prescribed. When the treatment involves the use of a pulse generator, there are several possible ways of fulfilling these requirements. The pulse generator can first of all be used to study the tachycardia by:

1. External control to generate a stimulation program and provoke the tachycardia (this can be achieved by programming the pacemaker to the triggered mode and then initiating external skin stimulation or by temporary programming techniques).
2. Incorporating memory capabilities that enable the pulse generator to be used as an implanted Holter and thereby record, on a long-term basis, data concerning the tachycardias.

The pulse generator can also be used to monitor and evaluate its own functional parameters such as battery status, current drain and characteristics of the pulse delivered, as well as parameters related to the pacemaker/patient interface, such as threshold and sensing characteristics.

Holter functions and memory capabilities

The Holter functions in such a pulse generator can be defined as the memory capabilities that are used to store data concerning the arrhythmia and the efficiency of the treatment used for its prevention or termination.

Memory technology has now reached such a stage of development, both in terms of size and current consumption, where memory can be incorporated in an implantable pulse generator. Pacemakers are now available with 2 kbytes of ROM (read only memory) and ¼ kbyte of RAM (random access memory), which is used as an active memory for the storage of data.

213

Furthermore, the continuing improvements in electronic technology have now already made it possible to go up to 8 kbytes of ROM memory and 2 kbytes of RAM memory.

To give an idea of the amount of information that can be stored in such a memory, we can take the example of a 1 kbyte memory – which can be used either for the storage of characters or for counting purposes. If it is used for character storage a maximum of 2000 characters can be stored. For a direct ECG recording, signals covering a period of up to 20 seconds, at a sampling frequency of 100 points per second, can therefore be stored in a 1 kbyte memory. However, for the proper interpretation of intracardiac signals, one should sample at a minimum frequency of 500 points per second, which, in the case of a 1 kbyte memory, represents a maximum ECG recording capacity of 4 seconds.

Alternatively, the memory can be split up, either into 512 counters, each of which has a counting capacity of up to 64 000, or 340 counters, each of which has a counting capacity of up to 16,000,000. This maximum value represents the number of cardiac cycles over a period of 6 months at a rate of 65 ppm. It can be concluded from these examples that a 1 kbyte memory is still too limited for the storage of ECG recordings, but that it allows for the incorporation of a wide range of counters with an extensive capacity.

Recording by means of counters implies processing of incoming data, by the ROM software, in order to select and store the correct information in the correct place. The amount of available ROM capacity is therefore an important factor in optimising the algorhythm for data recognition and data processing.

In addition, a careful selection of data to be stored has to be made in order to optimise the efficiency of the Holter functions.

The first demand placed on a Holter system specially designed to detect a particular arrhythmia is its ability to discriminate between this arrhythmia and any other normal or abnormal rhythm. In the case of an implantable pulse generator used for the automatic treatment of tachycardia, the recognition algorhythm is therefore very important, since it should not allow for:

1. tachycardias to go untreated,
2. tachycardia termination programs to be activated by a normal sinus rhythm,
3. misinterpretation of Holter monitoring data that have been distorted by oversensing or undersensing of the arrhythmia.

What information should be stored?

Assuming we have a good recognition algorhythm for tachycardias, the Holter should, in order to enable the physician to optimise the therapy, be able to provide data about the arrhythmia and the efficiency of the treatment employed to prevent or terminate it.

The efficiency of the treatment can be evaluated if the Holter can supply information relating to the tachycardia characteristics and to the results of the treatment used to prevent or terminate it. Such data should include information relating to the effectiveness of drug or pulse generator therapy in preventing and terminating the tachycardia by, for example, providing a cumulative indication of the number of tachycardias that have occurred in a given period. In addition, information should be included that gives the physician the tools to adapt and optimise the prevention treatment. This means that information relating to the type of tachycardia and to the events that lead up to it should be monitored whenever possible. Therefore a recording of the patient's cardiac rhythm outside the episodes of tachycardias, and of other arrhythmia such as premature beats should be made. Such additional information can be stored in histograms over a long period of time without any limitation due to memory capacity.

In a more acute stage, information regarding the onset of the tachycardia will be of invaluable assistance in determining methods of prevention. Since a patient may suffer from different types of tachycardia (different rates or a different A-V relationship), it will be necessary for the data related to tachycardias to be classified per type of tachycardia: this can include information relating to the onset, the rate or the A-V relationship. In addition, recording of the number of episodes and their duration will give detailed information on the effectiveness of the therapy employed. A differentiation can be made for all the different tachycardias and a preference can be given for a particular preventive treatment in relation to a given type of tachycardia.

After termination of the tachycardia one should be able to monitor the efficiency of the treatment. This efficiency can be measured quite simply by monitoring the mean duration of a tachycardia episode. The shorter the duration of the tachycardia, the more efficient the treatment becomes. Knowing the number of episodes of tachycardia and their cumulative duration gives extensive information about the efficiency of the treatment.

For treatment related data, the classification of tachycardias is very important, because of the fact that two different tachycardias may require different "stimulation programs" for interruption. Classification of the type of tachycardia allows for the storage, for every type of tachycardia, of the corresponding optimal "stimulation program" and thus avoids a search which delays the interruption of the tachycardia (see Figure 1). In this case, the Holter function is used not only to provide the physician with information about the treatment, but also to prevent the pulse generator from carrying out unnecessary search procedures in order to find the efficient "stimulation program".

The efficiency of the treatment can also be monitored by recording the number of unsuccessful programs, which reflects the duration of the search procedure before the tachycardia is stopped. A large number of unsuccessful programs could be an indication of a poorly adapted program and an attempt can then be made to improve it by using a better pacing sequence (e.g. by adding one stimulus to the program).

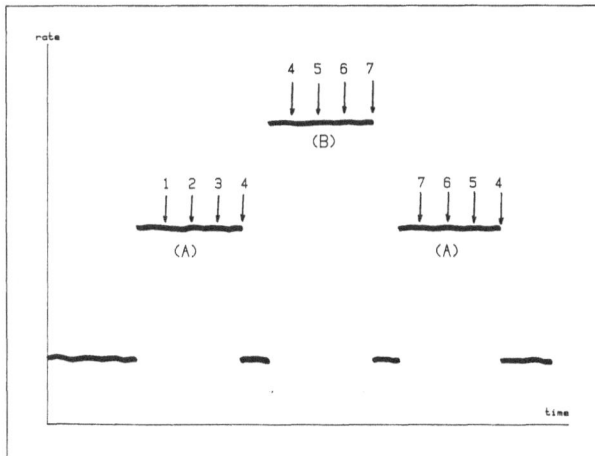

Fig. 1. Tachycardia A is interrupted by "program" 4 and tachycardia B is interrupted by "program" 7. If the pulse generator memorised only one „program", unnecessary search procedures would be initiated by the pulse generator and the interruption of both tachycardias would be delayed. Storage of the optimal "program" for each type of tachycardia would ensure optimal treatment by immediately selecting "program" 4 for tachycardia A and "program" 7 for tachycardia (B).

215

Unsuccessful attempts at termination should not only be analysed and memorised as a number. It is also important to know the consequences, on the arrhythmia, of an unsuccessful attempt at termination, i.e., is the tachycardia unchanged, or has it changed, for example, to a different rate, to a different A-V relationship, or has the termination attempt only succeeded in provoking another, possibly more serious, arrhythmia?

Such unsuccessful programs should be avoided, specially if the tachycardia is changed to another arrhythmia (see Figure 2).

The information related to the unsuccessful programs and to the arrhythmias generated should be stored in the pulse generator memory. They can be used by the physician to prevent the pulse generator from delivering dangerous stimulation programs by limiting the scope of the search algorhythm. This information could also by used be the pulse generator itself in deciding not to repeat a stimulation program that has already been seen to provoke a different arrhythmia.

Successful programs can also sometimes initiate transient arrhythmias which do not trigger a new program because they disappear spontaneously after a few complexes (see Figure 3).

Such programs should also be replaced by safer ones whenever possible.

The information to be stored by the Holter functions of an antitachycardia pulse generator can be summarised as follows:

Fig. 2. The ventricular tachycardia degenerates after the stimulation program.

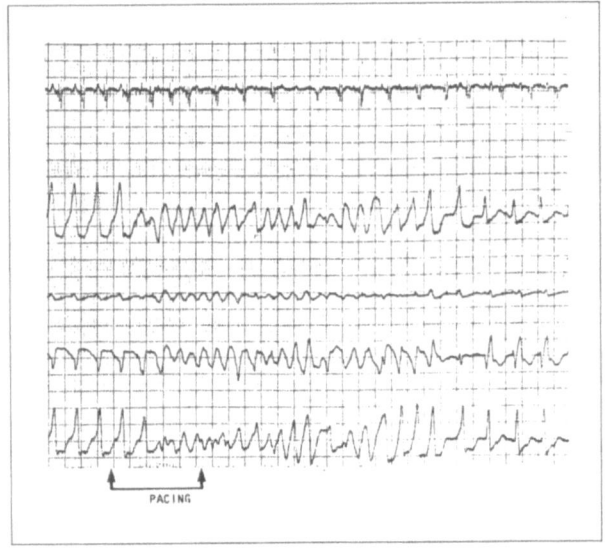

Fig. 3. Single stimulus program. The third attempt, which is successful, is followed by three ectopic beats.

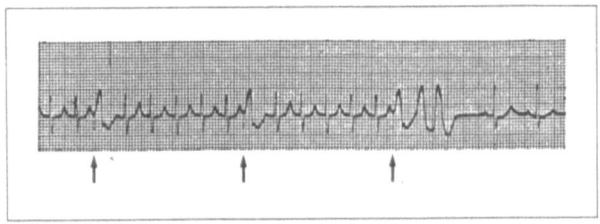

216

1. General rhythm information:

Spontaneous/paced rhythm outside tachycardia episodes.
Other arrhythmias (premature beats etc.).

2. Tachycardia classification:

Tachycardia rate.
A-V relationship.

3. Tachycardia prevention data:

Number of tachycardias.
Onset of the tachycardia.

4. Tachycardia treatment data:

Total duration of the tachycardia.
Most efficient termination program.
Number of unsuccessful programs.
Unsuccessful programs that triggered a different arrhythmia.
Successful programs that triggered a different, transient, arrhythmia.
Items 2, 3 and 4 should be repeated for every type of tachycardia.

How should the information be stored?

All of the information summarised above can be stored by means of counters and time interval data. The frequency of read-out of the counters will define their size, thus giving the option of having either a simple cumulative storage between two follow-ups or a more precise survey over a given period of time with preset intervals, for example: the last 24 hours in 24 sections of one hour for all data. The RAM memory capacity now available allows enough space for this kind of data processing and storage.

Storage of data in this way does present some inconvenience due to the fact that the information available is only a number of events or a time interval between detected cardiac activities. Proper interpretation of such information supposes that detection algorhythm of the stored event is reliable and does not accept any false positive or false negative counts. For correct analysis of the data concerning the onset of the tachycardia or the behaviour of the arrhythmia after delivery of a stimulation program, a recording of several cycles by means of interval time and A-V relation may not always be sufficient.

As mentioned earlier, direct storage of the intracardiac ECG would require a large memory. A compromise could possibly be reached by using sophisticated algorhythms in the pulse generator which process the intracardiac ECG and store, in addition to the interval time and A-V relationship, the type of rhythm concerned.

Conclusion

The Holter functions of an antitachycardia pulse generator should be oriented towards optimalisation of the prevention and the treatment of tachycardia, which can be used by the physician and also by the pulse generator itself. For this purpose, the data stored should include information concerning the onset of the tachycardia, its termination, possible rhythm complications due to the treatment, and the efficiency of the treatment itself. We have now arrived at a stage where sufficient RAM capacity can be made available, but this is of no use unless we also develop sophisticated algorhythms in order to be able to concentrate the information and optimise the recognition of arrhythmias. In this respect an increase in the ROM capacity and in the speed of microprocessors seems to be more important than a pure RAM capacity increase.

Finally it should be mentioned that any Holter pulse generator requires a fast and sophisticated communication system in order to handle the large amount of information in a simple and efficient way.

Authors' address:
Mr. Bernard Candelon
Product Manager
Vitatron Medical B.V.
Kanaalweg 24
P.O. Box 76
NL-6950 AB Dieren
The Netherlands

Antitachycardia Pacemakers – an Overview

A. W. Nathan*

Summary: A number of different methods of terminating tachycardia, using pacemakers, are available. These include underdrive, overdrive and the extrastimulus method. All have their complications, and the correct system must be chosen and carefully evaluated in each individual case. Advances in technology will expand the available range of devices.

Although early work in pacing concentrated on treating bradyarrhythmias, pacing has been used in the treatment of tachycardias. Initially it was used to prevent tachyarrhythmias by increasing the heart rate or by modifying the activation sequence.

Generally however, pacemakers have been more useful for tachycardia termination than prevention. In 1963 Moe et al. (1) described experimental intra AV nodal tachycardia in a canine model and noted that this arrhythmia could be terminated by single extrastimuli. Although paired pulse pacing had been used to control heart rate in arrhythmias by Chardack et al. (2), Haft et al. (3) are accredited with the first report of terminating an arrhythmia in man using pacing techniques, when they described the use of rapid atrial pacing to terminate atrial flutter. In the same year, Durrer et al. (4) described the use of premature beats for the same purpose. In 1968, Lister et al. (5) described the use of overdrive pacing to treat a variety of different arrhythmias, Hunt et al. (6) described the use of underdrive pacing for terminating a junctional tachycardia as well as atrial flutter, and Ryan et al. (7) described the use of a permanent demand pacemaker, together with a magnet to convert the pacemaker to fixed rate, for termination of a junctional tachycardia, again using the underdrive principle. Since then many different modes have been devised and used for antitachycardia pacing, but all fall into one of three basic categories.

Underdrive

Underdrive pacemakers deliver fixed rate (asynchronous) pacing during tachycardia at a rate less than that of tachycardia. In theory, therefore, a single stimulus is delivered throughout the tachycardia cycle which may, if it happens to be correctly timed, penetrate the circuit and effect tachycardia termination. Permanent pacemakers of two main types have been used for underdrive pacing. A conventional demand pacemaker may be patient or physician activated by the use of a magnet which converts the pacemaker to fixed rate (7), or an automatic unit may be used. Automatic underdrive systems include the upside-down pacemaker without bradycardia support (8), and dual-demand pace-

---

* Supported by the British Heart Foundation.

makers which have additional bradycardia back-up (9). Underdrive pacemakers should, in theory, deliver a series of single stimuli that occur throughout the tachycardia cycle (6). However, if tachycardia and pacing rates are harmonically related or if tachycardia is reset by paced beats and synchronised to the pacing rate, the tachycardia termination window may be missed. Stimulation may occur in the vulnerable period and unwanted and possibly more dangerous arrhythmias may be initiated. In addition, a single stimulus may be insufficient to penetrate the tachycardia circuit and may fail to terminate the tachycardia, even if the best practical electrode position is chosen (10).

Overdrive

Overdrive pacemakers allow capture of progressively more tissue until the tachycardia focus or circuit is penetrated, entrained and disrupted. It is a very effective form of tachycardia reversion (10), but very rapid rates may be necessary which can lead to the induction of more dangerous arrhythmias (11), or may cause haemodynamic embarrassment.
The earliest pacemakers of this type were radiofrequency systems, which consisted of an implantable inductive coil and electrode together with an external transmitter which is either patient or physician operated (12, 13). Similar units that require two-way communication for confirmation of tachycardia have been described, and recently fully implantable automatic units have been used (14). Older implantable burst pacemakers were non-adaptive, but newly available devices have adaptive capabilities.

Extrastimulus

In order to refine the underdrive technique and provide an adaptive system that was unlikely to cause haemodynamic deterioration or unwanted arrhythmias, Spurrell introduced the scanning extrastimulus pacemaker in 1975 (15). The tachycardia cycle is systematically scanned with one or two extrastimuli until tachycardia termination is achieved. Initially an external pacemaker connected to exteriorised permanent electrodes was used (15), but Critelli et al. (16) then introduced an external stimulator controlling, and communicating with, an implanted receiver using a radiofrequency link. More recently a fully implantable automatic system has been described (17).
Electrode position may be critical as theoretically the electrode should be positioned "on circuit". This is frequently not possible, particularly in patients with left sided accessory pathways. Although coronary sinus pacing may be used in such patients, pacing thresholds tend to be high and sensing is complicated by the complexity of the coronary sinus electrogram. Even in patients with junctional arrhythmias, right ventricular stimulation is frequently more effective than right atrial pacing (10), but is potentially more dangerous.
Stimulation in the vulnerable period may be responsible for the initiation of unwanted arrhythmias. The tendency to provoke such arrhythmias is increased by the use of high pacing energies, by multiple stimuli, by drugs such as digoxin, by electrolyte disturbances and by the presence of associated cardiac pathology, such as ischaemic heart disease. The vulnerable period for fibrillation and for repetitive extrasystoles is adjacent to the absolute refractory period of the paced tissue and usually the tachycardia termination window also lies adjacent to this. To minimise the risk of unwanted arrhythmias, stimulation

220

should occur as far away as possible from this vulnerable period, and in the case of the extrastimulus pacemaker used by the author (17), this is partially accomplished by a simple arithmetic decremental scan using progressively shortening coupling intervals. Other types of scan have been described including the original incremental arithmetic scan used by Spurrell (15). Sowton et al. (18) have described the geometric "hunting" scan and Vallin et al. (19) have suggested the centrifugal geometric scan, both of which have been designed to reduce the number of interventions required to find the termination window but their practical benefit has yet to be demonstrated. Under different conditions all these forms of scan may cause stimulation in the vulnerable period and the ideal method of scanning has yet to be determined.

In an effort to minimise the risks of closely coupled stimulation, the principles of both extrastimulus and burst pacing were combined by Nathan et al. (20) in the concertina method. This is a pacing mode using a small number of stimuli (usually up to seven), in which all pacing intervals are equal, including the initial coupling interval. If tachycardia is not terminated, all intervals decrement by a similar amount (for example six ms), until tachycardia is reverted. A relationship has been shown between the maximum effective coupling interval and the number of stimuli delivered – prescription of more stimuli allows the use of longer pacing intervals.

A totally automatic, completely implantable pacing system has obvious advantages over others that require an external component such as a magnet, a radiofrequency transmitter or an electrically coupled control box. With these systems, an external device must be carried by the patient to be used when tachycardia is appreciated. As experienced by patients in this series, use of this external device can prove difficult if hypotension, agitation or confusion are induced by tachycardia. The use of such a box certainly may have psychological disadvantages, as external activators have proved both inconvenient and embarrassing to some of the patients. Delay always occurs when terminating an arrhythmia with a manual system, and this may allow the development of compensatory cardiovascular reflexes, which may tend to perpetuate the arrhythmia.

If an automatic device is used, bipolar sensing is essential as unipolar sensing may cause false triggering from interference by myopotential activity (21). There is some theoretical advantage in the use of unipolar cathodal pacing, because anodal contact in a bipolar electrode may be more likely to precipitate unwanted arrhythmias. However, techniques of combined bipolar sensing and unipolar pacing are being evolved to overcome this. With the recent availability of high performance silicone and polyurethane as insulation materials for pacing leads, active and passive fixation bipolar electrode catheters are being developed, particularly for atrial use, which should facilitate lead implantation.

Most current automatic systems rely on rate alone, or high rate and rate of onset, as the trigger for intervention. This may not allow discrimination between different types of tachycardia, whether pathological or physiological, and a number of more sophisticated techniques for tachycardia discrimination are under investigation.

Many patients with ventricular tachycardias are unsuitable for automatic tachycardia reversion pacemakers because of the possibility of fatal, pacemaker induced, degeneration of the arrhythmia. This possibility exists, even if exhaustive pre- and post-implantation testing is performed, as the majority of patients with ventricular tachycardia have either coronary artery disease or a cardiomyopathy, and both of these tend to be progressive conditions with changing haemodynamic and electrophysiological substrates. In such patients, physician activated units may be preferable for use only when resuscitation facilities are available. However, even if physician operation is chosen, there is still a risk of spontaneous degeneration into ventricular fibrillation prior to pacemaker activation because of the inevitable delay in implementing therapy – the implantable defibrillator (or at least a device with defibrillation as a back-up) may offer a better alternative in patients with ventricular tachycardia.

Different patients have different electrophysiological substrates for their arrhythmias which require different methods of termination. There is a need for careful pre-implantation studies to define the mode of tachycardia termination which is most successful and which is most free from risk. However, even with careful studies requirements for tachycardia termination may change with time, but future advances in technology should help to overcome this problem by providing almost infinite flexibility within an implantable device.

Indications for permanent antitachycardia pacing now include the following:

1) arrhythmias refractory to medical or surgical treatment;
2) as an alternative to drug or surgical treatment in:
    A) patients with infrequent bouts of debilitating tachycardia
    B) women wishing to become pregnant who do not wish to be exposed to the teratogenic risk of drugs
    C) patients with poor ventricular function, which may be further impaired by antiarrhythmic agents, and in whom surgical therapy may carry a prohibitive risk
    D) patients with side effects from otherwise effective treatment;
3) possibly as treatment of first choice in many others.

Thus with advances in technology providing both flexibility and the possibility of using more complex and effective recognition and termination algorithms and with the encouraging clinical experience gained so far, antitachycardia pacing promises to be a major therapeutic option for large numbers of patients with a wide range of tachyarrhythmias.

References

1. Moe GK, Cohen W, Vick RL (1963) Experimentally induced paroxysmal A-V nodal tachycardia in the dog: a "case report". Am Heart J 65: 87
2. Chardack WM, Gage AA, Dean DC (1964) Slowing of the heart by paired pulse pacemaking. Am J Cardiol 14: 374
3. Haft JI, Kosowsky BD, Lau SH, Stein E, Damato AN (1967) Termination of atrial flutter by rapid electrical pacing of the atrium. Am J Cardiol 20: 239
4. Durrer D, Schoo L, Schuilenburg RM, Wellens HJJ (1967) The role of premature beats in the initiation and the termination of supraventricular tachycardia in the Wolff-Parkinson-White syndrome. Circulation 36: 644
5. Lister JW, Cohen LS, Bernstein WH, Samet P (1968) Treatment of supraventricular tachycardias by rapid atrial stimulation. Circulation 38: 1044
6. Hunt NC, Cobb FR, Waxman MB, Zeft HJ, Peter RH, Morris JJ Jr. (1968) Conversion of supraventricular tachycardias with atrial stimulation: evidence for re-entry mechanisms. Circulation 38: 1060
7. Ryan GF, Easley RM, Zaroff LI, Goldstein S (1968) Paradoxical use of a demand pacemaker in treatment of supraventricular tachycardia due to the Wolff-Parkinson-White syndrome: observation on termination of reciprocal rhythm. Circulation 38: 1037
8. Fisher JD, Furman S (1978) Automatic termination of tachycardia by an implanted "upside down" demand pacemaker. Clin Res 26: 231A
9. Krikler D, Curry P, Buffet J (1976) Dual-demand pacing for reciprocating atrioventricular tachycardia. Br Med J 1: 1114

10. Ward DE, Camm AJ, Spurrell RAJ (1979) The response of regular re-entrant supraventricular tachycardia to right heart stimulation. PACE 2: 586
11. Fisher JD, Mehra R, Furman S (1978) Termination of ventricular tachycardia with bursts of rapid ventricular pacing. Am J Cardiol 41: 94
12. Iwa T, Abe H, Sugiki K, Wada J (1970) Treatment of supraventricular tachycardia with inductive radiofrequency atrial stimulation. Progress in Medicine 74: 372
13. Fruehan CT, Meyer JA, Klie JH, Johnson LW, Obeid AI, Smulyan H, Eich RH (1974) Refractory paroxysmal supraventricular tachycardia: treatment with patient controlled permanent radio frequency atrial pacemaker. Am Heart J 87: 229
14. Griffin JC, Mason JW, Calfee RV (1980) Clinical use of an implantable automatic tachycardia-terminating pacemaker. Am Heart J 100: 1093
15. Spurrell RAJ (1975) Artificial cardiac pacemakers. In: Krikler DM, Goodwin JF (eds) Cardiac arrhythmias: the modern electrophysiological approach. WB Saunders, London, p 238
16. Critelli G, Grassi G, Chiariello M, Perticone F, Adinolfi L, Condorelli M (1979) Automatic "scanning" by radiofrequency in the longterm electrical treatment of arrhythmias. PACE 2: 289
17. Nathan AW, Camm AJ, Bexton RS, Hellestrand KJ, Spurrell RAJ (1982) Initial experience with a fully implantable, programmable, scanning, extrastimulus pacemaker for tachycardia termination. Clin Cardiol 5: 22
18. Sowton E, Elmqvist H, Hard af Segerstad C (1981) Two years' clinical experience with a self-searching tachycardia pacemaker. Am J Cardiol 47: 476
19. Vallin H, Hard af Segerstad C, Insulander P, Edhag O, Lagergren H (1983) Centrifugal geometrical scanning – an alternative concept in pacemaker treatment of tachycardias. PACE 6: A-14
20. Nathan A, Hellestrand K, Bexton R, Nappholz T, Spurrell R, Camm J (1982) Clinical evaluation of an adaptive tachycardia intervention pacemaker with automatic cycle length adjustment. PACE 5: 201
21. Hauser RG (1982) Bipolar leads for cardiac pacing in the 1980s: a reappraisal provoked by skeletal muscle interference. PACE 5: 34

Author's address:
Dr. A. W. Nathan
Department of Cardiology
St Bartholomew's Hospital
West Smithfield
London EC1A 7BE
England

Value and Limitations of the DPG-1 Pacemaker Anti-Arrhythmic Functions*⁾

G. Fontaine, R. Frank, J. L. Tonet, F. Fillette, and Y. Grosgogeat

Summary: The DPG-1 software pacemaker has some anti-arrhythmic functions. The report presents a new approach for the prevention of ventricular arrhythmias, based on a special lead arrangement used in combination with the "dynamic overdrive" function. One atrial lead is used for atrial pacing and sensing, a ventricular lead is used for ventricular sensing without ventricular pacing, because of the incorporation of a relatively high resistor. These two leads are connected to the output of the DPG-1 pacemaker. It is therefore possible to sense both atrium and ventricle and to pace the atrium only, as demonstrated by programming in the "triggered mode". It is therefore working in a "ADT" mode. After this, the pacemaker is reprogrammed in the inhibited "ADI" mode.

Prevention of extrasystole is performed by using the internal "dynamic overdrive" function. When the DPG-1 is normally connected to a single ventricular lead, a premature ventricular contraction leads to a premature pacing stimulus. With our particular arrangement a premature ventricular contraction leads to a premature atrial pacing stimulus which inhibits the appearance of a new extrasystole.

The software pacemaker is basically constituted by a microprocessor associated with random access memory (RAM), read only memory (ROM), and input/output circuits.

RAM memory enables the device to receive, store and erase data as often as required (1). These memories are therefore very flexible but have the disadvantage of a relatively limited capacity and relatively high energy consumption. RAMs can be erased intentionally by reprogramming or accidentally for example by a power failure. ROM memories contain prerecorded instructions which are fixed and cannot be changed. Their storage capacity is greater and they consume less electrical current than RAM (2, 3).

In addition, software pacemakers also have electronic circuitry designed to relay instruction of the external world to and from the microprocessor. The former include the sensing circuit for the detection of endocardial potentials, their amplification and analysis before introduction to the microprocessor's input circuit.

In laboratory oriented computers, signal analysis is usually carried out with an analogic/digital converter which rapidly digitilises the analogical signal for treatment. This solution is not yet available for use within a pacemaker. Conversion would have to be rapid and not require as much energy. Special electronic circuitry has therefore been developed which only analyses certain parts of the signal.

The latter basic circuit includes the output electronic circuitry which generates the electrical impulse based on data affecting impulse morphology, amplitude, duration, etc... for transmission to the pacing electrodes.

---

*⁾ Supported in part by grants from: Centre de Recherche sur les Maladies Cardiovasculaires de l'Association Claude Bernard.

The internal function of this type of pacemaker therefore depends on a set of instructions or programme which causes the microprocessor to react according to the different parameters contained in its ROM and also to certain data stored in its RAM. The larger the amount of data in the RAM, the greater the possibilities of "reprogramming", i. e. of changing the instructions influencing the microprocessor's function.

The theoretical main advantage of this new approach is to increase programmability, telemetry and modes of function. The most important characteristic is the possibility of changing the basic modes of function of the pacemaker by introducing new instructions into the RAM externally. These could be entirely different from those with which the pacemaker was originally programmed, providing the same organs of input and output are used (i.e. recording of endocavitary potentials and output of electrical impulses). For example, the DPG-1 can function like a conventional pacemaker but it could also theoretically be programmed to pace according to variations of the paced QT interval (adaptation to exercise). Although the DPG-1 pacemaker has not yet attained, practically speaking, this level of performance, it is, as far as we know, the most advanced unit of its type. To date, it has not been possible for reasons of safety and size of memory to construct an implantable pacemaker capable of changing its basic programme of function. However, advances in microchip technology have enabled the DPG-1 to be equipped with new anti-arrhythmic functions. Some of these functions have been studied in 7 patients based on our experience of both clinical pacing and clinical electrophysiology at the Department of Rhythmology of Jean Rostand Hospital. These 7 cases were selected from a series of 52 patients implanted with a DPG-1 pacemaker in which the main indication was the treatment of bradycardias. However, some patients also had attacks of tachycardia which enabled us to evaluate the anti-tachycardia function of this pacemaker.

"Automatic underdrive" function

This anti-arrhythmic function is based on the same principle as so-called "double demand" pacemakers in which the pacemaker functions in asynchronous rhythm when the spontaneous rhythm exceeds a given tachycardia limit, and also like an ordinary VVI pacemaker when the spontaneous cardiac rhythm is slower than the programmed pacemaker rhythm (4). This function has been improved in the DPG-1 pacemaker in that 1) the tachycardia rate which triggers the pacemaker, 2) the pacing rate after tachycardia detection and 3) the basal automatic rhythm can be programmed independently of each other.

An example of this mode of function is illustrated in Fig. 1, recorded after the implantation of the pacemaker in a patient presenting with attacks of narrow complex supraventricular tachycardia followed by sinus arrest giving rise to non-syncopal malaises suggesting the diagnosis of a "tachycardia-bradycardia syndrome" (5, 6). The ECG was recorded on a Hewlett-Packard 78225 computerised monitoring system. The "recall" function allows playback of abnormal variations of rhythm in 8 second strips from the disc memory. The ECG strip shows termination of a reciprocating tachycardia probably by the 7th pacemaker pulse. After a final atrial stimulation there is a pause followed by atrial pacing which prevents bradycardia due to the sinoatrial block.

Another example of the use of this function is shown in Fig. 2: this neurotonic patient had a WPW syndrome with attacks of reciprocating tachycardia related to a left posterior

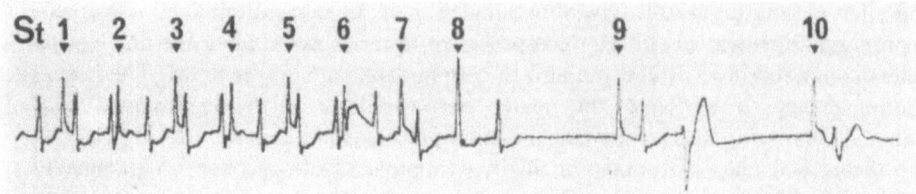

Fig. 1. Termination of a reciprocating SVT by the 7th atrial stimulation of the dynamic underdrive function of the DPG-1. Stimuli nos. 8 and 9 are eliciting a ventricular beat after an atrioventricular delay. However, due to the slow automatic pacemaker rhythm, a ventricular extrasystole arises. The supraventricular beat following stimulus no. 10 is probably a fusion between another idioventricular escape and the supraventricular activation. These extrasystoles will be easily suppressed by increasing the automatic rate.

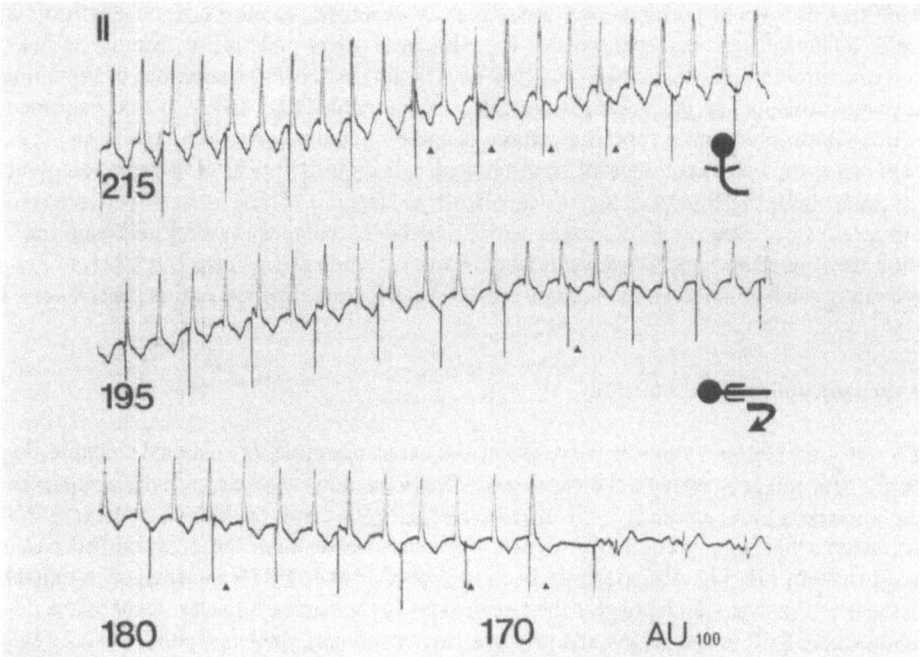

Fig. 2. SVT due to an intranodal reciprocating rhythm. The dynamic underdrive function in unable to terminate the episodes of tachycardia when the rhythm is relatively rapid (215 or 195/mn). On the other hand, when the patient lies down the rhythm of the tachycardia slows to 180 and then 170/mn and the arrhythmia is now terminated by the pacemaker. Arrows indicate the negative P waves during tachycardia.

paraseptal atrioventricular accessory pathway. The tachycardia rate varied with the patient's position mainly due to variations in the AV nodal conduction time (7). When standing, the tachycardia rate was 215/mn. Stimulation via a permanent right atrial pacing catheter was unable to terminate the attacks. This was also the case when the patient was sitting down despite a slower rhythm at 195/mn. When the patient lay down the tachycardia slowed to 180 and then 170/mn and underdrive pacing was able to terminate the attacks, and take over atrial command for 1 cycle before return to sinus rhythm.

This example illustrates the important role of the autonomic nervous system in terminating attacks of tachycardia which were psychologically very poorly tolerated in this young and active woman. It also demonstrates that several stimuli are sometimes required to terminate the arrhythmia. This was also poorly tolerated given the relatively rapid tachycardia rhythm. The arrhythmia became progressively more frequent with time (several attacks per day) and although the pacemaker always ended up by terminating the arrhythmia (in the recumbent position) the patient herself requested surgical interruption of the accessory pathway. This case also illustrates the variability of the conduction properties of the nodo-hisian pathway related to changes in sympathetic and parasympathetic tone. This probably explains the variation of 30 beats per minute of the tachycardia rhythm in this case.

Generally speaking, at a rhythm of over 200/mn, the time interval during which a stimulus would be effective is reduced. Therefore, it is important but sometimes difficult to position the pacing catheter as close as possible to the pathway of the circus movement. Another method is to use a burst of rapid stimulations to shorten the refractory periods of the paced zone. Beta blocker drugs can also be used to lengthen the period during which pacing could be effective. This was attempted in this patient but the secondary bradycardia and hypotensive effects of the drug during sinus rhythm were poorly tolerated and was not a practical solution.

Flywheel function

This function is designed to prevent abrupt variations in the decrease of cardiac rhythm. The principle is illustrated in Fig. 3. The central part of the diagram represents the spontaneous tachyarrhythmia which stops suddenly, the heart rate falling from 110 to 70/mn. This may be uncomfortable for the patient, especially if the basal rhythm is slower than that illustrated here. In these conditions the flywheel function will lead to the pacemaker taking over command at the termination of the tachycardia and progressively slowing the rate until the spontaneous basal rhythm is attained. The rate decrease is obtained by programming an increment of 1 to 10 ms to the preceding pacing cycle. Even when increments of 10 ms are used it takes several tens of seconds for the rhythm to return to the basal rate. In our opinion, this time is too long in most cases but the manufacturer has not yet been able to make the appropriate modifications.

This function is illustrated in Fig. 4. The patient had atrial extrasystoles which occasionally triggered atrial fibrillation. This event occurred in our case at an AAI pacing rate of 73/mn (period: 820 ms). The flywheel function is initiated and when an atrial extrasystole is detected, the pacemaker takes over command at a rhythm close to that determined by the preceding cycle, i.e. cycle length of 640 ms. The rate then slowly decreases with the pacing period increasing by 10 ms after each beat until the rhythm slows to the basal period of 820 ms.

Another example of the flywheel function used this time with ventricular pacing is shown in Fig. 5, in a patient with a regular ectopic atrial rhythm associated with single atrial extrasystoles and sometimes doublets. After programming the flywheel, an atrial extrasystole is detected with an interval of 390 ms between two consecutive ventricular com-

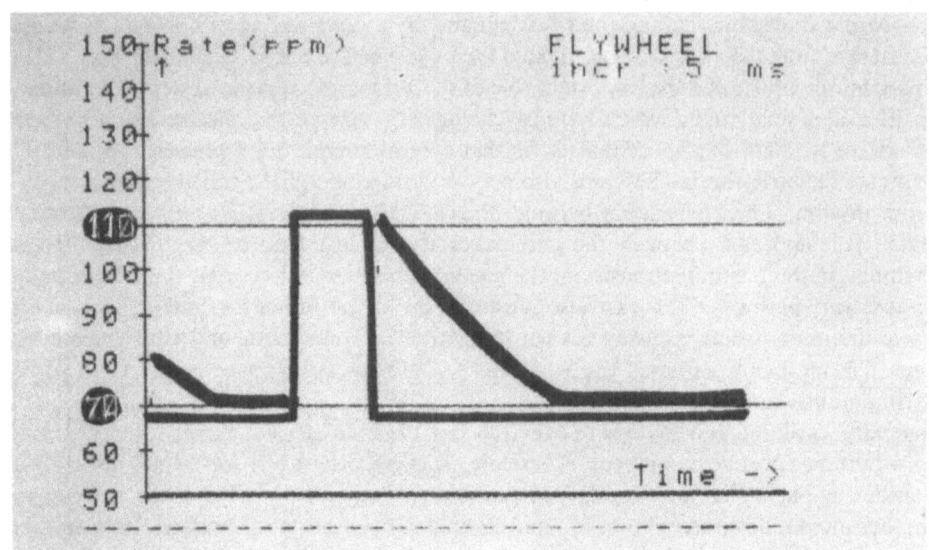

Fig. 3. Principle of the flywheel function. The patient's spontaneous rhythm is represented diagrammatically by the square graph and the curved and related line corresponds to pacemaker activity. After a sudden fall in the patient's rhythm the pacemaker takes over command and paces at a progressively slower rate until its programmed automatic rate is attained.

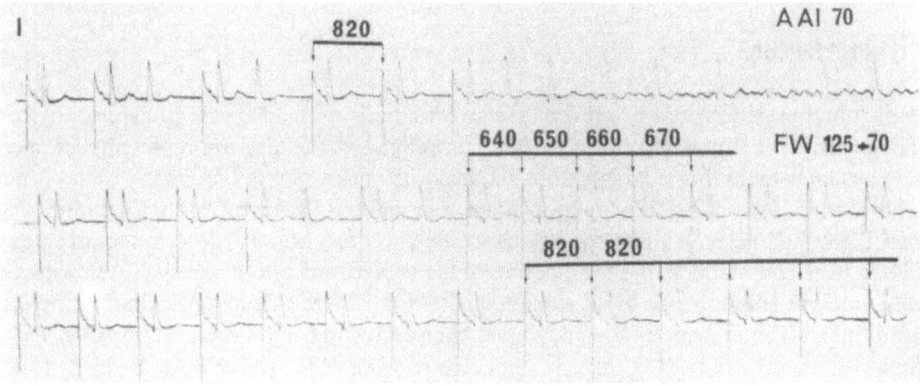

Fig. 4. Flywheel function in a patient with paroxysmal atrial fibrillation. The top strip shows the spontaneous initiation of atrial fibrillation by an atrial extrasystole. The middle strip shows two atrial extrasystoles shortening the cycle length. The second extrasystole triggers the flywheel function leading to temporary pacing at 125/mn (640 ms) followed by a progressive rate decrease until the basal period is attained (820 ms).

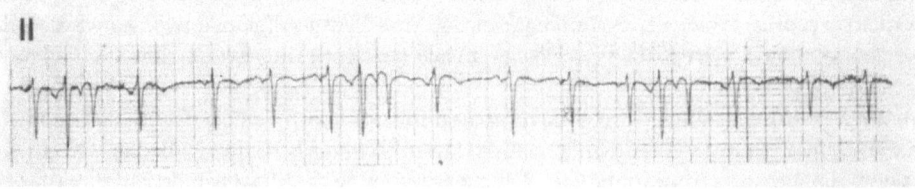

Fig. 5. A sequence of symptomatic atrial extrasystoles with 1/1 AV conduction.

228

plexes (Fig. 6). The pacemaker is triggered with an initial inter-spike interval of 488 ms. The rate then slowly decreases until the basal period is attained. Note that the interval between the ventricular complex following the atrial extrasystole and the first pacing artefact is 520 ms, i.e. longer than the first inter-spike interval. This is a normal property of the DPG-1 pacemaker. However, this relatively long diastolic period represents a sort of hysteresis which could favour the initiation of other arrhythmias. It would be better if the first interval after the extrasystole were 488 ms and not 520 ms. In the lower part of the same figure, two successive atrial extrasystoles are observed, the first of which triggers the flywheel function. The second extrasystole is not detected because of the pacemaker postdetection refractory period, despite being programmed at its lowest value (250 ms).

A rapid spontaneous rhythm could inhibit the pacemaker in flywheel function. However, at the detection of a long diastolic period, the pacemaker is triggered not in its automatic spontaneous rhythm but in the flywheel function (Fig. 7). In other words, the flywheel function, masked when the patient's spontaneous rhythm is faster than that of the flywheel rhythm, reappears after a relatively long diastole. This would seem to be a useful property especially in atrial pacing.

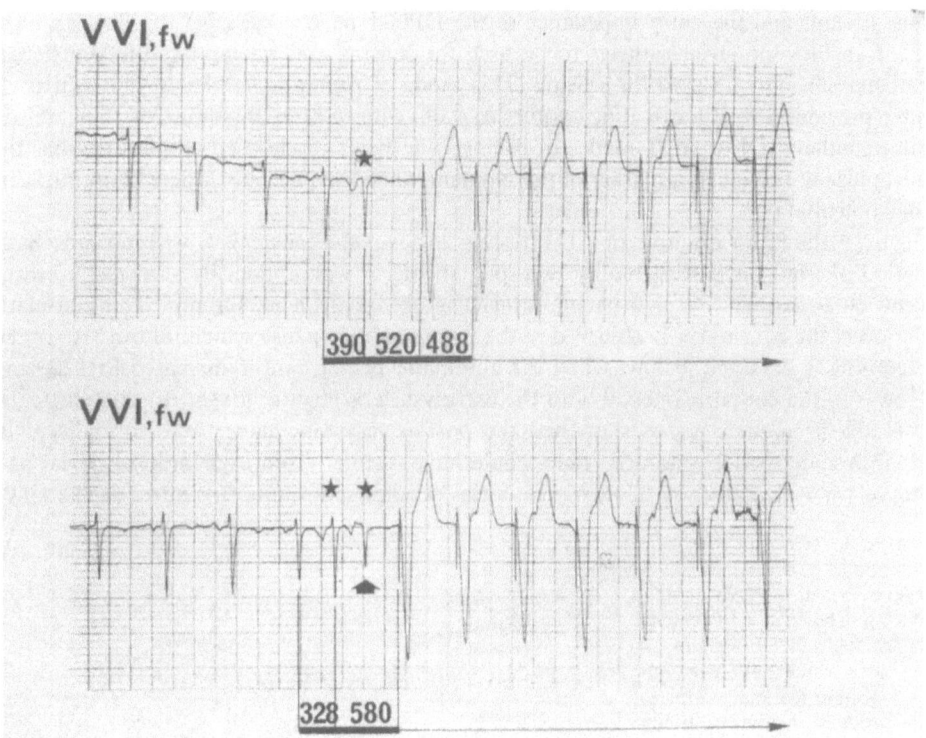

Fig. 6. Same patient as Fig. 5. Above: Triggering of the flywheel function after detection of the first atrial extrasystole underlined by a star leading to a faster rate of ventricular pacing before reversion to the pacemaker's automatic rhythm. Note that the 1st cycle following the extrasystole is inappropriately longer than the fast cycle of the flywheel function. Below: Two successive atrial extrasystoles. The first is sensed normally but the second is not detected. Therefore a better than expected flywheel function is obtained.

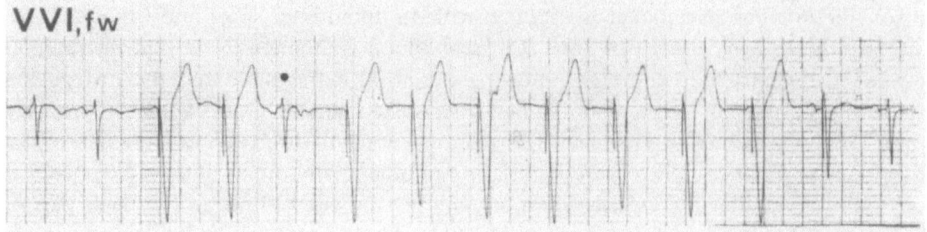

VVI,fw

Fig. 7. A premature supraventricular beat (point) temporarily inhibiting the pacemaker which restarts at the flywheel function period.

"Dynamic overdrive" function

We used this function in a special mode of pacing relaying the pacemaker to two endo-cavitary catheters, one in the atrium and the other in the ventricle but including a resistance in series with the latter with a value of 2 KOhms determined by the predicted rise in threshold of the electrode, the impedance measured with the endocardial lead selected for this attempt and the entry impedance of the DPG-1 pacemaker (Fig. 8). This arrangement enables the atrial catheter to be used for sensing and pacing but the ventricular catheter can only be used for sensing. This mode of pacing is similar to that which we have previously used for treating another case of ventricular extrasystoles (8). This set-up allows either ADI or ADT modes of pacing. The latter mode used temporarily has the advantage of serving as a marker of the moment when the pacemaker detects an intracar-diac potential (9).

Figure 9 shows an example of ADT pacing. Above, the pacemaker with an automatic period of 1480 ms is triggered by two spontaneous P waves, then by a correctly sensed ventricular extrasystole as a pacing artefact is observed on its summit. The automatic period of the pacemaker is observed in the compensatory pause which follows. A similar recording is obtained (below) when the automatic pacing rate is increased to 1200 ms. However, the coupling interval with the extrasystole is slightly longer. In this particular case the programming has shortened the post-extrasystolic pause and normalised the rhythm under better conditions than would have resulted from asynchronous atrial pacing or from the detection of retrograde atrial depolarisation after a ventricular extrasys-

Fig. 8. Set-up of ADI or ADT pacing. The atrial and ventricular pacing catheters are connected to the same pulse generator. A 2 KOhm resistance is placed in series with the ventricular pacing lead.

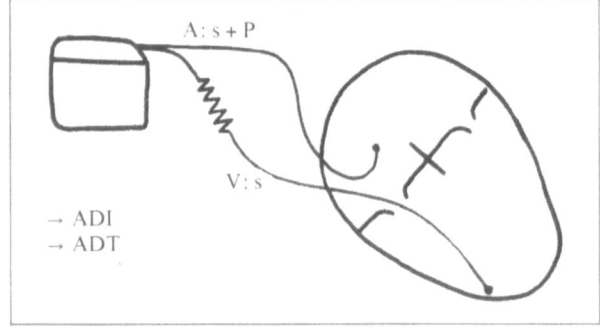

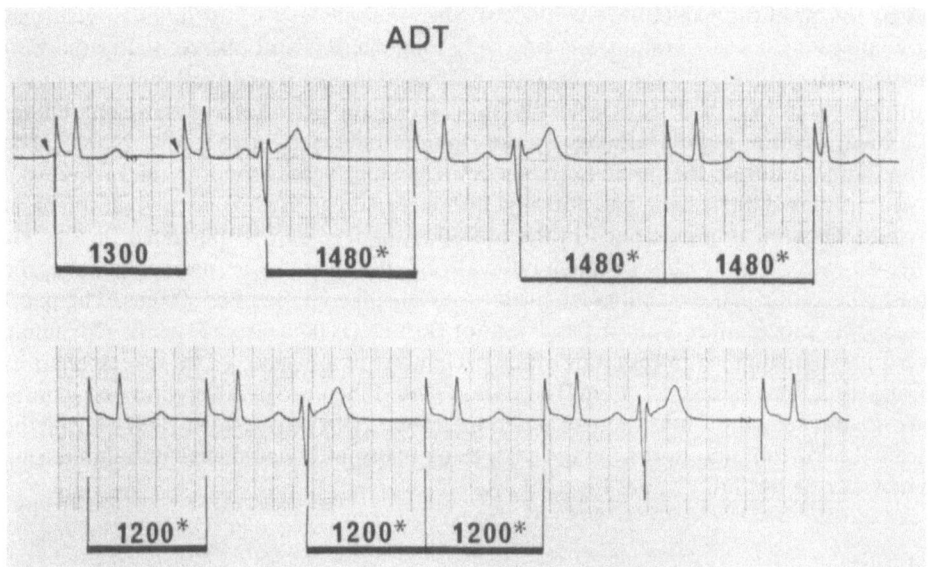

Fig. 9. DPG-1 functioning in ADT mode. Below: The pacemaker automatic period is 1200 ms. A ventricular extrasystole is correctly sensed and, as the pacemaker is programmed in the trigger mode, the spike falls on the QRS complex. Above: The pacemaker has now been programmed to a slower automatic rate (1480 ms). The first two spikes fall at the onset of spontaneous P waves separated by a basal sinus cycle of 1300 ms. The P waves have therefore been correctly detected.

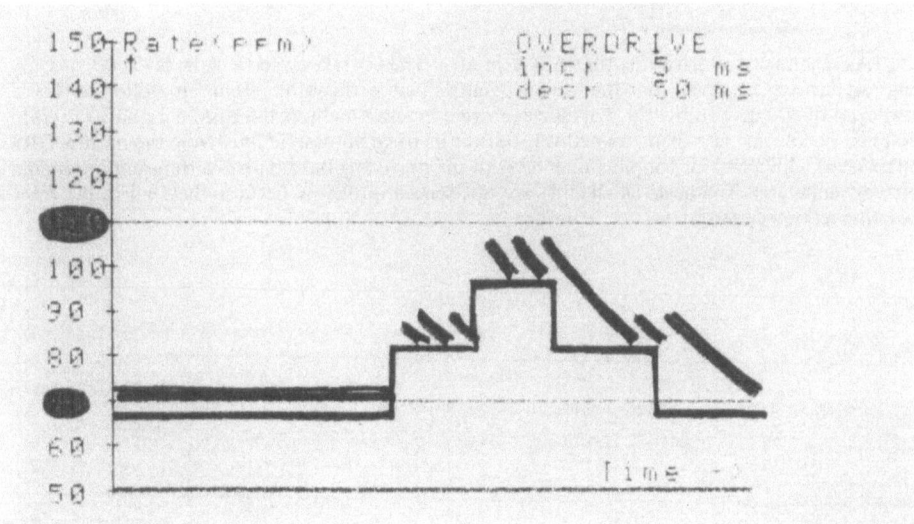

Fig. 10. Principle of the dynamic overdrive function of the DPG-1 pacemaker. The square lines represent the patient's spontaneous rhythm and the oblique lines indicate pacemaker function. The pacemaker reacts to every increment of the spontaneous rate by an even faster rate and finally decreases until the initial automatic rate is finally obtained. Therefore, the permanent rate acceleration imposed by the pacemaker only stops when the arrhythmia disappears, then the pacemaker reverts to its automatic rhythm.

tole by the atrial catheter (10). Nevertheless, when the sequence of the different ventricular complexes is closely examined, a relatively long pause is still observed after the ventricular extrasystole. To decrease this interval, the "dynamic overdrive" function is used as illustrated in Fig. 10. The patient's rhythm is schematically represented by square lines as a basal rhythm, a moderate tachycardia rhythm and a fast tachycardia rhythm. The oblique lines indicate the pacemaker function showing that as soon as the tachycardia rhythm is sensed, the pacing rate is always faster providing that it is faster than the basal rhythm. This function is applied in the preceding patient and is illustrated in Fig. 11. After an extrasystole with a coupling interval of 1000 ms with the preceding spike, the post-extrasystolic pause is shortened, the next atrial spike falling after 800 ms. The pacemaker was programmed with a basal rate of 60/mn (1000 ms) and so the "dynamic overdrive" function led to triggering of the pacemaker at a period of 200 ms less than its basal period, that is to say *800 ms*. The pacing period then progressively increases, unrelated to the premature beat (asterisk) and to undetected late extrasystoles (NS) slowing the pacemaker rhythm until it reaches the basal rate of 60/mn. It would have been interesting to increase the flexibility of this function by:

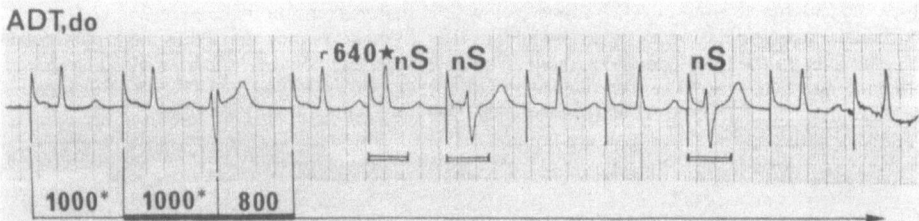

Fig. 11. Dynamic overdrive in the ADT mode. The basal cycle length is 1000 ms. A pacing artefact is observed on the sensed ventricular extrasystole. This is followed by a shorter cycle of 800 ms because the dynamic overdrive function reduces the basal pacemaker rhythm by 200 ms. The pacing rate then progressively falls to its basal automatic rate. Note the narrow QRS complex (star) with a 640 ms coupling interval with the preceding beat. This is a transient intranodal reentry phenomenon. The beats labelled nS are not sensed, probably because they fall in the post-stimulation refractory period.

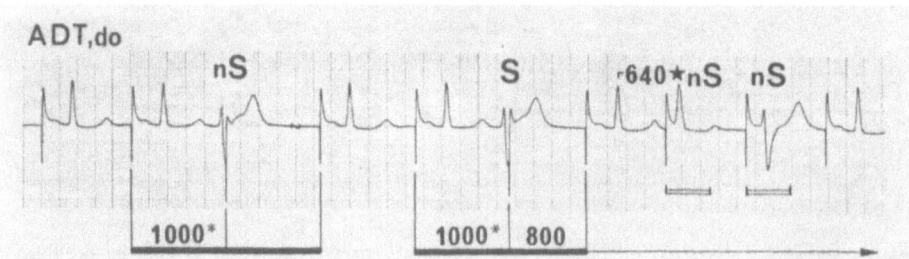

Fig. 12. The pacemaker automatic rate is still 1000 ms. The first ventricular extrasystole is not sensed because it is a little too late. The dynamic overdrive function is not initiated. However, the next extrasystole arises slightly earlier (note the slight difference in the shape of the QRS) and triggers dynamic overdrive with the same events at the beginning as described in Fig. 11.

232

- Increasing the range of programmable values of this interval.
- Having the option of adapting the coupling interval of the first pacemaker spike to the extrasystolic coupling interval as in the orthorhythmic pacemaker (11–13).
- Having the option of introducing a mathematical relation (possibly non-linear) between the coupling interval of the ventricular extrasystole and the premature stimulation.

The recording in Fig. 12 shows (right) an identical sequence to that shown in Fig. 11. However, on the left, a relatively late pacemaker escape complex at its automatic period is observed. In fact, the ventricular extrasystole was not sensed by the pacemaker which takes over command with an interval of 1000 ms corresponding to its own period. The spike on this complex corresponds simply to a pseudo-fusion phenomenon and not to a triggered stimulation.

Figure 13 shows the behaviour of the pacemaker whose basal rhythm has now been adjusted to 920 ms. After a supraventricular extrasystole (centre) a coupling interval of 759 ms is observed: this is unusual as one would have expected an interval of 920–200 ms =

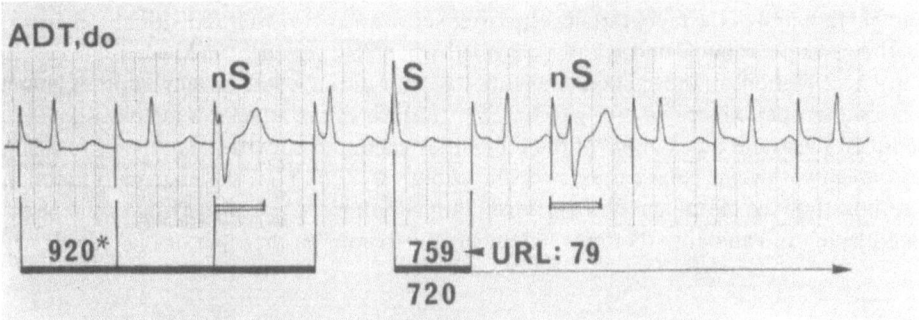

Fig. 13. The basal period of the pacemaker has been shortened to 920 ms. After the extrasystole (S) dynamic overdrive is initiated, not with a coupling interval of 720 ms as expected (920-200 ms) but with a longer period of 759 ms. This value corresponds to the upper rate limit (URL) which was programmed at 79/mn (= 759 ms).

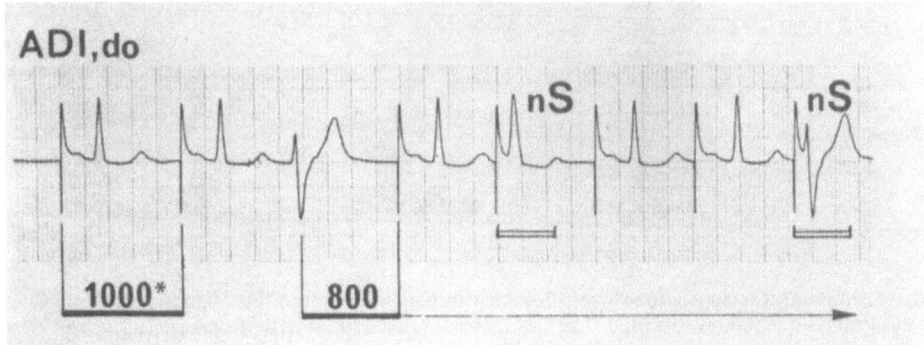

Fig. 14. The pacemaker has now been programmed in the ADI, do mode. Note disappearance of the marker spike on the ventricular extrasystole, but the dynamic overdrive functions as before.

720 ms. However, the value of the upper limit of the "dynamic overdrive" function which had been programmed at 79/mn has to be taken into consideration. This rate corresponds exactly to 759 ms. The sequence of progressive lengthening of the interspike intervals is respected thereafter.

Figure 14 shows the same function of this pacemaker in the ADI mode. In this mode, the ventricular extrasystole is no longer marked by the presence of the triggered spike.

Histogram function

The DPG-1 pacemaker possesses the unique property of analysing the spontaneous ventricular complexes with respect to time and of constructing a distribution histogramme. In addition, the user has the choice of each of the histogram window, expressed directly in beats/minute. In Fig. 15, this function was used over an 18 hour period in a patient with a spontaneous rhythm of 70 to 118/mn, corresponding to the main peak of the histogram. However, she also had episodes of paroxysmal tachycardia which explain the presence of rates of 138 to 214/mn. As there was a clear difference between the rates of sinus rhythm and of the tachycardias, the latter show up as two well individualised peaks, but this is the exception and is only observed when the period of analysis is relatively short. Accelerations of the spontaneous sinus rhythm during exercise and emotion giving rise to shorter periods are naturally recorded with those of the attacks of tachycardia (9).

Figure 16 illustrates an example of the difficulties encountered with this type of function in a patient with ventricular extrasystoles in whom we tried to use the histogram function to demonstrate the effectiveness of anti-arrhythmic therapy. The comparison of the histogram before (top) and after (bottom) treatments (histogram on the right of Fig. 16) clearly

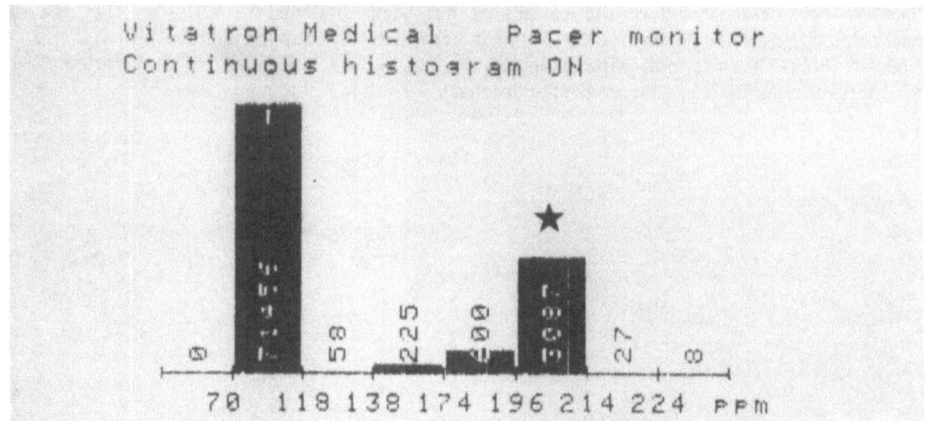

Fig. 15. Intranodal reciprocating rhythm recorded in patient in whom the diagnosis was confirmed by electrophysiological investigation. The rate increase related to the arrhythmia is clearly visible on the histogram situated in a range of 196 to 214/mn (star). However, this document is only valid for relatively short recording periods (about 8000 beats). During longer recording periods, variations of the sinus rhythm due to the influence of the autonomic nervous system may be recorded, confusing the results.

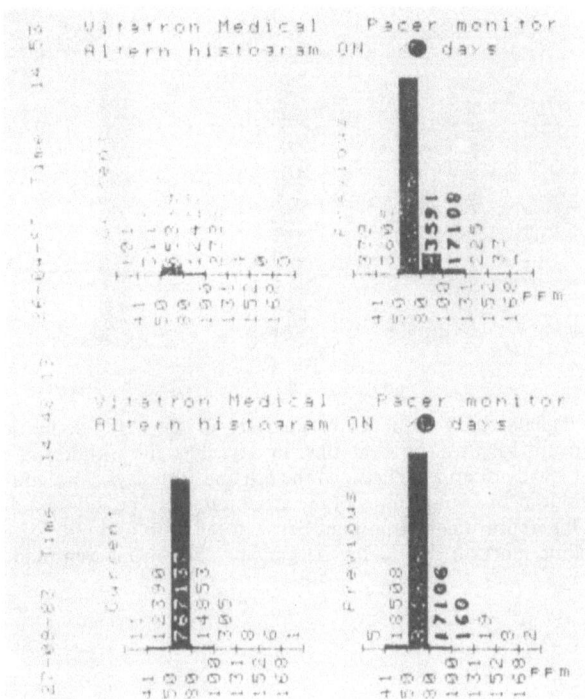

Fig. 16. Ventricular extrasystole before and after treatment. This figure illustrates the problems in evaluating the difference between two histograms.

shows a reduction of the columns corresponding to the short intervals. However, short intervals may also be due to accelerations of the sinus rhythm giving rise to appearances similar to those of the first histogram. In order to increase the value of this method there should be a system to discriminate between the spontaneous rhythm and extrasystoles, based on analysis of the width of QRS. Even so, bundle branch block widening the QRS could confuse the issue. A new solution to this problem has been found in dual software computerised pacemakers manufactured by the same company.

Analysis of a case of atrial fibrillation

The Holter function of the DPG-1 was used in a patient with the tachycardia-bradycardia syndrome to study paroxysmal atrial fibrillation using an atrial electrode. During atrial fibrillation, atrial potentials of sufficient amplitude and slope and intervals longer than the postdetection refractory periods are detected by the atrial electrode. The first histogram, Fig. 17 left, was recorded 5 days after withdrawal of digoxin. There are two main distributions, one corresponding to the spontaneous rhythm of 70 to 100/mn and the other to the atrial fibrillation with periods greater than 120/mn. Ten days later the shape of the histogram is quite different and the more rapid rates have almost disappeared with most rapid beats recorded between 100 and 120/mn. This change is thought to have been induced by the elimination of the digoxin which shortens the atrial refractory period and so favours shorter intervals during attacks of atrial fibrillation (14). The histogram re-

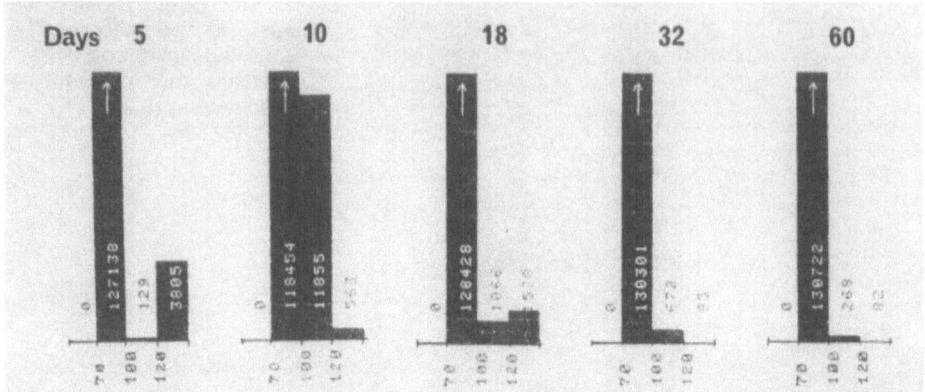

Fig. 17. Effects of withdrawal of digitalis in a patient by analysis of the "F" waves of paroxysmal atrial fibrillation. The horizontal figures show the time in days after the withdrawal of digitalis. A second peak at a fast rate gradually disappears between the 5th and 10th days. This could be due to the elimination of digitalis resulting in a lengthening of the atrial refractory periods and the suppression of the shortest periods. This improvement continues between the 18th and 60th days, probably because of better hemodynamic function due to the pacemaker normalising ventricular activity.

corded on the 18th, 32nd and 60th days show progressive disappearance of the shorter intervals. A gradual improvement in myocardial function could explain this evolution. The histogram function could therefore help the cardiologist in the choice and mode of administration of anti-arrhythmic therapy. However, in this case, difficulties were again encountered due to the relatively long post-detection refractory period even when programmed at its lowest value of 250 ms. Most of the f waves of the faster rhythm could have not been detected.

Conclusion

The DPG-1 pacemaker offers a wide choice of anti-arrhythmic functions, not only in ventricular but also in atrial pacing; its active intervention may prevent some arrhythmias, other pacing functions terminate attacks and it also provides quantitative data for the assessment of anti-arrhythmic therapy. These functions were demonstrated in a series of patients in which the indication for pacing was essentially the implantation of a multi-programmable pulse generator for the treatment of bradycardia. The episodes of tachycardia were associated with bradycardia in most cases and tachycardia alone was not the indication for pacemaker implantation. Nevertheless, the clear-cut advantages of a programmable pacemaker have been demonstrated, especially when designed in collaboration with clinicians who know how to extract the maximum performance from the potentially very rich functions of the device and when new functions can be entered non-invasively. In this field, the DPG-1 pacemaker represents a first step and a significant advance in the assessment and treatment of cardiac arrhythmias.

236

References

1. Gordon PL, Calfee RV, Baker RG (1982) Multiprogrammable pacemaker technology. In: The third decade of cardiac pacing, Barold SS, Mugica J (eds), Futura Publications, New York, P 127
2. Hartlaub J (1982) Pacemaker of the future: Microprocessor based on custom circuit? In: The third decade of cardiac pacing, Barold SS, Mugica J (eds), Futura Publications, New York, P 417
3. Buffet J, Meunier JF, Gautier JP, Jacquet JP (1982) Technology and reliability of microprocessor used in pacemaking. In: The third decade of cardiac pacing, Barold SS, Mugica J (eds), Futura Publications New York, P 429
4. Krikler DM, Curry P, Buffet J (1976) Dual-demand Pacing for reciprocating atrioventricular tachycardia. Br Med J: 1114–1116
5. Slama R, Waynberger M, Motte G, Bouvrain Y (1969) La maladie rythmique auriculaire. Etude clinique électrique et évolutive de 43 observations. Arch Mal Coeur 62: 297
6. Moss AJ, Davis RJ (1974) Brady-tachy syndrome. Progr Cardiovasc Dis 16: 439
7. Furman S, Fisher JD, Pannizzo F (1982) Necessity of signal processing in tachycardia detection. In: The third decade of cardiac pacing, Barold SS, Mugica J (eds), Futura Publications, New York, P 265
8. Fontaine G, Beneton H, Frank R, Guiraudon G, Grosgogeat Y, Facquet J (1975) Préventtion de la tachycardie ventriculaire après infarctus du myocarde par pacemaker intracorporel. Arch Mal Coeur 68: 961
9. Barnay C, Coste A, Medvedowski JL (1984) Stimulateur anti-arrhythmique a logiciel. Premiers résultats cliniques en stimulation auriculaire. Stimucoeur 12: 9
10. Langendorf R, Pick A, Winternitz M (1955) Mechanisms of intermittent ventricular bigeminy. I-Appearance of ectopic beats dependent upon the length of the ventricular cycle, the rule of bigeminy. Circulation 11: 422
11. Zacouto F, Guize L, Fontaine G, Gerbaux A (1974) Improved control of recurrent tachycardias by automatic orthorhythmic pacing. Circulation 50, Sup III: 226
12. Guize L, Zacouto F, Lenegre J (1971) Un nouveau stimulateur du coeur: le pacemaker orthorhythmique. Presse Med 79: 2071
13. Guize L, Zacouto B, Meilhac B, Le Pailleur C, Di Matteo J (1974) Stimulations endocardiaques orthorhythmiques. Intérêt diagnostique et therapeutique. Nouv Presse Med 3: 2083
14. Hordof AJ, Spotnitz A, Mary-Rabine L, Edie RN, Rosen MR (1978) The cellular electrophysiologic effects of digitalis on human atrial fibers. Circulation 57: 223

Authors' address:
Professor G. Fontaine
Service de Rhythmologie et de Stimulation Cardiaque
du Professeur Y. Grosgogeat
Hôpital Jean Rostand
39 rue Jean Le Galleu
94200 Ivry, France

237

Use of Flywheel, Automatic Underdrive and Dynamic Overdrive in Atrial Pacers

C. Barnay and J. L. Medvedowsky

Summary: Atrial pacing is now easy due to recent improvements in leads and pacers and microprocessor based pacers offer more flexible possibilities for antiarrhythmic stimulation. This paper reports preliminary results obtained with the Vitatron DPGl pacemaker in this field.

DPGl is a multiprogrammable pacemaker with analysis functions, Holter functions (premature beat counter, tachycardic episodes counter and cumulated duration of the accesses, inhibited and paced beats counter, number of inhibition to stimulation transitions) and three special pacing modes: automatic underdrive: (asynchronous pacing to stop reentry tachycardias); dynamic overdrive: (overdriving rate permanently adjusted to the underlying spontaneous rhythm of the patient); flywheel: (escape rhythm of the pacer permanently adjusted to the spontaneous rhythm of the patient).

These antiarrhythmic pacing modes were used in the following situations.

Intractable paroxysmal *junctional tachycardia* associated with severe sinus bradycardia: the patient was paced in the atrium to perform automatic underdrive interruption of the attacks of tachycardia. The result was excellent on the attacks but undesired detections of R and T waves led to false diagnosis of tachycardia and inappropriate automatic underdrive pacing, which finally initiated episodes of reciprocating tachycardia. This example illustrates some limitations of automatic underdrive pacing at the atrial level. However, although some difficulties of atrial sensing are not completely solved, some analysis functions of the DPGl, like the intracardiac signal amplitude measurement, allow more accurate positioning of the atrial lead.

Atrial extrasystoles: one patient was affected with near permanent atrial begemeny, intractable by drugs, with long compensatory cycles, involving exercise dyspnea and severe asthenia which disappeared when dynamic overdrive permitted to maintain a regular and not too rapid rate.

Sinus node dysfunction: in patients affected with sino atrial block or atrial extrasystoles the suppression of abrupt changes in the cycle length was obtained with flywheel pacing. Six patients had documented brady-tachy-syndrome; with flywheel pacing the episodes of tachycardia disappeared in 2 patients without additional drug treatment, whereas three patients needed additional antiarrhythmic drug treatment. Besides the haemodynamic advantages of atrial pacing in sinus node disease there is a possibility for the episodes of tachycardia to disappear after suppression of the bradycardia. Furthermore, flywheel pacing, by avoiding abrupt changes in the heart rhythm, which are supposed to favour discrepancies between refractory periods of adjacent fibers and induce arrhythmias, could significantly reduce the incidence of tachycardic episodes.

With the exception of AV block, the atrium is the key of many cardiac arrhythmias, both of the tachycardic and bradycardic types. Therefore, atrial pacing is a "new frontier" for pacemakers, now accessible due to recent improvements in the technology of leads and pacers (1). Furthermore, new special pacing modes, permitted by microprocessor based pacers, offer more flexible and varied possibilities for antiarrhythmic stimulation than former simple demand devices. This paper reports the preliminary results obtained with the Vitatron DPGl in this field.

Methodology

The DPGl is a microprocessor based pacer, whose programming is performed using the HP 85 desk computer. Special functions are available, including bidirectional telemetry,

Holter functions and antiarrhythmic modes. The programmable parameters include pacing frequency, impulse duration, output voltage, sensitivity (1 to 10 mV), hysteresis, sensing refractory period and pacing refractory period. This makes the pacer a good one for atrial pacing, as well as analysis functions (amplitude of the intracardiac signal, measurement of the critical impulse duration, of the voltage threshold and of the lead impedance). Furthermore, two particular features are especially useful for antiarrhythmic purposes:
– Holter functions
– Special pacing modes.

a) Holter functions

Four types of data can be obtained from the pacer through the HP 85 computer:
– Premature beat counter (with adjustable criteria of prematurity: 12.5 or 25%).
– Tachycardic episodes counter (over an adjustable rate threshold) and cumulated duration of the accesses.
– Inhibited and paced beats counter, also giving the number of inhibition to stimulation transitions.
– RR interval histograms, either continuous (recording data continuously) or alternate (two histograms, one active (recording current data for a period of time) the other inactive, keeping data from the preceding period). The duration of the cycle with the alternate histograms and the limits of the classes are adjustable by the user.
All the counters can be interrogated or reset to zero at any moment.

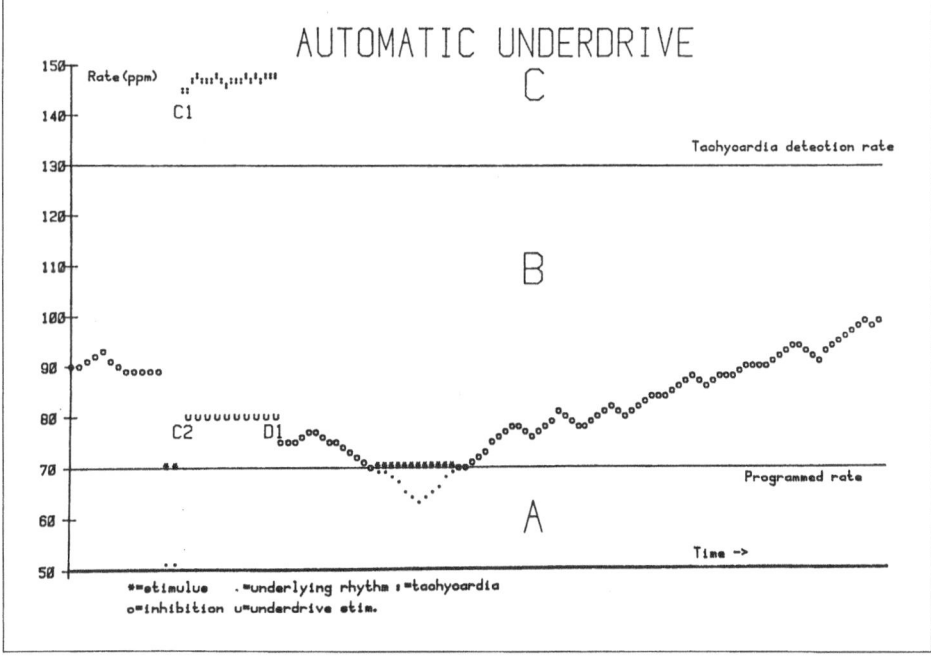

Fig. 1. See text.

b) Special pacing modes

Antiarrhythmic functions

Three antiarrhythmic modes can be activated: automatic underdrive, dynamic overdrive, and flywheel.

Automatic underdrive

With the automatic underdrive mode, if the spontaneous frequency of the patient exceeds a given value (tachycardia detection rate), an asynchronous pacing occurs at a rate (frequency of the tachycardia/2–10%) realizing a scanning of the cardiac cycle over 5 to 10 beats. In addition, usual demand pacing is still operating. Thus, three zones of frequency exist (Fig. 1): demand pacing (under the programmed rate) inhibition (between programmed rate and tachycardia detection rate) and automatic underdrive (above tachycardia detection rate). The asynchronous scanning pacing is capable of stopping reentry tachycardias rapidly.

Dynamic overdrive

Overdrive pacing is supposed to suppress the spontaneous rhythm of the patient by pacing well above his frequency, in order to avoid abrupt changes in the rhythm or extrasystoles.
This could lead to exceedingly rapid rates, not acceptable by the patient. On the other hand, with dynamic overdrive, the pacing rate is permanently adapted to the underlying spontaneous rhythm of the patient (Fig. 2). When a spontaneous beat occurs, the escape interval of the pacemaker is decreased by a preadjusted decrement interval (10 to 200 ms) in such a manner that the pacer captures the heart. The pacing interval then progressively increases by a preadjusted increment interval (1 to 10 ms), until the spontaneous rhythm reappears, restarting the same process. This pacing mode operates between a lower rate limit, where continous pacing occurs, and an upper rate limit, above which the pacer is inhibited (or can function in automatic underdrive mode if the two modes an associated). After the first spontaneous beat, if the reduction of the escape cycle is not sufficient to control the heart rhythm (for example if there is a second extrasystole with a shorter coupling interval than the escape cycle) the pacing cycle is again reduced by the decrement interval and so on until the upper rate limit is reached. This pacing mode produces a permanent control of the heart rhythm at a frequency slightly faster than the patient's.

Flywheel

The role of the flywheel mode is to avoid abrupt changes in the heart rhythm. To attain this purpose, the escape rhythm of the pacer is not fixed like usual demand pacers, but permanently adapted to the spontaneous rhythm of the patient (112.5% of the sponta-

240

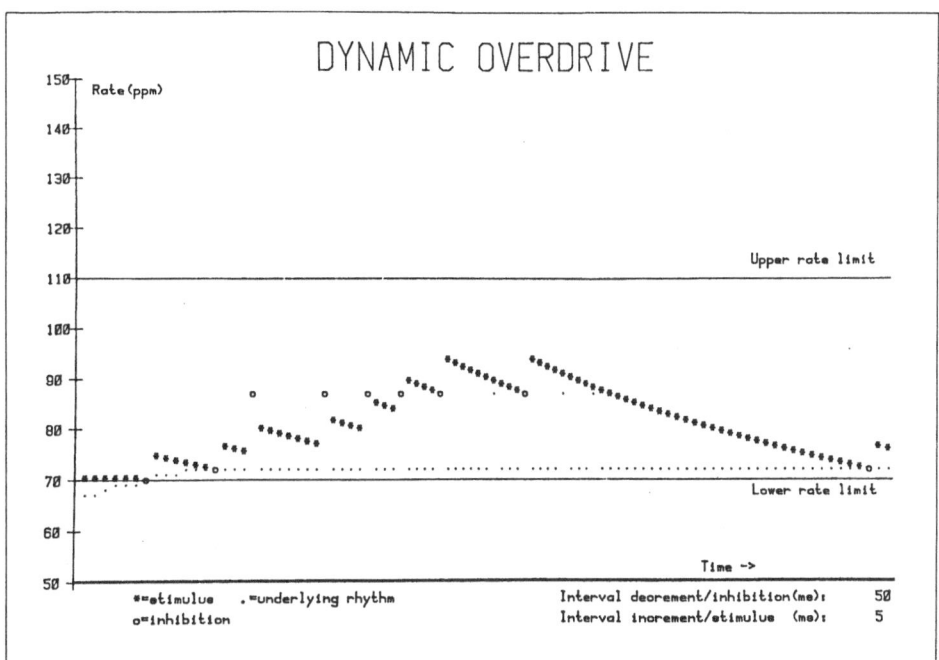

Fig. 2. See text.

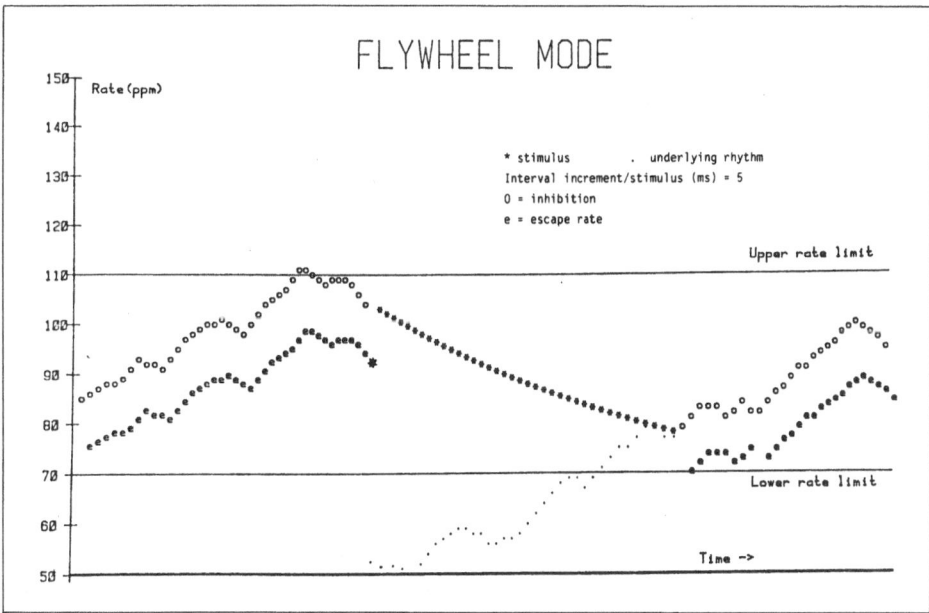

Fig. 3. See text.

neous cycle (Fig. 3)). If this condition occurs, the pacer delivers an impulse, then increases the pacing cycle after each impulse with an adjustable interval (increment inter-

241

val), until the spontaneous rhythm reappears. This process operates between a lower rate limit under which a continuous pacing is delivered, and an upper rate limit above which the pacer is inhibited.

Like dynamic overdrive, flywheel can be combined with automatic underdrive to associate prevention and treatment of tachycardic episodes.

Patients

Ten patients (Table 1), 8 women and 2 men, aged 67 to 89 years, received a DPG in our division between September 1982 and January 1984. Eight had sinus node dysfunction, with sinoatrial block in 2 cases and documented bradycardia-tachycardia syndrome in 6. In all these patients, atrial pacing was decided after AV conduction had been found normal on the basis of normal QRS, PR AH and HV intervals within normal limits and a Wenckebach point above 130/mn. None of the patients developed AV conduction disorders during the follow-up. In one case, severe sinus bradycardia was associated with intractable paroxymal junctional reciprocating tachycardia, and in one case, the pacer was implanted because of permanent atrial bigeminy refractory to drug treatments and producing a bradycardia responsible for marked asthenia and exercise dyspnea.

The results in the patients with brady-tachy syndrome were evaluated by symptoms and Holter functions of the pacer, particularly with histograms and premature beat counter.

Table 1. Clinical data.

Case No.	Name	Age	Sex	ECG	Pacing mode	Follow-up (months)
1	LOD	76	F	BTS	FW	19
2	FER	89	F	BTS	FW	19
3	REV	67	M	PJT	AV	17
4	LOM	76	F	BTS	FW	15
5	LAN	87	F	BTS	FW	12
6	POU	81	F	BTS	FW	12
7	BOS	70	F	AE	DO	12
8	COS	74	F	SAB	FW	11
9	ART	78	F	BTS	FW	7
10	DEL	75	M	SAB	FW	1

SAB: sinoatrial block; BTS: bradycardia-tachycardia syndrome; PJT: paroxysmal junctional tachycardia; AE: atrial extrasystoles; FW: flywheel; DO = dynamic overdrive; AU: automatic underdrive.

Results

Junctional tachycardia

One of our patients (case 3) had been suffering for several years from disabling attacks of reciprocating junctional tachycardia.

Severe symptomatic sinus bradycardia was associated, hindering drug treatment of the tachycardia and indicating pacemaker implantation.

After an electrophysiological study the patient was implanted by DPGl with an atrial lead to perform automatic underdrive interruption of the attacks of tachycardia. This had excellent results on the attacks, which were quickly interrupted by the pacer, but they were more frequent than before implantation. On the ECG (Fig. 4) the behaviour of the pacer was surprising, exhibiting chaotic pacing cycles whatever the programmed rate. The use of triggered mode explained this phenomenon (Figs. 5–6), showing undesired detection of R wave and T wave. Prolongation of the refractory period suppressed R wave detections but it was not possible to avoid T wave sensing which lead to false diagnosis of tachycardia by the pacer and inappropriate automatic underdrive pacing, which finally initiated true episodes of reciprocating tachycardia. This example illustrates some limitations of automatic underdrive pacing at the atrial level.

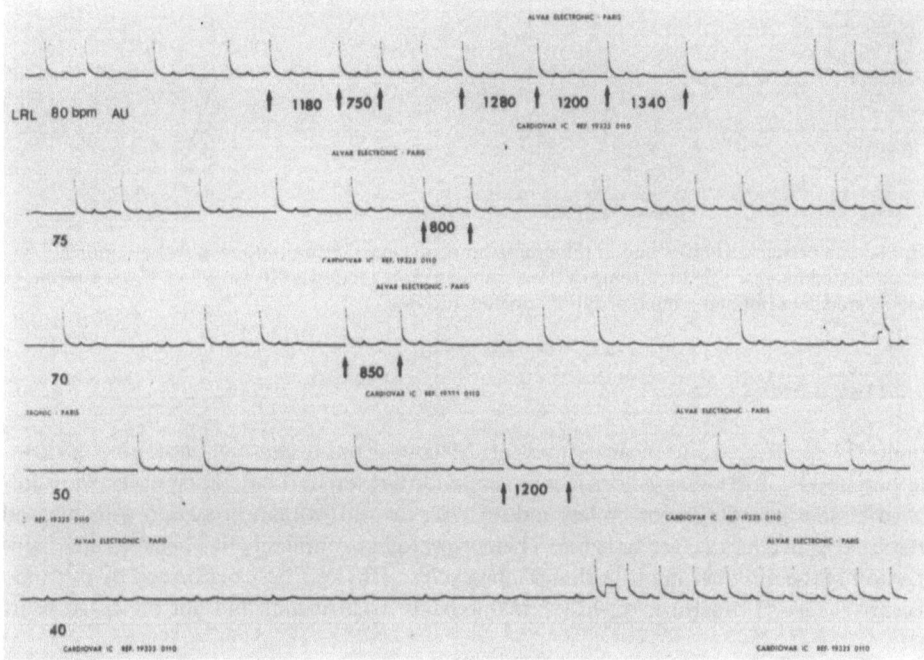

Fig. 4. Chaotic behavior of an atrial pacer with automatic underdrive mode. The pacing cycle is variable, irrespective of the programmed values. Lower strip: automatic underdrive triggering without any tachycardia.

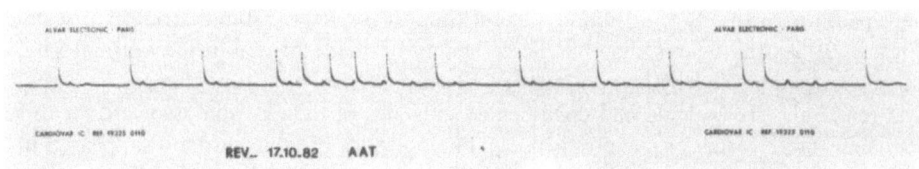

Fig. 5. Same patient as Fig. 4, triggered mode. Sensing of R wave and T wave.

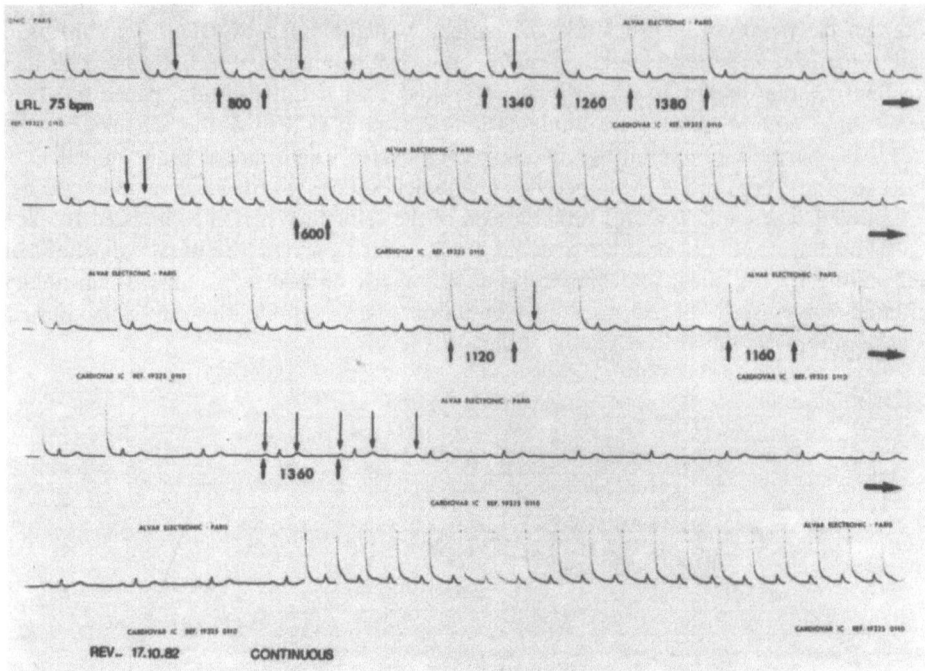

Fig. 6. Same patient as Figs. 4 and 5: the programmed cycle is 75/mn (800 ms). Arrows indicate undesired detections resetting the pacing cycle. Second strip: detection of R wave and T wave mimicks a tachycardia and initiates a burst of automatic underdrive.

Atrial extrasystoles

Patient 7 was affected with near permanent, 24-hour atrial begeminy, remaining intractable despite all of the various drug treatments administered. The extrasystoles were followed by long compensatory cycles, and this 70 year old woman presented with marked exercise dyspnea and severe asthenia. These symptoms completely disappeared after suppression of the alternation of short and long cycles. This was best performed by dynamic overdrive (Fig. 7) which permitted the maintenance of a regular and not too rapid heart rate.

Sinus node dysfunction

Two patients affected with sino atrial block without evidence of tachycardia episodes were paced with the flywheel mode. One of them (case 10) exhibited atrial extrasystoles (Figs. 8, 9). As the figures show, a choice had to be made to obtain the optimal rate: a narrow range of cycle length variations and the suppression of abrupt changes.
The remaining six patients had documented episodes of tachycardia associated with severe sinus bradycardia or sinoatrial block. The episodes of tachycardia disappeared in 2 patients without additional drug treatment. Three patients needed antiarrhythmic drugs to be completely free of tachycardic episodes. The last patient had persisting episodes of

244

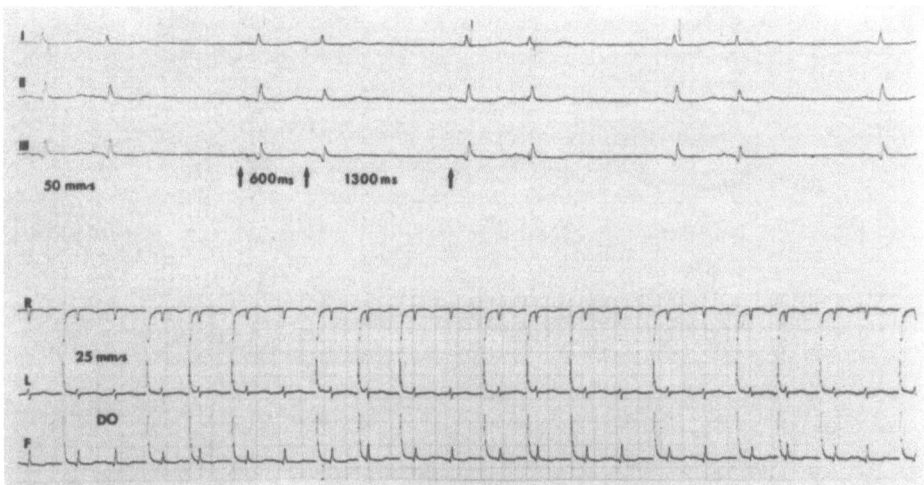

Fig. 7. Upper strip: atrial bigeminy with alternating short and long cycles. Lower strip: dynamic overdrive is used after the extrasystole and drives the heart rate, progressively decreasing until a spontaneous beat (another extrasystole) reappears.

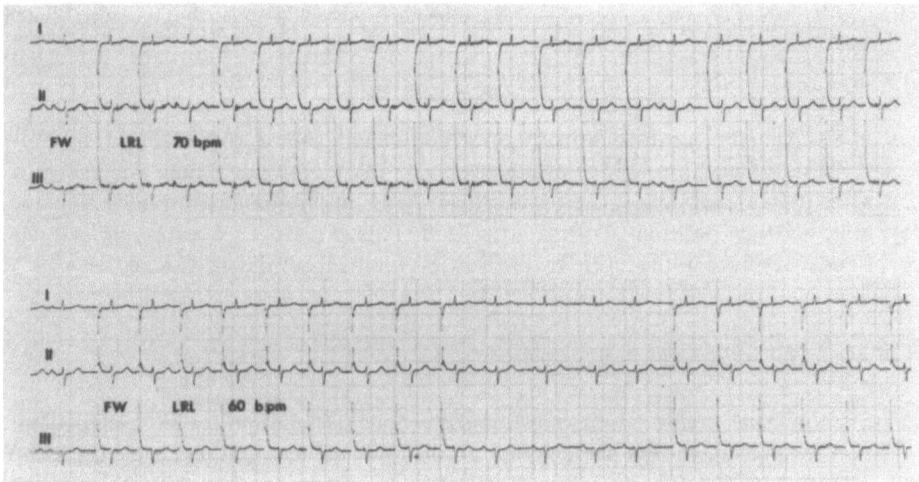

Fig. 8. Sinoatrial block with AAI pacing. Persistence of an irregular rhythm due to atrial extrasystoles.

tachycardia despite associated drug treatment; however these episodes were less frequent than previously.

Comments

Atrial sensing with the DPG

Atrial sensing is always a difficult problem because of the weak intracavitary atrial signal and the risk of lack of detection or, conversely, false detection of other signals like R

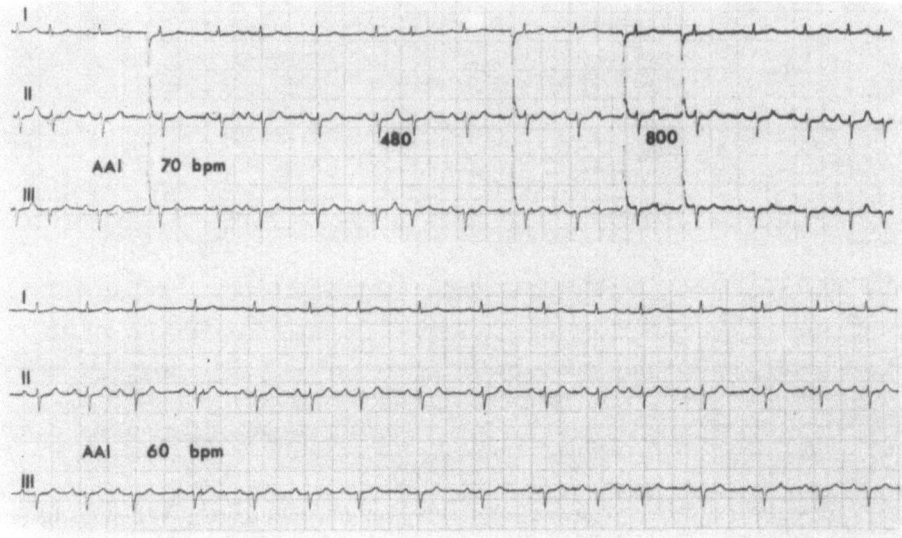

Fig. 9. Same patients as Fig. 8, with flywheel: with a LRL of 70 bpm, after an extrasystole, the atrium is either paced or not according to three parameters: preceding cycle, coupling interval and escape interval.

wave or T wave. None of these difficulties are completely solved in the DPGl (especially because the minimum threshold is not inferior to 1 mV). However, some analysis functions of the device, particularly the intracardiac signal amplitude measurement function, allow more accurate positioning of the atrial lead. This is mainly a question of lead, and may be better resolved in the future by further developments of the atrial leads.

Atrial pacing for sinus node dysfunction

The benefit of atrial pacing is well known in sinus node dysfunction (2). In these patients, it has been demonstrated that pacing does not improve the survival, but only the symptoms. This may be due to heart failure, frequent in the disease, and frequently aggravated in sinus node dysfunction by ventricular pacing because of retrograde AV conduction. Retrograde AV conduction is not altered and the sinus node function is depressed, which favours retrograde capture of the atrium (3). The haemodynamically deleterious effects of retrograde VA conduction are well demonstrated (4).

On the other hand, conservation of the atrial systole with a normal AV sequence can considerably improve the haemodynamic result of pacing. This conclusion had lead to the diffusion of dual chamber pace-makers, because of the risk of associated AV conduction disorders in sinus nodal dysfunction. This association is really frequent, as several authors have reported (5, 6). However, little is known about the natural history of the disease, i.e. about the incidence and rate of development of AV conduction disorders in patients affected with sinus node dysfunction who have a normal AV conduction at the date of discovery of the disease. In our experience, the development of such AV conduction disorders during the course of the disease is extremely rare and slow. This authorizes atrial pacing in patients affected with SN dysfunction if AV conduction has been found normal after careful electrophysiologic study.

Antiarrhythmic pacing in the brady tachy syndrome

In the brady-tachy syndrome, sinus node failure is associated with episodes of tachycardia, usually atrial fibrillation or atrial tachycardia. Although the physiopathologic mechanism of this association is still subject to controversy, there is a possibility for the episodes of tachycardia to disappear after suppression of the bradycardia (7). However, this is not often the case with usual demand pacers, perhaps because the heart rhythm remains irregular with the differences between sinus rhythm, sinus pauses and paced rhythm. Flywheel could be a solution to this problem, by avoiding abrupt changes in the heart rhythm, which are supposed to favour discrepancies between refractory periods of adjacent fibers and induce arrhythmias.

In our series, only two patients in six have become completely free of tachycardic episodes after atrial pacing with flywheel mode alone, whereas three of the six needed additional drug treatment. However, one cannot come to a conclusion with so few patients and it would be interesting to continue these investigations in a larger series, perhaps after external Holter or electrophysiological studies, in order to predict more exactly the conditions of onset of tachycardic episodes in such patients.

References

1. Barold S, Mujica J (1982) The third decade of cardiac pacing. Futura Publications, New York
2. Lekieffre J, Medvedowsky JL, Thery C (1979) Le noeud sinusal normal et pathologique. Sandoz, Paris, p 170
3. Medvedowsky JL, Barnay C (1973) Etude sur la conduction retrograde. Coeur 4: 363
4. Daubert JC, Roussel A, Langella B, Besson C, Gouffault J (1983) Haemodynamic consequences of ventriculo-atrial conduction in man. In: Levys S (ed) Recent Advances in Cardiac Arrhythmias. J Libbey, London, pp 387–391
5. Narula OS (1971) Atrioventricular conduction defects in patients with sinus bradycardia. Circulation 44: 1096
6. Medvedowsky JL, Barnay C, Vincey JC, Jouven JC (1977) Dysfonctionnement sinusal et troubles conductifs nodo-hisiens. Indications de la stimulation cardiaque définitive. Arch Mal Coeur 70: 981
7. Coumel P, Attuel P, Lavallee JP, Flamang D, Leclerq JF, Slama R (1978) Fibrillation auriculaire d'origine vagale. Arch Mal Coeur 71: 645

Authors' address:
Dr. C. Barnay
Service de Cardiologie
Centre Hospitalier
Avenue des Famaris
F-13100 Aix-en-Provence, France

Description and Efficacy of PASAR Algorithms

A. W. Nathan*, A. J. Camm*, and R. A. J. Spurrell

Summary: An automatic, fully implantable, scanning pacemaker was developed and has been used for tachycardia termination in man. Since January 1982, 22 patients have had this pacemaker implanted at St Bartholomew's Hospital and over 125 devices have been used throughout the world. Clinical results have been encouraging, especially with the second generation device.

The use of precisely timed extrastimuli for the termination of reentrant tachycardias is now well accepted (1, 2). In 1982 the first use was reported of a fully implantable automatic scanning pacemaker for the termination of reentrant tachycardias (3, 4). In this review the updated clinical experience of two automatic implantable antitachycardia pacemakers (Telectronics PASAR 4151 and 4171**) is reported.

Descriptions of pacemakers

PASAR 4151

The Telectronics 4151 is a bipolar lithium powered pacemaker which is fully implantable and requires no external control device. Figure 1 diagrammatically illustrates its mode of action. Following four consecutive cardiac cycles at a rate faster than a programmed tachycardia trigger rate, an extrastimulus is emitted with a preset coupling time (programmable from 200 ms to 390 ms). If tachycardia continues then a further extrastimulus is emitted every four cycles but the coupling time is reduced by 6 ms (Figure 1A). In this way 90 ms of the cardiac cycle can be scanned.
If tachycardia is terminated no further stimuli are emitted. If after 15 decrements the tachycardia continues, the pacemaker recycles and the same scan is repeated. A second stimulus (Figure 1B) can be selected with a fixed coupling interval programmable from 100 ms to 370 ms (125 ms to 380 ms in earlier devices). A memory function is incorporated to retain successful sequences to use at the onset of the next tachycardia. If, however, on this occasion tachycardia is not terminated then the scan is continued. Other programmable features include tachycardia trigger rate, pulse width and sensitivity.

PASAR 4171

All features of the PASAR 4151 are incorporated in the PASAR 4171. There are however important additional features.

---

* Supported by the British Heart Foundation.
** Telectronics Pty Ltd, Sydney, Australia.

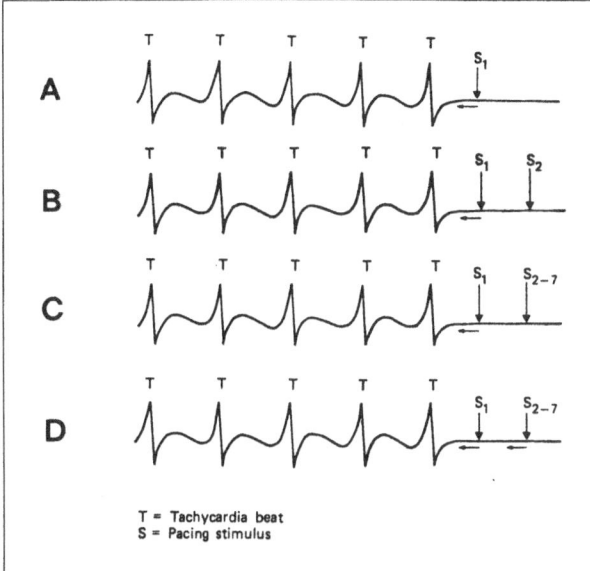

Fig. 1. The diagram shows the operation of model 4151 (panels A and B) and model 4171 (all panels). Panel A shows a single scanning extrastimulus, and B demonstrates a second, fixed stimulus. Panel C represents the shifting burst mode, and panel D, the scanning burst (concertina) mode. T = tachycardia beat, S = pacing stimulus.

1. Shifting burst mode (Figure 1C):
Up to seven extrastimuli can be programmed. The coupling interval between the last sensed tachycardia beat and the first extrastimulus (S1) is independently programmable (200 to 395 ms), but all subsequent stimulus coupling intervals (S2 to S7), although also programmable, are equal (105 to 375 ms). When three or more stimuli are programmed, the minimum coupling interval of S2 to S7 is limited to 220 ms. After four cycles of tachycardia, the stimuli are generated and if tachycardia continues only the first extrastimulus is scanned (6 ms decrements) with the subsequent intervals remaining fixed with respect to S1. A total of 15 decrements may occur.

2. Scanning burst (concertina) mode (Figure 1D):
This mode is similar to the shifting burst, but if the first intervention is unsuccessful, the coupling interval of all stimuli in the burst decrements by 6 ms. When two pulses are programmed the initial S2 interval may be programmed from 220 to 275 ms, but when three or more stimuli are used the minimum initial S2 to S7 coupling interval is limited, for safety reasons, to 300 ms.

3. Bradycardia support (60 bpm) is available on this unit particularly to provide rate support for those patients who exhibit post tachycardia sinus suppression.

Patients and methods

At the time of writing, over 125 patients throughout the world have been treated with PASAR antitachycardia pacemakers. However this paper will concentrate on the experience relating to those patients who have been treated in the Department of Cardiology at St Bartholomew's Hospital, London.

A total of 22 patients (nine males) had PASAR systems implanted, 19 with the 4151 version and eight with the 4171 unit (five of whom had previously had 4151s implanted). Their ages, at implant, ranged from 12 to 73 (mean 45) years. Nine patients had intra AV nodal reentrant tachycardias, usually due to functional duality of AH conduction (one also with a bystander accessory pathway), and 12 had atrioventricular reentrant tachycardias, three due to concealed accessory pathways and nine in association with the Wolff-Parkinson-White syndrome (WPW). One had ventricular tachycardia. Tachycardia cycle length varied from 275 to 430 (mean 335) ms. One patient had Ebstein's anomaly and another had coronary artery disease. The length of history varied from two to 40 (mean 14) years. The frequency of attacks ranged from four episodes per year to 15 episodes per day (mean 1.4 per day), and lasted from a few minutes to 24 hours (mean four hours). Nine patients had been treated with three or less drugs and were not considered resistant to medical therapy, but the remainder had taken up to eight different drugs and were considered to be drug refractory. The mean number of drugs taken (for the whole group) was four. Six patients had previously had other tachycardia reversion pacemakers implanted, one with a patient activated ventricular underdrive unit and five with patient activated rapid atrial pacing systems.

Prior to implant all patients had a full electrophysiological study performed in order to: a) determine the electrophysiological basis of the arrhythmia, including accessory pathway characteristics if present; b) to test the efficacy of this form of tachycardia reversion pacing; c) to ensure other factors contraindicating or complicating tachycardia reversion pacing were not present; and d) to ensure atrial and ventricular stability (lack of repetitive firing) to maximal stimulation protocols, including scanning down to the myocardial refractory period, as well as to the intended antitachycardia pacing algorithm. If all was suitable and the patient was agreeable, further testing was carried out using one or more temporary electrodes left positioned at a site suitable for permanent use. Stimulation was tested on many occasions in a variety of postures including the supine and upright postures and also during upright exercise. In each case, an external version of the intended implantable unit was used in order to exactly simulate the operation of the permanent system. Exercise testing was also performed to determine the maximum sinus rates achieved in each patient.

Pacemakers were implanted using conventional operative techniques, usually under local anesthetic. Endocardial electrodes were used throughout.

Repeat electrophysiological testing after implant (usually after 48 hours) enabled proper "set-up" of the pacemakers. Care was taken to evaluate tachycardia termination in a variety of postures. Exercise testing was also completed at this stage as was ambulatory ECG monitoring.

Results

PASAR 4151

Atrial pacing (double stimuli) was used in four of the patients, and ventricular pacing in 15 (initially four with single and 11 with double extrastimuli).

Initially, all patients had very satisfactory results, with almost immediate termination of tachycardia in each case. A variety of medical and technical problems occurred, and to clarify the results, the patients can conveniently be divided into four groups:
1) Patients currently using a pacemaker with satisfactory results;
2) Patients with satisfactory results until their pacemakers developed technical problems;
3) Patients in whom the pacemakers were deactivated or removed;
4) Patients who have died since implantation.

Group 1

As of May 1984, only eight of the patients still utilise normally functioning 4151 pacemakers. Follow-up ranges from 28 to 40 (mean 36) months. The clinical results in these patients are excellent, both symptomatically and as monitored by ambulatory ECG recordings and by repeat exercise and electrophysiological testing.

One patient is symptomatically free of arrhythmias despite ambulatory monitoring evidence of tachycardias which are almost immediately terminated by the pacemaker. In the other seven patients, tachycardias are symptomatically terminated in two to 120 (mean 29) seconds. Five require no antiarrhythmic medication, but one takes flecainide to prevent exercise induced atrial fibrillation, one takes disopyramide to prevent pacing induced atrial fibrillation and one takes metoprolol to facilitate termination in the upright posture (by broadening the tachycardia termination window).

Group 2

Five patients received pacemakers which developed a batch-related technical defect, now identified and corrected in later units.

Following this, all had the more versatile 4171 unit implanted. Prior to the defect, which manifested itself by oversensing, all five enjoyed rapid termination of their arrhythmias, although four had required additional antiarrhythmic drugs to enable termination under all physiological conditions.

Group 3

Three patients have had their pacemakers deactivated. One of these had excellent results from his pacemaker without additional drug therapy, but one year after implant required coronary artery bypass grafting. At the time of surgery the concealed accessory pathway was ablated and the pacemaker was deactivated. Another, who had frequent arrhythmias (mean 450 episodes per month) for many years, became asymptomatic without recordable arrhythmias. An electrode problem developed (Medtronic 6972*) and the pacemaker was deactivated. The third patient had occasional episodes of presyncope occurring at the onset of spontaneous tachycardia. He had failed drug therapy and had initially declined

---

* Medtronic Inc, Minneapolis, USA.

surgery. A decision was made to implant the pacemaker and although it terminated tachycardias very rapidly in all postures, further presyncope occurred and the patient eventually underwent successful ablation of an accessory pathway and the pacemaker was deactivated.

One further patient has had the pacemaker explanted. A man suffering from paroxysmal ventricular tachycardia, on the basis of coronary disease, became arrhythmia free and the pacemaker was removed because it was uncomfortable.

Group 4

Two patients with WPW died suddenly. Drug therapy had been unsuccessful in both, and neither would accept surgery. Both had left free wall pathways, one with an anterograde effective refractory period of 265 ms (shortest preexcited RR interval during atrial fibrillation of 310 ms), the other with anterograde refractoriness of 270 ms (atrial fibrillation not inducible). As tachycardia termination was most effective from the right ventricle, both had ventricular systems implanted, programmed to deliver two stimuli in each case. One died suddenly whilst at rest, 22 months after implant, and the other died whilst cycling slowly, after 12 months of successful pacing. Post-mortem examinations were unremarkable, as was pacemaker analysis in the one patient in whom the device was recovered.

PASAR 4171

Eight patients have had 4171 pacemakers implanted, seven with electrodes in the atrium and one with an electrode in the ventricle. Follow-up has been from two to eight (mean five) months.

The ventricular system replaced a defective 4151 and used the preexisting electrode. It operates in burst scanning (concertina) mode utilising two stimuli, and the patient no longer needs additional antiarrhythmic drug therapy (which had been necessary with the 4151 unit in which only the first stimulus was capable of scanning).

Six patients have had atrial systems programmed in the concertina mode, five with seven stimuli and one with four stimuli. An additional patient has an atrial electrode with the pacemaker operating in the shifting burst mode with seven stimuli.

All patients experience almost immediate termination of tachycardias, and only one has required any additional antiarrhythmic drug therapy (flecainide to prevent spontaneous atrial fibrillation).

Discussion

Although most regular tachycardias may be both initiated and also terminated by appropriately timed electrical stimuli (2), tachycardias vary according to the physiological status of the patient (5).

Therefore adaptable pacemakers are required and the PASAR 4151 was the first automatic fully implantable pacemaker to be capable of such adaptation. The model 4171 has increased these capabilities further.

Overall, the pacemakers have performed well and patients' symptomatology has dramatically improved in most of the cases. The results are all the better when the otherwise refractory nature of some of the patients' arrhythmias is considered.

However, a number of problems were encountered in this clinical study and these require further examination.

Additional antiarrhythmic therapy was required in several patients. Although this need was identified in occasional patients prior to implant, the number of patients eventually needing such therapy exceeded initial expectations. The most common factor associated with the need for drug therapy was shrinking or disappearing tachycardia termination windows on standing. However, the ability of the 4171 model to introduce more stimuli has reduced this problem. In addition, occasional patients had atrial arrhythmias, either spontaneous or induced by the pacemaker, and these were not always anticipated by the pre-implant testing, and it must be appreciated that such testing cannot predict all events in an ongoing form of therapy.

Although no new major engineering concepts were employed in these pacemakers, the circuitry is necessarily complex. A batch-related manufacturing problem caused several units (model 4151) to develop sensing problems necessitating explantation. It is hoped that such problems will not be encountered in later units.

The occurrence of syncope or presyncope early in an episode of tachycardia must be considered a relative contraindication to such pacemakers. The one patient who suffered from presyncope prior to implant, presumably due to the sudden onset of tachycardia, did not have this symptom alleviated, even though the pacemaker terminated tachycardia rapidly. Any adaptive system may take a few seconds to operate effectively and this is usually too long to prevent such syncope.

The two deaths are a cause of great concern. The exact mode of the deaths will remain unknown and the patients may have suffered either spontaneous or pacemaker-induced arrhythmias. Although there is little definitive data to establish whether or not an accessory pathway is "safe", Klein et al. (6) studied 25 patients with WPW, all of whom had been rescusitated from ventricular fibrillation preceded by atrial fibrillation. All had a shortest preexcited RR interval during atrial fibrillation of 250 ms or less (mean 180 ms), a statistically significant from controls who had not suffered ventricular fibrillation. Measurement of the anterograde refractory period was less discriminatory. We have now made an arbitrary decision not to pace patients with accessory pathways capable of preexcited RR intervals of 300 ms or less (whether atrially paced or during atrial fibrillation), nor those with an anterograde accessory pathway refractory period of 300 ms or less. If ventricular pacing is necessary in any patient, those requiring coupling intervals within 20 ms of the ventricular myocardial effective refractory period are also excluded now. Testing to ensure ventricular stability is performed at high energy (20 mA) as well as at more conventional outputs, and in addition is carried out during exercise and during isoproterenol infusion. Atrial stimulation is used where possible, although the relative safety of atrial and ventricular pacing in patients with WPW is difficult to establish.

The use of up to seven stimuli in the 4171 model has certainly allowed a greater use of atrial stimulation, and also permits the use of longer coupling intervals. Nathan et al. (7) have demonstrated a relationship between the maximum effective coupling interval and the number of stimuli used to terminate tachycardia, and only experience will determine whether more stimuli of longer coupling intervals are in fact safer than fewer, more closely coupled stimuli. Although there is the ability in the model 4171 to introduce bradycardia support pacing, this has not been found necessary in any of the patients.

With refinements in tachycardia recognition, together with even more versatile reversion algorithms including back-up defibrillation, tachycardia reversion pacing will continue to evolve as a highly acceptable therapy for patients with a variety of tachycardias.

References

1. Spurrell RAJ (1975) Artificial cardiac pacemakers. In: Krikler DM, Goodwin JF (eds) Cardiac arrhythmias: the modern electrophysiological approach. WB Saunders, London, p 238
2. Wellens HJJ, Bar FW, Gorgels AP, Muncharaz JF (1978) Electrical management of arrhythmias with emphasis on the tachycardias. Am J Cardiol 41: 1025
3. Nathan AW, Camm AJ, Bexton RS, Hellestrand KJ, Spurrell RAJ (1982) Initial experience with a fully implantable, programmable, scanning, extrastimulus pacemaker for tachycardia termination. Clin Cardiol 5: 22
4. Spurrell RAJ, Nathan AW, Bexton RS, Hellestrand KJ, Nappholz T, Camm AJ (1982) Implantable automatic scanning pacemaker for termination of supraventricular tachycardia. Am J Cardiol 49: 753
5. Curry PVL (1979) The hemodynamic and electrophysiological effects of paroxysmal tachycardia. In: Narula OS (ed) Cardiac arrhythmias: electrophysiology, diagnosis and management. Williams and Wilkins, Baltimore, p 364
6. Klein GJ, Bashore TM, Sellers TD, Pritchett ELC, Smith WM, Gallagher JJ (1979) Ventricular fibrillation in the Wolff-Parkinson-White syndrome. N Engl J Med 301: 1080
7. Nathan AW, Cochrane T, Bexton RS, Spurrell RAJ, Camm AJ (1983) Relationship between pacing cycle length and duration of pacing for the termination of reentrant tachycardias. Circulation 68-III: 313 (Abstract)

Authors' address:
Dr. Anthony W. Nathan
Department of Cardiology
St Bartholomew's Hospital
West Smithfield
London EC1A 7BE
England

Clinical Results with the Tachylog P43

E. Sowton, R. J. Wainwright, and J. C. P. Crick

Summary: Tachylog is an implantable unit with four anti-tachycardia modes (in addition to dual demand). It will distinguish physiological from pathological tachycardias, and can be fully automatic or patient activated. An interactive mode allows non-invasive EPS to be performed and its memory can be interrogated at any time. In VVI mode Tachylog performs as a multiprogrammable Siemens Model 668.

The first implant was in December, 1982 and 17 patients have now been treated at Guy's Hospital. Ten had WPW, two A–V nodal tachycardia and three VT. All were refractory to drug therapy alone. Ten have complete control of tachycardias without any drugs and four have complete control with additional drugs. Two patients developed AF with ventricular rates up to 300/minute and required surgical division of the accessory tract and one is awaiting replacement with a bipolar unit because of myopotential sensing.

Thirteen of the 14 patients have a self-searching programme capable of finding the termination window automatically by monitoring the electrophysiological response of the heart to stimulation and one has a four beat burst overdrive to the atrium.

Twenty-five per cent. of the patients can be controlled with a single stimulus, but electrode position is critical and most require two beats. Tachycardias are usually controlled within a few seconds, and patient acceptance is very high.

Introduction

Tachylog* is an implantable, conventionally sized, single chamber stimulator capable of functioning as a multiprogrammable VVI bradycardia pacemaker or as an anti-tachycardia device which can be activated automatically or by the patient (Fig. 1). It has the capability to distinguish between physiological and pathological tachycardias and to update its memory according to the results during the last tachycardia. In addition it can be interrogated to display the number of tachycardias terminated, the method of termination, the number of failures, and the parameters of the current programme. An interactive mode is available which allows the physician to perform non-invasive electrophysiological studies using chest wall stimulation. Any number of stimuli between one and 256 can be delivered and all searches can be carried out using multiple stimuli. Early units were unipolar but current production can be programmed to unipolar or bipolar modes. When programmed for anti-tachycardia functions four modes of termination are available:

1. Critical timed stimulation

The pre-programmed number of stimuli are delivered after a programmable delay from the QRS and with programmable intervals which can be varied.

If several stimuli are programmed this mode provides burst overdrive termination.

---

* Siemens Elema AB, Stockholm, Sweden.

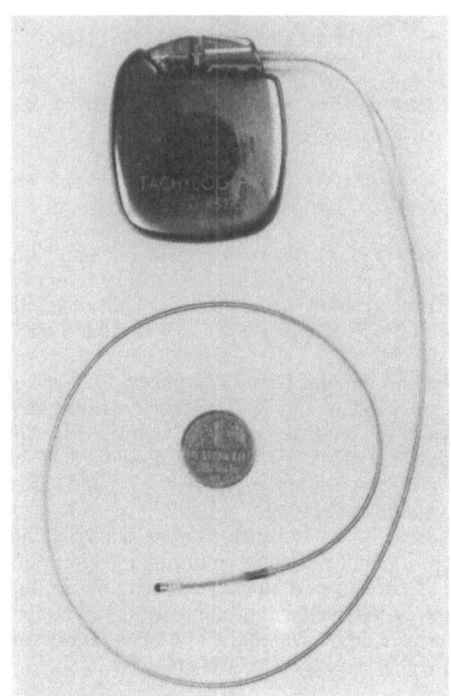

Fig. 1. Tachylog P43 generator.

2. Self-searching

In this mode the response of the pacemaker is not pre-ordained but is dependent upon the electrophysiological response of the heart to the previous stimulus. If the tachycardia is reset but not terminated then the next stimulus will be moved earlier; if no reset is obtained it will be moved later. Each increment is reduced in subsequent cycles until the termination window is identified and the setting will then update the memory and be used for the initial attempt in the next episode of tachycardia. This mode is not applicable where no reset can be obtained and this has been found to be critically dependent upon electrode position. The self-searching mode can be used with multiple stimuli.

3. Adaptive table scanning

Up to five sets of timing for stimuli can be entered by the physician and when a tachycardia is detected Tachylog will deliver impulses with the first set. If this fails it will proceed to the second set and so on down the table. If the final timings also fail to terminate the tachycardia a search will be initiated until successful timings are found. When the tachycardia is terminated the successful timings will be entered at the top of the table and the bottom data deleted. In this way Tachylog updates its memory with every successive tachycardia and by using successive lines in the table is theoretically capable of dealing with several different tachycardias in the same patient.

256

4. Centrifugal scanning

This programme also uses a table of coupling intervals and chooses the first one accord-ing to a programmable calculation based upon cycle length. If this fails the next attempt will be from the row above the first and the subsequent attempt from the row below. This sequence is then repeated. It is possible in this programme for the search to be carried out with a single stimulus followed by double stimuli, then by treble (or more if necessary) until the tachycardia is terminated.

In addition to these formal anti-tachycardia programmes the Tachylog is capable of per-forming as a dual demand pacemaker in the usual way.

Failure of termination

If the Tachylog fails to terminate the arrhythmia after the programmed number of at-tempts the anti-tachycardia functions become quiescent, although the pacemaker contin-ues to perform as a VVI unit. The anti-tachycardia programme will be re-activated by a spontaneous termination of the arrhythmia or by the temporary application of a magnet over the unit.

Programming

This is carried out with an HP 85 computer and a Siemens interface. Programmable fea-tures include the rate at which the anti-tachycardia programme is initiated, the type of search, the limits of the search, the number and timing of stimuli, and the number of at-tempts to be made. In addition all the functions of the Siemens Model 668 can be pro-grammed in the usual way.

The HP 85 is also used to interrogate the memory.

Patients

The first implant was carried out in December, 1982 and a total of 17 patients have re-ceived Tachylogs at Guy's Hospital. All had proved resistant to drug therapy including amiodarone and verapamil. Before implantation all had extensive electrophysiological investigation. The tachycardias ranged from 190–330 bpm with a mean for the group of 220 bpm and the patients were experiencing up to 25 attacks daily, some lasting several hours.

There were nine male and eight female patients with an age range of 19 to 64 years (mean 37). Twelve patients had Wolff-Parkinson-White syndrome, two had reciprocating AV nodal tachycardia and three had ventricular tachycardias.

The mean follow-up time is approximately 25 months, and the longest is 33 months.

Results

Fourteen of the 17 patients have had all episodes of tachycardia terminated by their Ta-chylog, usually within a few seconds (often less than five seconds). In ten of these patients no anti-arrhthymic drugs at all have been necessary. Amiodarone has been used in one patient with ventricular tachycardia and verapamil has been used in three patients to prevent rapid antegrade conducton down the accessory pathway during episodes of atrial fibrillation.

In three patients electrical treatment has not been completely satisfactory although in all cases multiple attacks of re-entry tachycardia have been terminated (Fig. 2). Two of these three patients developed atrial fibrillation with very rapid ventricular rates (in excess of 300 bpm) and both have had the accessory pathway divided surgically. In the third patient sensing of skeletal muscle potentials results in inappropriate stimuli from his Tachylog which produces iatrogenic episodes of tachycardia (which are then terminated) and so replacement with a bipolar Tachylog is planned.

Electrodes

Nineteen Siemens Elema carbon tip tined electrodes were used in these 17 patients. Two patients had bipolar electrodes and two further patients had unipolar replaced with bipolar. Sixteen of the electrodes were positioned in the right ventricle, usually at the conventional position near the apex, and two were in the atrium. One electrode was placed in the coronary sinus and successfully terminated all tachycardias with single

Fig. 2. Termination of tachycardia episode.

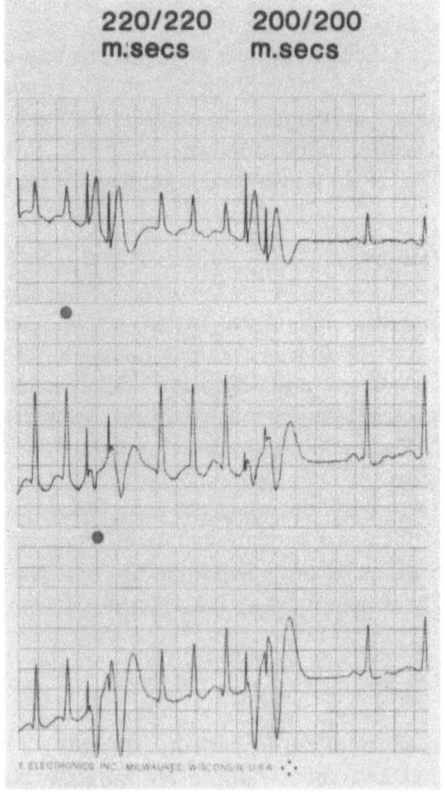

258

stimuli. However, the electrode became displaced to the right ventricle and a single stimulus was then ineffective. Complete control of the tachycardias was regained by reprogramming Tachylog to double stimuli.

Memory function

In each termination mode the successful timing of the stimuli updates the memory and these values are then used for the initial attempt at stopping the next episode of tachycardia. This results in most tachycardias stopping extremely quickly but it is not yet established whether this feature is of universal value since the tachycardia window need not remain constant, particularly under different physiological conditions (see later). If an antitachycardia pacemaker has a pre-ordained scan and the remembered timing from the previous tachycardia is inappropriate for the next episode then the stimulator may have to scan through its entire cycle to reach the correct timing. This may well take longer than starting from a pre-programmed value. This disadvantage does not apply to the self-searching programme since Tachylog is designed to move the stimuli in the correct direction if the first attempt fails.

The second memory function is similar to a Holter monitor and can be interrogated to determine a wide variety of information. The readout will display the number of episodes of tachycardia occurring since the memory was last cleared together with the number of attempts and the final success rate. The actual values in the memory are also displayed together with the last changes in the search.

Electrophysiological studies

Non-invasive electrophysiological programmed stimulation can be carried out with the Tachylog in interactive mode since it will then respond to skin stimuli. These can be delivered from a conventional programmable stimulator and will be faithfully followed by Tachylog which delivers stimuli to the heart at the external timing. An extensive programme of investigation has been carried out in this way and will be presented in detail elsewhere. The clinically important conclusions relate to alterations in the tachycardia window over long periods of time and in different postures as well as when anti-arrhythmic drugs are taken. It is almost universal that the tachycardia window becomes very much narrower when a patient changes from supine to erect position and it often narrows further on exercise. In a recent study from Guy's Hospital by Schmidinger (1) 274 episodes of tachycardia were started and terminated in eight patients with Tachylogs. The duration of the tachycardia window decreased by 46% when the patients changed from supine to erect position and in two patients it vanished completely. It is apparent that when this phenomenon occurs electrical termination of a tachycardia cannot occur until the patient lies down and the window reappears. An alternative is to attempt to lengthen the window by anti-arrhytmic drugs. In extreme cases the burst overdrive mode could be used instead of critical timed stimulation. The phenomenon is probably associated with an electrode position where the tip is some distance from the anatomical re-entry circuit. The reduction in tachycardia window is largely due to movement of the right hand end (i.e. late stimuli) rather than the left hand end (early stimuli).

Complications

The commonest problem has been episodes of iatrogenic tachycardia caused by inappropriate stimuli in response to sensed myopotentials. Although the Tachylog then correctly terminated the episode of tachycardia the patient nevertheless experiences a considerable increase in the number of attacks each day and soon learns that particular arm movements are likely to induce tachycardias. This complication has affected eight of our 17 patients at some time and for this reason we now recommend that only biopolar systems are implanted. The unipolar mode is still programmable for particular applications such as the easy identification of stimuli on an ECG, for example in the vario cycle to determine threshold.

The possibility of dangerous arrhythmias being triggered by anti-tachycardia pacemakers has received close attention and in exploring the limits of the left hand edge of the window with triple stimuli we have produced VT in one patient who previously had been documented only as having SVT. The Tachylog correctly stopped the episode of VT and reprogramming the search limits prevented this complication. No further such incident has occurred over the year since this iatrogenic arrhythmia. There have heen no incidents of infection, perforation or other complications in patients with implanted Tachylogs.

Patient acceptance

Four of these patients had previously been treated with the patient-activated P23 system, both with fixed timing (2, 3) and also during the development of the self-searching algorithm (4, 5). They are delighted with the success of a fully implanted system which frees them from all external apparatus. A significant advantage of electrical stimulation is appreciated by the ten patients who have been freed from the necessity to take any drugs at all. This is particularly important in women patients who may wish to become pregnant, but in all patients it avoids the problems of long-term side effects, inability to control tachycardias, malabsorption or the difficulty of drug schedules.

Conclusion

Our first year's experience with implanted Tachylogs demonstrates that this is a viable alternative treatment to anti-arrhythmic therapy or accessory path surgery. In this highly selected group of 17 patients who were resistant to drug therapy 14 out of 17 (83%) have complete control of their tachycardias, and only four of these need drugs. The problems identified relate mostly to sensing, and improvements in the apparatus can be expected to provide even better results as the apparatus is refined in the future.

References

1. Schmidinger H (1983) Unpublished observation
2. Kappenberger L, Sowton E (1979) A method for control of tachycardia by long-term programmed stimulation. Proceedings of the British Cardiac Society Autumn Meeting. Br Heart 41: 371

3. Kappenberger L, Sowton E (1981) Programmed stimulation for long-term treatment and non-invasive investigation of recurrent tachycardia. Lancet 1: 909–914
4. Sowton E, Elmqvist H, Hard af Segerstad C (1981) Two years' clinical experience with a self-searching tachycardia pacemaker. Am J Cardiol 47: 476
5. Sowton E (1981) A self searching tachycardia pacemaker. Proceedings of the British Cardiac Society Autumn Meeting. Br. Heart 45: 340–341

Authors' address:
Dr. E. Sowton
Director Cardiac Department
Guy's Hospital
St Thomas Street
London SE1 9RT
England

The Antitachycardia Capabilities of Symbios

W. A. Kaiser

Symbios is the family name of the fourth generation of Medtronic dual chamber pace-makers. They are basically anti-brady systems whereby one of the bipolar Symbios (7008) has additionally two well-known antitachy modes incorporated in it (burst and dual demand).

There are many devices made by Medtronic for treating and diagnosing tachycardiac rhythm disturbances (Spectrax combined with a patient activator (a "burst" antitachy device), the "Interactive AntiTachy System", consisting of the SP 503, SP 500 and SP 501 and the external Cardioverter and Defibrillator SP 5350 and the implantable Cardioverter 7210).

The Symbios 7008 has nevertheless a notable position amongst these devices. It is the first DDD pacemaker which incorporates antitachy modes, and it is intended to be used as a DDD antibrady pacemaker in the presence of episodes of atrial and supraventricular tachycardias. Up till now, the occurrence – even intermittent – of atrial and supraventricular arrhythmias has been a contra-indication for DDD pacing due to the danger of conducting the high atrial rate into the ventricles, and thus perhaps starting a severe ventricular tachycardia. Symbios 7008 is the first antibrady DDD pacemaker operating in a truly bipolar fashion, and is designed to automatically interrupt those tachycardias. The 7008 has telemetry which besides interrogating and programming the system in a multi-programmable mode, serves diagnostic functions by transmitting in a real time fashion intracardiac electrograms of the atrium and ventricle, respectively, or the "Medtronic inherent Marker Channel signals".

An essential prerequisite in the operation of a DDD system is the prevention of conducting the high atrial rates into the ventricles and at the same time to distinguish between physiological and pathological rate increase. In order to achieve this, the Symbios 7008 has a unique feature not present in any current pacemaker – the AV-block mode. This mode is only accessible if the 7008 is programmed to a DDD mode with one of the antitachy modes (i.e. "burst" or "dual demand"). As soon as one P-P interval is recognized as being shorter than the corresponding programmed "upper rate", serving as "tachycardiac detection" interval, the AV-block mode is activated. In case this "upper rate" counter has not elapsed within an AV interval of 25 ms following the sensed P-event, the ventricular output will be blocked, thus preventing the conduction of the P-wave. The next P-wave – provided the "upper rate" counter has elapsed – will be conducted with a 25 ms AV interval. This mode will continue until five consecutive P-P intervals, which are shorter than the corresponding programmed "upper rate" intervals are detected by the logic of the system. Only if this criterion is met will the selected "antitachy mode" be applied.

Parallel with this, an internal modification of the atrial refractory period, which is programmable in the Symbios, will be switched to either 135 ms following an atrial sense, or to an AV interval of 25 ms plus the programmed atrial refractory period after an atrial pace, thus opening a wider window for detecting high atrial rates.

262

Of special interest in this context is that the AV-block mode does not behave in a Wenckebach fashion, i.e. the ventricular output can only take place if the programmed upper rate has elapsed, but first after the next P-sense and then with the 25 ms AV interval. The system is therefore not pacing at the upper rate like an ordinary DDD pacemaker would. The incorporation of this AV-block feature opens new horizons in DDD treatment of patients with tachy-brady problems.

Author's address:
W. A. Kaiser, M.D.
Medtronic GmbH
Kieler Straße 208
2000 Hamburg 54
West Germany

Clinical Long-Term Experiences with High Rate Antitachycardia Stimulation (Cybertach 60)

D. W. Behrenbeck, V. Hombach, H.-W. Höpp, A. Osterspey, U. J. Winter, and H. H. Hilger

Summary: Several investigators have judged the burst overdrive pacing mode to be effective in tachycardia termination during right ventricular programmed stimulation. The aim of the study was to investigate the long-term results of burst overdrive pacing by means of an implanted, programmable burst pacemaker (Intermedics Cybertach 60) in the treatment of drug-refractory supraventricular (n = 3) and ventricular (n = 3) tachycardias. Therefore 6 patients were repeatedly controlled during a follow-up period of up to 3 years. In 4/6 patients the parameters of the burst stimulation had to be changed within the first 6 months after the implantation. All 6 patients needed an additional antiarrhythmic drug treatment for the tachycardia conditioning. Due to a significant reduction of the tachycardias and hospitalisations all patients could normalize their lives. In a 20 year old man the batteries ran out after a 2 year period of excellent antitachycardia function. The patient was hospitalised due to continuous burst pacing, even during sinus rhythm or premature ventricular beats.

In conclusion, long-term burst pacing in patients with recurrent supraventricular or ventricular tachycardias by means of implantable antitachycardia pacemakers is a helpful therapeutic alternative. Additional antiarrhythmic drug treatment and programmability of the antitachycardia device are necessary prerequisites for a successful long-term application.

Introduction

With increasing knowledge of ventricular arrhythmias and improved arrhythmia recognition during recent years, the development of tachycardia-activated, self-activated or automatic antitachycardia pacemakers became possible. Thus patients with rapid ventricular tachycardias (V. Tach.) having severe hemodynamic side effects, where a rapid, patient-independent onset of antitachycardia pacing was necessary, could also be treated. Recent types of these closed-loop pacemakers have incorporated complex antitachycardia pacing modes.

Pathogenesis of ventricular tachycardias

According to recently presented data, 37% of V. Tach. have a focal origin, 29% are associated with a macroreentry around a scar and 34% are of uncertain pathogenesis (1). The detection of reentry tachycardias is based on the assumption (for clinical purposes) that tachycardias which are capable of sudden initiation and termination by distinct events (premature depolarisation) are reentrant tachycardias (2). The basic understanding of electrical termination of V. Tach. is such that premature depolarisations are delivered in the exitable gap of the reentry circuit, cause a dispersion of depolarisation and repolarisation and that the unidirectional block (due to partially refractory myocardium) stops the running wave front. Fast V. Tach. rates indicate a small reentry circuit, polymorphic V.

Tach. different reentry circuits. The so-called "point of earliest ventricular activation", which was inaugurated by M. E. Josephson, is difficult to define in a reentry circuit (3) and cannot always be recorded during endocardial mapping in patients with V. Tach. (1). Wellens and Brugada proposed parameters which can help to define reentrant tachycardias during programmed ventricular stimulation (4). However, recurrent V. Tach. in patients with cardiomyopathy, long QT-syndrome are not yet completely understood.

Principles of antitachycardia pacing

There are three main principles of antitachycardia pacing, namely underdrive, overdrive and extrastimulus stimulation. *Underdrive pacing* means a stimulation with a rate lower than the spontaneous rate. *Overdrive pacing* is a stimulation where the rate is higher than the spontaneous rate. *Extrastimulus stimulation* means a stimulation with one or more premature depolarisations. *Burst pacing* is a special type of overdrive pacing, a high rate pacing. In the *scanning mode,* first inaugurated by Spurrell (2), the coupling interval of the extrastimulus is progressively and automatically reduced by small decrements until the refractory or termination zone is reached. Recently, Zipes at al. (citation by (5)) proposed a method of transvenous, endocardial, low energy cardioversion via a special electrode catheter with the poles at the vena cava superior and at the right ventricular apex.

Pathophysiology of ventricular tachycardias amenable for tachycardia terminating pacing

J. Fisher (6) was one of the first investigators who showed "the bad and the good" of TTP. In 390 well-tolerated V. Tach. the tachycardia termination rate could be increased from 57% (1 extrastimulus) to 59% (2 to 3 extrastimuli) and 96% (burst pacing). But the tachycardia acceleration rate also increased from 0.4% (1 extrastimulus) to 2.2% (2 to 3 extrastimuli) and to 4.4% (burst pacing). This and other experiences pointed out that the clinical effectiveness of the highly sophisticated antitachycardia pacemaker can be modified by the pathophysiological circumstances in the patient. The successful electrical termination of reentry tachycardias is dependent on (2): 1. the tachycardia rate or the diameter of the reentry circuit (inverse relationship); 2. the distance between the stimulation place and the reentrant loop; 3. the electrophysiological characteristics of the conducting myocardium between the stimulation place and the reentry circuit; 4. the difference between refractory time and conduction time in the pathological pathway; 5. the change of the refractory time and conduction time due to the electrical induced cardiac actions.

Intensive clinical investigations showed that the tachycardia termination zone becomes significantly shorter from the lying via the standing to the exercise condition. The tachycardia termination zone for a single ventricular premature beat is 30 ms long at a cycle length of 340 ms in supine position. Upon standing the cycle length decreases to 270 ms and the termination zone disappears. Supine exercise has the same effect (2). Prolongation of the termination zone is achieved by practolol, flecainide or a combination of both (2). Since most of the recently developed antitachycardia pacemakers are triggered by a rate increase or a minimum rate criterion is satisfied the additional antiarrhythmic drug therapy with substances which reduce heart rate may also alter the effectiveness of the implanted device.

265

Objective

The aim of the study was to investigate the clinical long-term efficacy of high rate stimulation for the treatment of drug-resistant tachycardias by means of an implanted, automatic burst pacemaker (Intermedics Cybertach 60).

Patients and methods

Patients

A total of 6 patients (3 ♀, 3♂, 16 to 59 years) had to be hospitalized due to recurrent, drug-resistant tachycardias. Three patients had supraventricular tachycardias (WPW syndrome) and 3 patients ventricular tachycardias (COCM, CHD, VSD).
One young female suffered from frequent attacks of atrial tachycardias of long durations (up to 1–2 h). Another young female had frequent attacks of WPW re-entry tachycardias, which lasted several hours (up to 6 h). In both patients antiarrhythmic drugs like digitalis, beta-blockers, verapamil, prajmaliumbitartrate and propafenone were ineffective. Three male patients had drug-resistant ventricular tachycardias (myocardial instability due to congestive cardiomyopathy in one patient, in the second due to coronary heart disease with the tachycardias occurring 5 years following aneurysmectomy, and following surgical correction of ventricular septal defect and pulmonary stenosis in a 16-year-old male).

Methods

The tachycardia type, etc. was studied in each patient by programmed atrial and ventricular stimulation, before or during antiarrhythmic drug therapy. The patients were followed up for 3 years (mean duration) with frequent controls of the pacemaker functions (using regular pacemaker control) and Holter monitoring as well as pacemaker-Holter ECG.
In the 3 patients with supraventricular tachycardias the arrhythmias were initiated using magnetically induced constant rate stimulation (Figure 1). The ventricular tachycardias in the 3 patients were provoked by programmed, right ventricular stimulation via a temporary lead (Figure 2). This procedure was repeated several times in order to check the reproducibility and safety of electrical termination.

Pacemaker

The Cybertach 60, Model 262-01 (Intermedics) is a single chamber, adjustable, automatic burst pacemaker with a back-up antibradycardia pacing mode. The programmable options are as follows: pacing mode, rate of the stand by pacing (60 ppm; 80 ppm), sensitivity (0.5 to 3.0 mV), impulse width (0.15 to 2.29 ms), tachycardia recognition rate (137 bpm; 180 bpm), high rate burst stimulation (140/206/360/480/720/1440 per minute) and duration of the burst pacing (0.33/1.3/2.7/4.0/5.3 sec). Since the Cybertach 60 is a bipo-

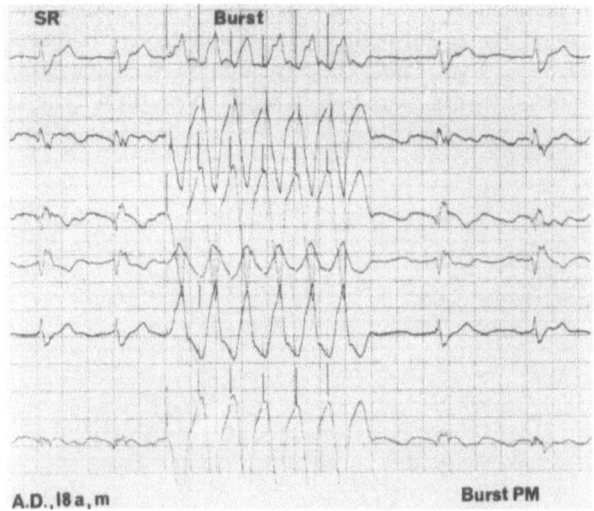

Fig. 1. Reproducible, successful termination of a supraventricular tachycardia by means of burst stimulation (tachycardia conditioning by verapamil).

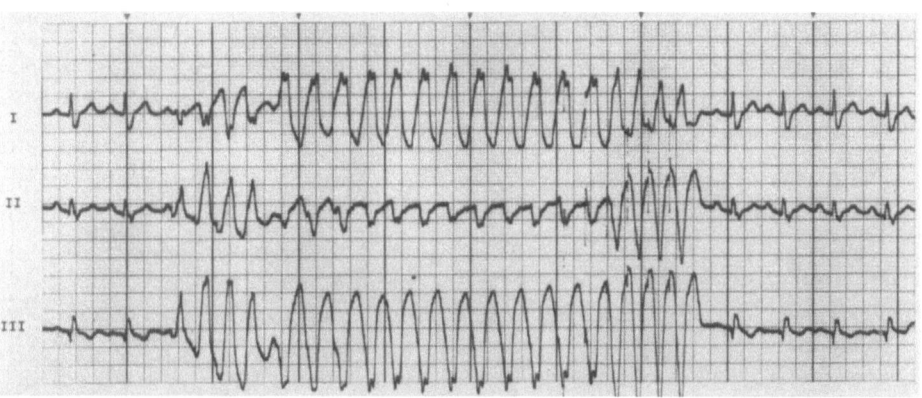

Fig. 2. Reproducible, successful termination of a ventricular tachycardia by means of burst stimulation, 240 ppm and 1.3 sec (electrode positioned in the coronary sinus), 5 days after the correction of a ventricular septum defect.

lar pacemaker, two intracardiac electrodes (Helifix, Vitatron) had to be positioned in the right atrium or ventricle.

Results: Patient follow-up

In 4/6 patients the burst stimulation characteristics and the sensitivity had to be changed within the first 6 months, according to the different modes of tachycardia initiation and termination during repeated programmed stimulation. All patients were on antiarrhythmic drugs in order to condition the tachycardia for a more successful electrical termination. Since by these means the tachycardias could be controlled in all patients the significant reduction in the number and duration of the tachycardias meant that they could normalize their daily activities. In one 20 year old man who had undergone 3 surgical operations in order to correct a VSD, about 2 years after the implantation, the pacemaker delivered continuous bursts during sinus rhythm or rare monomorphic VES (EOL criteria reached: Figures 3 and 4).

Fig. 3. After more than 2 years of correct functioning the burst pacemaker showed signs of energy depletion. During normal sinus rhythm, repetitive bursts were delivered.

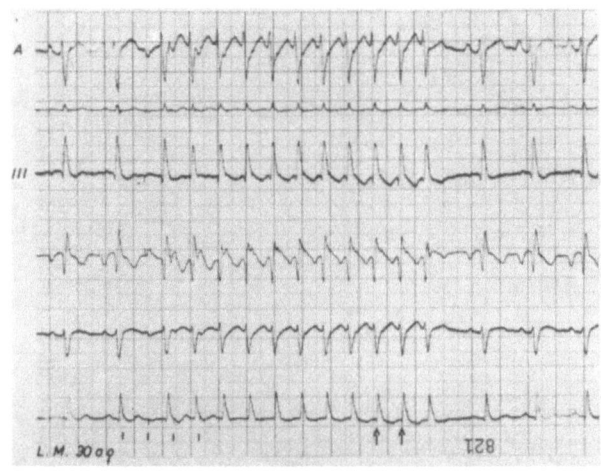

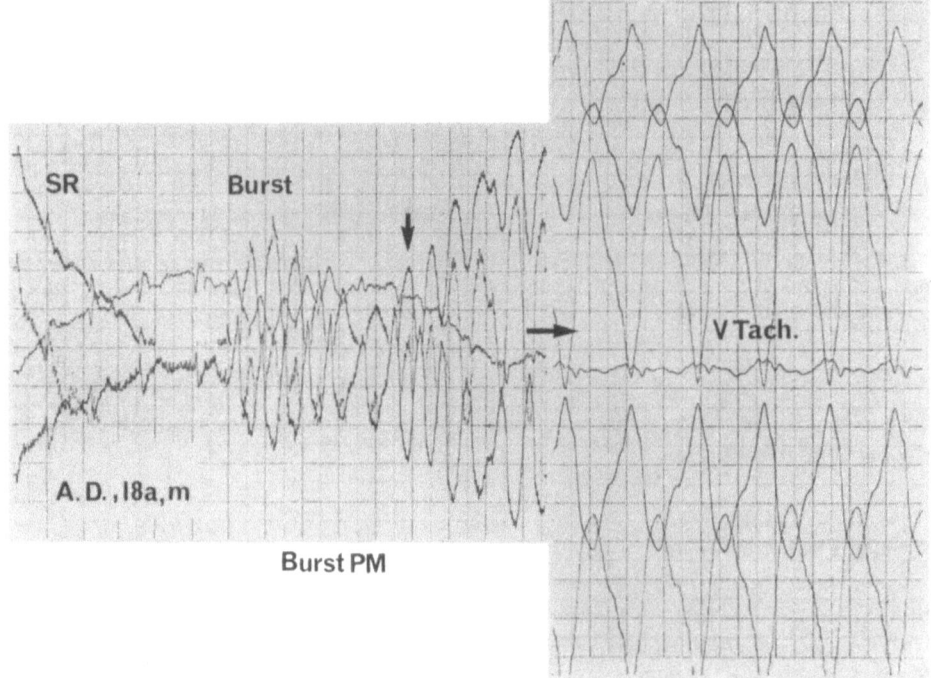

Fig. 4. Repetitive bursts during sinus rhythm led to ventricular tachycardia and hospitalisation (burst pacemaker: "end of life" criteria reached).

Discussion

In our series of 6 patients with drug-resistant supraventricular (n = 3) and ventricular (n = 3) tachycardias this type of antitachycardia pacemaker was implanted after careful electrophysiological intracardiac evaluation of the initiation-termination mechanisms of the tachycardias. In each patient the possible degeneration of ventricular tachycardia to ventricular flutter/fibrillation or acceleration of ventricular tachycardia by rapid ventricular burst pacing was tested.

Based on previous reports and our own experience, we suggest the following criteria when considering the implantation of an automatic antitachycardial pacemaker: 1) Prior to implantation careful intracardiac mapping and pacing should be performed in order: a) to demonstrate reproducible termination of the tachycardia; b) to evaluate the optimal lead position of intracardiac pacing electrodes; c) to evaluate the optimal pacing mode for termination, and d) to test the influence of antiarrhythmic drugs, particularly on the initiation and termination mechanisms of the tachycardia. 2) In the case of ventricular tachycardias different burst rates and burst durations have to be tested to evaluate: a) whether acceleration of the tachycardia or degeneration to ventricular flutter/fibrillation will ensure; b) at which burst rate and burst duration this will occur; c) whether antiarrhythmic drugs will alter the response of ventricular tachycardias to burst stimulation. 3) In the case of WPW-supraventricular tachycardia one has to test whether atrial burst stimulation during tachycardia will result in atrial fibrillation, and if so, whether this fibrillation will result in high A-V conduction rates. 4) The long-term efficacy of the implanted antitachycardial pacemaker has to be tested at regular intervals by: a) Holter ECG and pacemaker Holter ECG in patients with spontaneously occurring tachycardias; b) induction of supraventricular tachycardias by the pacemaker, using magnetically-induced fixed rate pacing; c) initiation of ventricular tachycardia using temporary transvenous programmed right ventricular pacing and testing whether the pacemaker implanted will reproducibly terminate the tachycardia.

In many patients symptoms can be reduced by slowing the tachycardia rate by β-blocking drugs. Furthermore the effectiveness of antitachycardia pacing has improved since the tachycardia pacing termination zone has been prolonged. Pacemaker malfunctions can occur if the rate increase criterion cannot be satisfied due to reduced rate increase (2). Disopyramide is recommended for the treatment or prevention of atrial fibrillation which very often misleads the tachycardia detection system (2).

In our patient population the following drugs were (either alone or in combination) partly ineffective in controlling the tachycardias: lidocaine, mexiletine, prajmaliumbitartrate, propafenone, and amiodorone. These drugs were helpful in conditioning the tachycardias and were therefore necessary.

References

1. Mason J (1984) Management of intractable ventricular tachycardia. Clinical Tutorial, NASPE meeting, New York, May 1984
2. Camm, JA, Ward D (1983) Pacing for tachycardia control. Teletronics Publications
3. Scherlag B (1984) Personal communication

4. Wellens HJJ, Brugada P, Vanagt EJDM, Ross DL, Bär FW (1981) New studies with triggered automaticity. In: Harrison DC (ed) Cardiac arrhythmias, a decade of progress. GK Wall Publishers, Boston, Massachusetts, pp 601–610
5. Fisher J (1984) Antitachycardiac devices. Meet the experts, NASPE meeting, New York, May 1984

Authors' address:
Professor D. W. Behrenbeck
Medizinische Universitätsklinik III
Josef-Stelzmann-Straße 9
5000 Köln 41
West Germany

Endo-Epicardial Cardioversion-Defibrillation for Termination of Drug-Refractory Ventricular Tachyarrhythmias

V. Hombach, H. W. Höpp, A. Osterspey, A. Hannekum, D. W. Behrenbeck, T. Eggeling, B. Herse, U. J. Winter, H. Dalichau, and H. H. Hilger

Summary: Long-term treatment of patients with recurrent attacks of ventricular tachycardia (VT) and an increased risk of sudden death may be crucial, since in some patients antiarrhythmic drugs may be ineffective or may induce serious side effects. Thus, endo-epicardial cardioversion-defibrillation seems an attractive alternative for short-term, and probably also long-term treatment of recurrent VT and ventricular fibrillation (VF).

We have evaluated the efficacy and safety of both methods in 31 patients with recurrent attacks of VT-VF and various cardiac diseases: coronary heart disease (CHD): 22 patients; congestive cardio-myopathy: 4 patients; hypertrophic-non-obstructive cardiomyopathy: 1 patient; Löffler's endocardi-tis: 1 patient; QT syndrome: 2 patients; and surgically corrected Fallot-tetralogy: 1 patient. In 39 pa-tients endocardial cardioversion (ECV) was considered prospectively for termination of inducible VT, and in 19 patients with spontaneously occurring or inducible VT ECV was tested for VT ter-mination. A total of 87 cardioversion shocks with energies of 0.03–20.0 joules were delivered via a special cardioversion electrode with two pairs of electrodes located within the RV apex and the su-perior vena cava-right atrial junction. 37/47 VT episodes were directly terminated by ECV, and 8/47 VT episodes indirectly by slowing of VT and spontaneous termination shortly thereafter. Cardiover-sion threshold without antiarrhythmic drugs was 3.46 ± 5.3 joules, and with antiarrhythmic drugs 0.8 ± 0.60 joules. One patient with spontaneous attacks of VT-VF and cardiac resuscitation (three times successfully) was provided with the automatic intracardiac cardioverter-defibrillator (AICD), which was functioning quite well when tested intraoperatively and just prior to discharge (induction of VT-VF during general anesthesia and testing of the efficacy of the first AICD shock). In concord-ance with the experiences in the literature and these preliminary results we conclude that the con-cept of endo-epicardial cardioversion-defibrillation seems to be very safe and promising for the short and long-term treatment of patients with recurrent attacks of drug-resistant VT-VF.

Introduction

Complex ventricular arrhythmias, such as multiform ectopic beats, ventricular couplets and ventricular tachycardias, seem to be of important prognostic significance in deter-mining the risk of sudden cardiac death, particularly in patients with coronary heart dis-ease and impaired left ventricular function (1, 2, 3). In the clinical setting it is rather diffi-cult to determine the individual risk of a given patient and to predict long-term efficacy of oral antiarrhythmic drug therapy in preventing the deleterious event of sudden ar-rhythmic death, and there are contradictory results regarding success rates of medical prophylaxis against sudden death (4, 5, 6). In most patients with ventricular tachyar-rhythmias basic initial management is antiarrhythmic and antifibrillatory drug therapy. However, due to failure of drugs to prevent repetitive forms of ventricular arrhythmias or due to patient non-compliance or severe side effects of these drugs, in a certain number of patients alternative methods for tachyarrhythmia control, like electrical or surgical the-rapy, may be advocated. There are principally two types of electrical therapy of regular ventricular tachycardias and/or ventricular tachyarrhythmias: antitachycardia pacing in the former case, or endocardial cardioversion/defibrillation in the former and latter case

(7, 8, 9). The most recent attractive methods of tachycardia termination seem to be endocardial cardioversion or epicardial cardioversion/defibrillation, either in the external mode or with the implantable and fully automatic devices, which were particularly developed for the high risk group of patients prone to recurrent attacks of ventricular tachycardia/fibrillation. We report our initial experiences with both types of tachycardia termination, the bedside application of endocardial cardioversion and the implantation of an automatic intracardiac defibrillator.

Patients

A total of 31 patients, 5 females and 26 males, aged 25–63 years were studied either prospectively during programmed ventricular stimulation (n = 28 individuals) or with ventricular tachycardia running during the cardioversion study (n = 3 patients). In 10 patients external DC-cardioversion had been necessary to terminate ventricular tachyarrhythmias (one to five times), and 3 of these individuals had been resuscitated from sudden cardiac tachyarrhythmic events. The following cardiac diseases were found: in the group of 19 patients with spontaneous or induced ventricular tachycardias: coronary heart disease (CHD): 15 (LV aneurysm in 11 patients, in 10 with anterior wall aneurysm, in 1 with posterior wall aneurysm); congestive cardiomyopathy: 1 patient; hypertrophic non-obstructive cardiomyopathy: 1 patient; Löffler's endocarditis: 1 patient; and operated Fallot's tetralogy: 1 patient; in the group of 12 patients without inducible ventricular tachycardias: CHD: 7 patients (LV aneurysm 4 patients, anterior wall 4 patients); congestive cardiomyopathy: 3 patients; QT-syndrome: 2 individuals. In one patient with congestive cardiomyopathy and three episodes of ventricular tachycardia-fibrillation with successful resuscitation and drug resistant ventricular tachyarrhythmias the automatic intracardiac cardioverter/defibrillator (AICD) has been implanted to terminate further attacks of ventricular tachyarrhythmias. The patients were instructed in detail about the procedure and the possible risks and gave their written consent. The electrophysiological evaluations were performed late in the morning or in the early afternoon at the coronary care unit.

Methods

In local anesthesia the special cardioversion electrode (Medtronik No. 6880) was introduced either via the left subclavian vein (in 25 patients), the right subclavian vein (in 2 individuals), or via the right femoral vein (in 4 patients) by use of a special introducer system (Littleford/Spector Introducer, Cordis), advanced to the right ventricle and finally positioned with its tip within the right ventricular apical region close to the interventricular septum (Figure 1). The proximal pair of electrodes was located at the superior vena cava-right atrial junction, or at the level of the high right atrium. This cardioversion electrode was connected with the external cardioversion/defibrillation device (Medtronik 2326) for receiving the intraventricular ECG signals, for programmed ventricular stimulation, and for delivery of the endocardial microshocks. The cardioversion device provides a marker impulse from the intracardiac ECG which serves as the indicator of the trigger point of the microshock relative to the QRS complex (the microshock is regularly

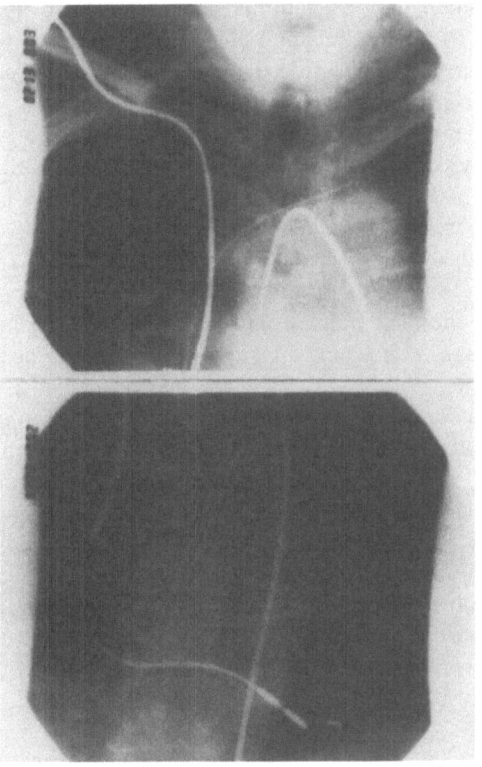

Fig. 1: Chest X-ray showing the position of the special endocardial cardioverter electrode. The electrode is introduced via the right subclavian vein (upper half), and its tip is located within the right ventricular apex at the interventricular septum (lower half). The patient had previously been provided with a conventional permanent VVI pacemaker, whose electrode is seen introduced via the left subclavian vein and positioned within the right ventricular apex.

delivered during the first third of the QRS complex). Conventional Einthoven leads I-III were recorded from the patients together with the marker impulse on a six-channel ink jet recorder (Siemens-Elema, Mingograph).

The cardioversion catheter is a No. 10F, with two bipolar pairs of stainless steel electrodes with a surface area of 2.5 cm²/pair. The distal electrodes located at the tip are separated by 5 mm and provide bipolar sensing of ventricular depolarisation to synchronize the microshock. The proximal electrodes with a separation of 5 mm are located 100 mm, 130 mm or 150 mm from the catheter tip. When the shock is delivered, the two distal electrodes are coupled together to form the cathode and the two proximal electrodes are coupled together to form the anode (7).

The external cardioverter delivers truncated exponential waveforms of 2 ms, 6 ms and 12 ms duration (according to the tilt values of 27%, 63%, and 87%) at 36 energy levels of 0.03 to 28.0 joules. A programmable unit is interfaced within the cardioverter, providing the sensing and timing for the cardioversion shocks during tachycardia. The energy of the initial shocks which were failing to terminate the VT was increased stepwise to determine the cardioversion threshold, which is defined as the minimum energy required to terminate the ventricular tachycardia.

The automatic intracardiac cardioverter/defibrillator (AICD) monitors the patient's cardiac electrical activity. If it detects ventricular tachycardias of fibrillation above a pre-set rate, it applies electrical defibrillatory pulses to the heart through implanted leads in an attempt to restore an effective rhythm. The rate cut-off is nominally set at 160 beats/

min. The total elapsed time from onset of malignant arrhythmia to the delivery of the first pulse is 10 to 30 seconds, depending on the arrhythmia and pulse energy to be delivered. The AICD's logic requires 5 to 15 seconds to diagnose the malignant arrhythmia and another 5–15 seconds to store the energy in its output capacitors.

The initial pulse is nominally 25 joules, and if the tachycardia persists, a second 25 joule pulse is delivered after another detection and charging time of 10 to 30 seconds. If the tachyarrhythmia still persists, a third pulse of 25 joules and eventually a fourth pulse of approximately 30 joules are delivered. This fourpulse sequence lasts approximately two minutes. If the arrhythmia is terminated with the first, second or third microshock, a 35 second recycle time is required, i.e. if the first pulse terminates the tachyarrhythmia which then recurs in less than 35 seconds, the next pulse would behave as the second pulse, but if the arrhythmia recurs more than 35 seconds after the first pulse the next pulse would be the first of a new sequence.

The total cardioversion-defibrillation system comprises two patch electrodes, two sensing electrodes, the battery-operated pulse generator, and the AICD-check equipment. In our patient a medial sternotomy and pericardial incision was performed for positioning one (the larger) patch electrode over the LV-apical and posterobasal regions, and the second (the smaller one) patch electrode over the anterior free wall of the right ventricle. Both patch electrodes were sutured to the epicardium for safe connection to the myocardium, after testing the optimal position of the patch electrodes with minimal pulse energies to terminate ventricular fibrillation. Another set of two sensing electrodes (screw-in type) were attached to the right ventricular free wall myocardium. The four leads were tunneled under the skin and connected to the pulse generator implanted in a left paraumbilical pocket (Figure 2).

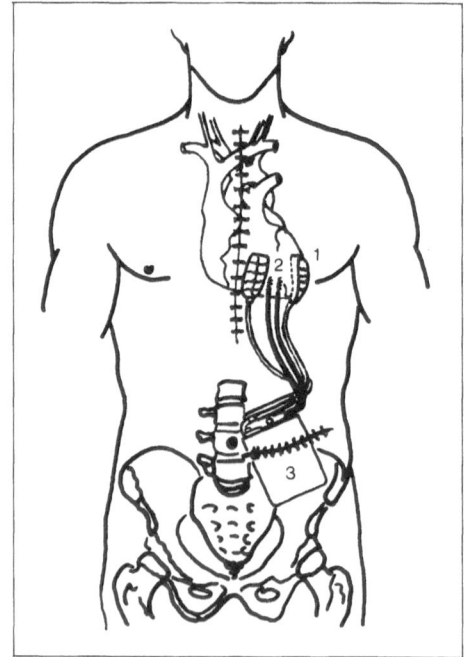

Fig. 2: Schematic drawing of the implantation procedure of the automatic implantable cardioverter/defibrillator (AICD). Following a medial sternotomy and pericardial incision, two patch electrodes are placed epicardially, one behind the posterior wall of the left ventricle and over the LV apex, and the other over the anterior RV free wall (1). Two screw-in sensing electrodes (2) serve for continuous detection of cardiac rhythm and the occurrence of ventricular tachycardias and/or fibrillation and for triggering the cardioversion-defibrillation unit (3), which is placed in a subcutaneous abdominal pocket after tunneling the electrode-wires subcutaneously.

Results

In 12 patients endocardial cardioversion was prospectively considered for termination of VT, however, in these patients the tachycardia could not be induced by programmed right ventricular stimulation. In 19 patients ventricular tachycardias were observed spontaneously or induced by programmed ventricular stimulation (basic driven rhythms of 100, 120, 140 and 160 stimuli/min with one or/and two extrastimuli with steadily decreasing coupling interval down to the effective refractory period of the right ventricle), and could be treated by the endocardial cardioversion (ECV) method. In these 19 patients a total of 47 episodes of ventricular tachycardias were observed, and a total of 87 microshocks with energies of 0.03 to 20.0 joules were delivered via the cardioversion electrode (Table 1). 37/87 microshocks delivered were successful in terminating the tachyarrhythmia (Figure 3), and 37/47 VT episodes were immediately and safely terminated by ECV,

Table 1. Summary of the overall cardioversion results.

Number of patients with VT (spontaneous, induced):	19 Patients
Number of patients without VT:	12 Patients
Number of VT episodes observed:	47 Episodes
Number of shocks delivered:	87 Shocks
Termination rates related to number of shocks:	37/87 Shocks
Termination rate related to VT episodes (direct):	37/47 Episodes
Termination rate related to VT episodes (indirect):	8/47 Episodes
Termination rate on antiarrhythmic drugs (VT episodes)	30/36 Episodes
Termination rate without antiarrhythmic drugs (VT episodes)	8/11 Episodes
Severe acceleration of VT on microshock:	3 Episodes
External DC shock required (V flutter not related to cardioversion)	2 Episodes
Cardioversion threshold without antiarrhythmic drugs:	3.46 ± 5.3 joules
Cardioversion threshold with antiarrhythmic drugs:	0.80 ± 0.60 joules

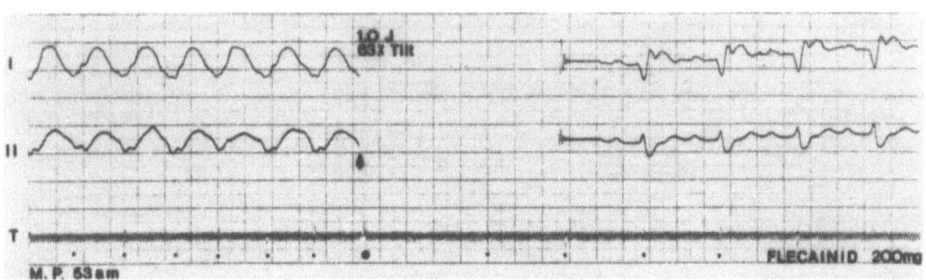

Fig. 3: Termination of a run sustained ventricular tachycardia in a 53 year old male with large anterior wall aneurysm by a low energy endocardial microshock of 1.0 joules to sinus rhythm. The patient was set on chronic oral therapy with flecainide.

I and II: Einthoven leads I and II, T: test or sensing impulse which indicates proper sensing of the external cardioversion unit and identifies the correct timing of the microshock within the first third of the tachycardia QRS complex (arrow).

8/47 VT episodes were indirectly terminated by ECV by slowing down of the VT rate, and in 2/47 VT-V flutter episodes external DC-shock was required to terminate the ventricular tachyarrhythmia. In 2 patients a severe acceleration of VT was induced by low energy cardioversion pulses, and both ventricular tachycardia episodes were terminated by a 15.0 joule and 10.0 joule defibrillation shock. In a third patient severe acceleration of VT occurred following ventricular burst pacing in an attempt to terminate the tachycardia, and in this case a 20.0 joule defibrillation pulse terminated the ventricular flutter episode.

Of the 87 microshocks 65 were delivered when the patients were set on chronic oral antiarrhythmic drug therapy. In 8/22 microshocks delivered in patients without antiarrhythmic drug therapy these microshocks were successful in terminating the VT, as compared to 30/65 successful microshocks in patients on oral maintenance drug therapy. 36 VT episodes were observed in patients with drug therapy, and in 30 instances VT was immediately and successfully terminated by ECV, as compared to 8/11 successful terminations of VT episodes in patients without antiarrhythmic drug therapy (Table 2). The cardioversion threshold for ventricular tachycardias was 0.80 ± 0.60 joules in patients with chronic oral antiarrhythmic drug therapy, compared to a cardioversion threshold of 3.46 ± 5.30 joules in patients without antiarrhythmic drug therapy.

In general, cardioversion shocks with energies of 1.5 to 2.0 joules were well tolerated, with patients reporting mild to moderate discomfort due to the microshocks. However, shocks with levels of 5.0 joules and more were reported to be painful, and patients who

Tab. 2a. Comparison of the efficacy of microshocks without and with antiarrhythmic drugs in a total of 87 microshocks delivered.

	Successful	Not successful	Total
Without AAD	8	14	22
With AAD	30	35	65
Total	38	49	87
	$x^2 = 1.10$	$p = 0.29$	

AAD: antiarrhythmic drugs.

Tab. 2b. Comparison of the overall efficacy of microshocks without and with antiarrhythmic drugs, as related to VT episodes.

	Successful	Not successful	Total
Without AAD	8	3	11
With AAD	30	6	36
Total	38	9	47
	$x^2 = 1.489$	$p = 0.22$	

AAD: antiarrhythmic drugs.

required higher energy cardioversion-defibrillation shocks were immediately anesthetized (in 3 instances).

In one patient with recurrent episodes of ventricular tachycardia/fibrillation and successful resuscitation electrophysiological testing revealed that for termination of VT episodes cardioversion energies of more than 5.0 joules were necessary, and this individual was considered for implantation of the AICD device. After placing the two patch electrodes at the left and right ventricular site, as described above, the lowest defibrillation threshold was determined, and was found to be 11.0 joules after definite electrode position (Figure 4). One further episode of ventricular fibrillation was induced intraoperatively, and the implanted AICD immediately detected this fibrillation episode and successfully terminated ventricular fibrillation by a 25 joules pulse. Three weeks postoperatively the patient experienced a shock episode while walking in the ward, but this episode was not monitored by conventional or Holter ECG recording. Therefore an electrophysiological study was performed prior to discharge of the patient, and the ventricular tachycardia-flutter episode, as induced by programmed ventricular stimulation, was again immediately recognized by the AICD device and successfully terminated by the first 25 joules shock delivered.

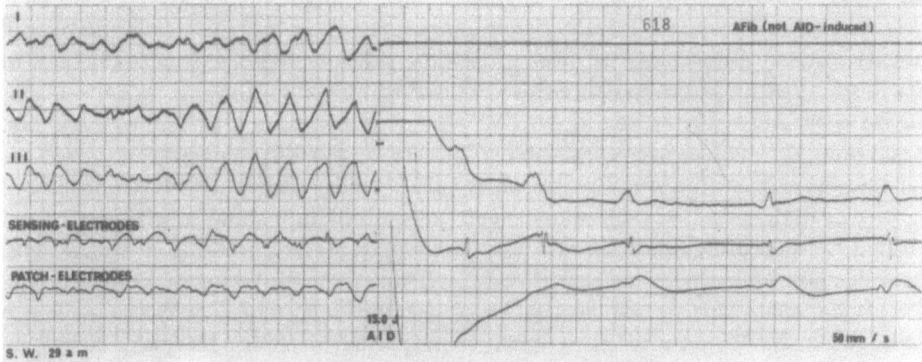

Fig. 4: Intraoperative testing of the efficacy of the implantable cardioverter/defibrillator to terminate ventricular tachyarrhythmias. The heart has been fibrillated by an AC fibrillator (left panel), and after sensing of this tachyarrhythmia the defibrillation pulse is delivered by the defibrillator, resulting in prompt termination of ventricular flutter/fibrillation (right panel). The post-shock rhythm is atrial fibrillation, which had initially been induced by AC-fibrillation in order to facilitate AC-fibrillation of the ventricles.
I-III Einthoven leads I-III, AID: automatic implantable defibrillator.

Discussion

Coronary heart disease patients with complex ventricular arrhythmias and impaired ventricular function carry a 2-3-fold risk of sudden arrhythmic death as compared to the normal population, at least in the first year after myocardial infarction. In more than 80% of sudden death victims ventricular tachycardia-flutter-fibrillation seems to be the primary cause of death. In the case of recurrent attacks of ventricular tachycardia/fibrillation antiarrhythmic drugs may fail to prevent this deleterious event, and electrical methods are considered for short and long-term treatment of these arrhythmias. Historically anti-tachycardia pacing was first tested for its efficacy and safety of terminating regular and sustained forms of ventricular tachycardias (9). Although different pacing modes have been applied e.g. most recently rate responsive antitachycardia pacing, and in a more recent study the efficacy of antitachycardia burst pacing has been reported to be as effective as endocardial cardioversion (13), there is still the potential danger of accelerating the tachycardia or of primary induction of ventricular fibrillation by antitachycardia extrastimulus or burst pacing at the ventricular site. Therefore the new methods of endocardial cardioversion/defibrillation seem to be a very attractive alternative to the ventricular pacing procedure (7, 8, 12, 14).

According to the initial reports by Kallok and Zipes et al. (7), the conversion rate of VTs to sinus rhythm was relatively high in our series (direct conversion of VT to sinus rhythm in 36/47 VT episodes = 76.6%, indirect conversion by slowing of the VT in 8/47 episodes = 17.0%), and so far only 3/47 VT episodes have required endocardial defibrillation with pulse energies of 10.0 to 20.0 joules. It is also interesting to note that in our series the success rates with endocardial cardioversion were higher with antiarrhythmic drugs (30/36 episodes = 83%) than without antiarrhythmic therapy (8/11 VT episodes = 72.7%), and that the cardioversion threshold was lower with antiarrhythmic drugs (0.8 ± 0.6 joules) than without antiarrhythmic therapy (3.46 ± 5.3 joules), these differences were not, however, statistically significant because of the relatively small number of patients studied without antiarrhythmic oral drug therapy. Similar conversion rates of VTs to sinus rhythm were reported in a recent multicenter study (14), i.e. an 84% success rate in 36 patients with 188 episodes of VT with a cardioversion threshold of 0.8 joules. In addition, 397/402 episodes of unstable VTs were successfully terminated by endocardial cardioversion with a mean pulse energy of 6.2 joules, and finally 9/10 episodes of ventricular flutter and 19/27 episodes of ventricular fibrillation could successfully be terminated by endocardial microshocks of pulse energies of 19.0 joules as a mean. Thus, based on these experiences endocardial cardioversion seems to be an effective and relatively safe method for repeated termination of sustained ventricular tachycardias. It also seems reasonable to improve the termination rates and to reduce the pulse energy required for termination by treating the patient with antiarrhythmic drugs in order to condition the tachycardia for the termination procedure.

Since the implantable cardioverter provides cardioversion pulses of 2.0 joules as a maximum, this device does not seem to be of use for chronic treatment of patients with recurrent attacks of ventricular tachyarrhythmias like VT/V flutter or ventricular fibrillation. Since the initial clinical investigations, as initiated by Mirowski et al. in February 1980, in more than 200 patients with ventricular tachyarrhythmias the automatic intracardiac defibrillator was implanted in its initial (AID®) or more recent versions (AID®-B, AID®-BR). Follow-up data of more than 100 individuals provided with the AID revealed a 22.9% one-year mortality, and a 52% decrease from the 48% mortality, which would be expected in the same group of patients without the device (15), and the mortality attributed to the ventricular tachyarrhythmia only was found to be 8.5%. It was concluded that the automatic cardioverter/defibrillator can reliably identify and terminate potentially lethal ventricular tachyarrhythmias, and thus, may lead to a substantial increase in survival in properly selected high risk patients. This was the reason why one young patient was provided with at least 3 episodes of VT/fibrillation and resuscitations with the AID, after thorough testing of antiarrhythmic drugs' efficacy with programmed stimula-

Table 3. Comparison of the different criteria of the implantable cardioverter and the automatic intra-cardiac cardioverter/defibrillator (AICD).

Criterion	Endocardial cardioverter	AICD
Implantation procedure	Simple, like pacemaker implantation	More complicated thoracotomy, subxiphoidal incision
Temporary mode	+	–
Low energy cardioversion	+	–
Intracardiac defibrillation	– (Only with external device)	+
Back-up pacing	+	–
Acceleration of VT	(+)	(+)
Programmability of implantable device	+	–
Shocks painful with defibrillation	+++	+
Relative costs of the implantable device	Lower	Higher

tion (more than 6 drugs and 3 drug combinations were ineffective) and the possibility of terminating the tachyarrhythmias by endocardial cardioversion (ineffective with 5.0 joules without antiarrhythmic drug therapy). The function tests of the AID intra- and postoperatively revealed a proper sensing and delivery function of this device.

There are some important differences between the endocardial cardioversion and defibrillation methods (Table 3). The implantation procedure of the implantable cardioverter is simpler than of the AID, it can be used in a temporary mode for emergency or elective termination of VT during programmed stimulation (cardioversion and defibrillation), and in its implantable unit the cardioverter provides back-up VVI pacing as opposed to the AID. On the other hand, the implantable AID provides defibrillation properties and seems to possess the highest probability and safety for termination of ventricular fibrillation, be it spontaneously occurring or induced by lower energy cardioversion. Due to different topical delivery of the cardioversion/defibrillation pulses, the cardioversion system seems to require higher pulse energies than the AID, whose electrodes are more closely placed to the left ventricular myocardium, where most pathological re-entrant VTs are located (16). In addition, the microshocks from the cardioversion unit may be more painful than from the AID due to the larger area of the AID system's patch electrodes, although to date no direct comparison has been made with both techniques in the same patients. However, recent experiences with sequential microshock application have shown that the pulse energies required for successful termination of ventricular flutter-fibrillation can be considerably reduced by this procedure (17, 18).

In conclusion, the new methods of intracardiac cardioversion or cardioversion/defibrillation (AID) constitute an important step forward in the treatment of patients with recurrent attacks of life-threatening ventricular tachyarrhythmias, both in the external bedside and in the chronic implantable mode. Further intensive studies have to be performed in order to properly select patients suitable for this treatment, to improve the electrode design and pulse delivery mode (perhaps sequential pulse delivery), and to prolong the longevity of the batteries, to incorporate back-up pacing and perhaps antitachycardia pacing in these devices as the initial mode for termination of an eventually regular type of VT, and perhaps to decrease the size of the implantable units.

References

1. Lown B (1980) Cardiovascular collapse and sudden cardiac death. In: Braunwald E (ed) Heart Disease, A Textbook of Cardiovascular Medicine. W. B. Saunders, Philadelphia, London, Toronto, p 778
2. Hombach V, Höpp HW, Osterspey A, Winter U, Deutsch H, Hilger HH (1984) Ambulatory ECG monitoring in the detection of patients at risk of sudden cardiac death. Herz 9: 6
3. Moss A, De Camilla J, Davis HT. Clinical significance of ventricular arrhythmias recorded at different time periods after myocardial infarction. In: Hombach V, Hilger HH (eds) Holter Monitoring Technique. FK Schattauer-Verlag, Stuttgart, New York (in press)
4. Myerburgh R, Conde C, Mayorga-Cortes A, Castellanos A (1980) Mortality after survival from pre-hospital cardiac arrest might be influenced by the use of membrane-active antiarrhythmic drugs. In: Rapoport E (ed) Current Controversies in Cardiovascular Disease. WB Saunders Company, Philadelphia, London, Toronto, p 351
5. Cobb L, Hallstrom A (1980) Mortality in survivors of out-of-hospital ventricular fibrillation is not improved by the routine use of quinidine or procainamide. In: Rapoport E (ed) Current Controversies in Cardiovascular Disease. WB Saunders Company, Philadelphia, London, Toronto, p 359
6. Lown B, Lampert S. Protecting the patient at risk for sudden cardiac death. In: Hombach V, Hilger HH (eds) Holter Monitoring Technique. FK Schattauer-Verlag, Stuttgart, New York, (in press)
7. Zipes DP, Jackman WM, Heger JJ, Chilson DA, Browne KF, Naccarelli GV, Rahilly GT, Prystowsky EN (1982) Clinical transvenous cardioversion of life-threatening ventricular tachyarrhythmias. Low energy synchronized cardioversion of ventricular tachycardia and termination of ventricular fibrillation in patients using a catheter electrode. Am Heart J 103: 789
8. Mirowski M, Reid PR, Watkins L, Weisfeldt ML, Mower MM (1981) Clinical treatment of life-threatening ventricular tachyarrhythmias with the automatic implantable defibrillator. Am Heart J 102: 265
9. Fisher J, Mehra R, Furman S (1978) Termination of ventricular tachycardia with bursts of rapid ventricular pacing. Am J Cardiol 41: 94
10. Myerburgh RJ, Kessler KM, Estes D, Conde CA, Luceri RM, Zaman L, Kozlovskis PL, Castellanos A (1984) Long-term survival after prehospital cardiac arrest: Analysis of outcome during an 8 year study. Circulation 70: 538
11. Camm AJ, Ward D (1983) Pacing for Tachycardia Control. Telectronics, Australia
12. Hombach V, Höpp HW, Behrenbeck DW, Osterspey A, Jansen W, Winter U, Tauchert M, Hilger HH (1984) Endocardial cardioversion: a new method for the treatment of recurrent ventricular tachycardias. Deutsch Med Wochenschr 109: 1433
13. Saksena S, Shah Y, Boccadamo R, Rothbart ST (1984) Comparative efficacy of transvenous cardioversion and pacing in ventricular tachycardia: A prospective randomized cross-over study. Circulation 70 (Suppl II): 1625
14. Kallok MJ, Fisher JD, Fletcher RD, Hartzler GO, Kehoe RF, Klein GJ, Prystowsky EN, Ruffy R, Zipes DP (1983) Intracavitary cardioversion and defibrillation. A multicenter study. Circulation 68 (Suppl III): 88
15. Mirowski M, Reid PR, Mower MM, Watkins L Jr, Platia EV, Griffith LSC, Juanteguy JM (1983) Treatment of ventricular tachyarrhythmias with implantable automatic cardioverter-defibrillator. In: Steinbach K, Glogar D, Laszkovics A, Scheibelhofer W, Weber H (eds) Cardiac Pacing, Proc VIIth World Symp on Cardiac Pacing, Vienna 1983. Steinkopff Verlag, Darmstadt, p 815
16. Naumann D'Alnoncourt C, Eingartner C, Lüderitz B (1984) Defibrillation energy requirements using implantable patch electrodes and/or endocardial leads in different positions. Circulation 70 (Suppl II): 1627

17. Zipes DP, Kallok MJ, Gill RM, Kammerling JM (1984) Efficacy of sequential electrical shocks to terminate ventricular fibrillation in dogs after myocardial infarction. Circulation 70 (Suppl II): 1626
18. Bourland JD, Tacker WA, Wessale JL, Graf JE, Kallok MJ (1984) Energy reduction for implantable defibrillation using a sequential-pulse method to decrease generator size and increase safety. Circulation 70 (Suppl II): 400

Authors' address:
Professor V. Hombach
Medizinische Universitäts-Klinik III
Josef-Stelzmann-Straße 9
5000 Köln 41
West Germany

Single-Beat Stimulation and Train of Stimuli Method for Prevention of Reentrant Tachycardia

K.-H. Kuck, K.-P. Kunze, M. Schlüter, and W. Bleifeld

Summary: Eleven patients with an atrioventricular accessory pathway were studied by programmed electrical stimulation to determine if reentrant tachycardia can be prevented in these patients by delivery of a single atrial extrastimulus, applied at a critical time after the tachycardia-initiating stimulus (or stimuli), or by delivery of a train of stimuli. In all 11 patients, reentrant tachycardia could reproducibly be induced from high right atrium with a single premature beat, and in all patients initiation of tachycardia could be prevented from the same site by a second premature beat. This second extrastimulus was effective if delivered within a zone which began 10 ms outside the effective refractory period of the tachycardia-initiating stimulus, and averaged 61 ms in width. It was termed the "preventive zone". In 7 patients the effect of train stimulation to the high right atrium was studied. In all 7, results were concordant with those obtained by single-beat stimulation. Any train to achieve single atrial capture within the preventive zone was effective in preventing tachycardia. Prevention was always possible with a single atrial extrastimulus or with single-capture train stimulation, whereas termination of an ongoing tachycardia required at least 2 atrial extrastimuli, or stimulation from the right ventricle.

Introduction

The initiation and termination of reentrant tachycardia by programmed electrical stimulation of the heart are well-known electrophysiologic techniques (1). It has recently been shown that termination of sustained tachycardia can be achieved more effectively by short bursts (trains) of extrastimuli than by critically timed single stimuli (2). Implantable antitachycardia pacemakers have been developed which incorporate various pacing modes to terminate such arrhythmias either automatically (3) or by patient-activated systems (4). The mode of action of these systems always implies recognition and subsequent termination of a spontaneously initiated arrhythmia.

Critically timed premature beats and trains of extrastimuli, applied immediately after the extrastimuli which initiated the arrhythmia, should work as preventive modes in circus movement tachycardia by interfering with the reentrant wavefront. Therefore, the purposes of this investigation were: first, to determine if initiation of a reentrant tachycardia can be prevented by a single well-timed premature beat following the arrhythmia-initiating stimulus (or stimuli); and second, should the single-beat mode turn out to be effective, to determine if prevention can be less critically achieved by rapid trains of extrastimuli.

Methods

Eleven patients (7 men and 4 women, aged between 17 and 64 years, mean 31 years) with an atrioventricular accessory pathway were studied. Eight patients had Wolff-Parkinson-White (WPW) syndrome and 3 had a concealed left-sided accessory pathway. They had been off any medication for 72 hours prior to the investigation. All patients gave informed written consent before entering the study.

For the electrophysiologic study 4 electrode catheters were introduced from both femoral veins, using the Seldinger technique. Quadripolar catheters were placed in the high right atrium and in the coronary sinus, and bipolar catheters were placed across the tricuspid valve, to record His bundle potentials, and in the right ventricle. The stimulation protocol included stimulation of high right atrium, coronary sinus and right ventricle with 1 or 2 extrastimuli during basic drive pacing. Details of the stimulation protocol have previously been given (5).

First, the tachycardia zone during which atrial extrastimuli (S_2) elicited an atrioventricular reentrant tachycardia was determined during basic pacing (S_1S_1) of the high right atrium. Then, an extrastimulus (S_2) in the center of the tachycardia zone was delivered after every 8th beat of basic pacing and was tested at least 5 times to ascertain reproducibility of tachycardia initiation. The tachycardia-initiating coupling interval S_1S_2 was held constant for the entire study.

Termination of tachycardia was then attempted from the high right atrium with a single atrial premature beat delivered at a coupling interval 100 ms less than the tachycardia cycle length. This coupling interval was progressively decreased in 10 ms steps until either tachycardia was terminated or atrial refractoriness was reached. When the single stimulus failed to terminate the arrhythmia, a second and, maximally, a third termination stimulus was delivered. When completion of this atrial stimulation protocol also failed, stimulation of the right ventricle was started, following the same pattern as for atrial stimulation, with a maximum of 2 ventricular premature beats.

Subsequently, programmed electrical stimulation was used to determine the preventive zone (Fig. 1, panel A). A second atrial premature beat (S_3) was delivered at the same anatomical site (high right atrium) as the tachycardia-initiating S_2 stimulus, and was timed 100 ms earlier than the expected retrograde right atrial depolarization (A_T) by the initial tachycardia beat. The S_2A_T interval was termed "initial tachycardia interval". The S_2S_3 coupling interval was progressively shortened by 10 ms decrements until refractoriness of S_2 was reached. Programmed stimulation was terminated when the S_2S_3 interval was 50

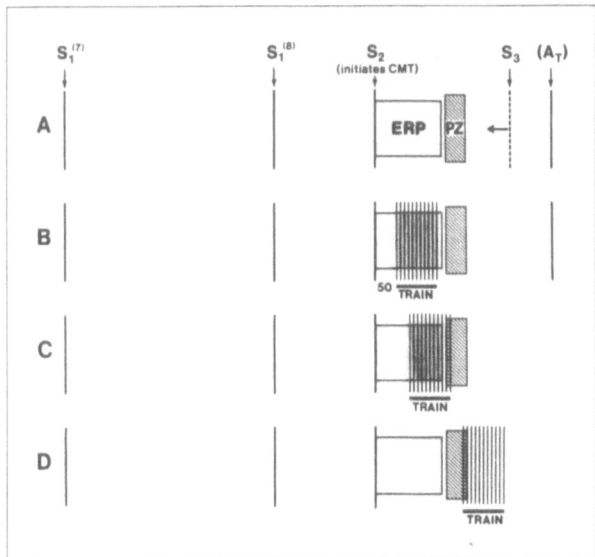

Fig. 1. Panel A: Schematic diagram illustrating the determination of the preventive zone by single-beat stimulation of high right atrium. See text for details. Panel B: Delivery of a 100 Hz train of 10 extrastimuli (10×10 ms) 50 ms after S_2. Duration of train is completely within ERP. Atrial capture does not occur and tachycardia is not prevented. Panel C: Delay of train delivery results in single atrial capture within PZ. Tachycardia is prevented. Panel D: Further delay of train delivery still prevents tachycardia as long as first train stimulus falls within PZ. Abbreviations: A_T = retrograde atrial depolarization by initial tachycardia beat; CMT = circus movement tachycardia; ERP = atrial effective refractory period of S_2 stimulus; PZ = preventive zone; $S_1^{(7)}S_1^{(8)}$ = last paced interval.

283

ms within the refractory period of S_2. The longest S_2S_3 interval for which S_3 prevented the initiation of a circus movement tachycardia represents the upper limit of the preventive zone, whereas the shortest S_2S_3 interval represents the lower limit.

Following the determination of the preventive zone with single stimuli, a 100 Hz train, consisting of 10 extrastimuli with a 10 ms interval between successive stimuli, was delivered to the high right atrium in 7 patients, starting with a coupling interval of 50 ms between S_2 and the first train stimulus (Fig. 1, panel B). The train therefore covered the zone from 50 to 150 ms which, in these patients, was always within the atrial effective refractory period of S_2. Thereafter, delivery of the train was delayed by additional 10 ms, until single atrial capture was obtained (Fig. 1, panel C). The train was further shifted towards diastole in 10 ms increments (Fig. 1, panel D), until the first train stimulus was 50 ms outside the preventive zone.

Programmed single extrastimuli used in the investigation were provided by the Biotronik ERA-S-His stimulator. Trains of stimuli were provided by the Medtronic SPO503 MKIV stimulator. Stimulus amplitude was twice diastolic threshold (1.2–4.3 mA) and stimulus duration was 0.5 ms. Three surface leads (II, V_1, V_6) and 5 intracardiac leads were recorded on a 16-channel electrocardiographer (Siemens) at a paper speed of 100 mm/s. Electrocardiographic surface leads were filtered at 0.1 to 20 Hz and signals from intracardiac leads were filtered at 40 to 500 Hz.

Statistical analysis was performed using linear regression analysis and Student's t-test.

Results

In all 11 patients orthodromic circus movement tachycardia could be initiated during right atrial stimulation with a single atrial extrastimulus. The electrophysiologic data are listed in Table 1. The S_1S_2 interval which reproducibly initiated tachycardia averaged 251 ms, with a range between 230 and 290 ms. Mean cycle length of circus movement tachycardia was 312 ms, ranging from 240 to 400 ms.

Termination of circus movement tachycardia was achieved in 7 patients from the high right atrium, and in 4 patients from the right ventricular apex.

In each patient, a temporal range of S_3 stimuli was found during which S_3 reproducibly prevented the initiation of circus movement tachycardia. The mean width of this preventive zone was 61 ms (S_2S_3, on average, ranged from 196 ms to 257 ms). Differentiation of our patient group into those with a right-sided accessory pathway (cases 1, 2, 5 and 11) and those with a left-sided accessory pathway yielded mean widths of the preventive zone of 88 ± 52 and 46 ± 10 ms, respectively. This difference, however, was statistically not significant. In all patients the lower limit of the preventive zone was 10 ms outside the effective refractory period of S_2.

In the 7 patients studied with 100 Hz trains of stimuli, responses to these trains were found to be concordant with those of single stimuli. Each train extending the effective refractory period of S_2 by at least 10 ms led to single atrial capture, reproducibly preventing circus movement tachycardia. Train stimulation maintained effectiveness in tachycardia prevention as long as the first train stimulus was still within the preventive zone (Fig. 1, panel D). When the train began outside the preventive zone, single atrial capture resulted in resetting of tachycardia.

284

Table 1. Electrophysiologic data of 11 patients with an atrioventricular accessory pathway.

Patient	Localization of AP	Mode of CMT initiation		CMT		Mode of CMT termination		AERP of S_2	Preventive zone		Train stimulation
		BCL (S_1S_1)	CI of APB (S_1S_2)	S_2A_T	CL	Site of stim	Number of ES (CL)		$S_2S_3{}^{min}$–$S_2S_3{}^{max}$	Width	
1	RS	510	250	430	340	HRA	2 APBs (210/220)	160	170–220	50	yes
2	RS	640	240	380	240	RV	2 VPBs (170/200)	170	180–230	50	yes
3	LS	640	250	420	290	HRA	2 APBs (220/190)	200	210–250	40	yes
4	LS	760	270	570	370	HRA	2 APBs (240/220)	210	220–260	40	yes
5	RS	440	250	320	300	RV	1 VPB (200–220)	170	180–270	90	yes
6	LS	510	240	360	290	RV	1 VPB (200–220)	190	200–240	40	yes
7	LS	510	230	430	280	HRA	3 APBs (190/180/200)	190	200–240	40	no
8	LS	640	250	480	320	HRA	2 APBs (210/200)	200	210–270	60	no
9	LS	640	240	420	330	HRA	2 APBs (220/200)	210	220–260	40	no
10	LS	760	250	370	270	RV	2 VPBs (200/200)	180	190–250	60	no
11	RS	640	290	570	400	HRA	2 APBs (200/250)	170	180–340	160	yes
			251 ±16	432 ±81	312 ±46		(200/250)	196 ±17	196– 257 ±17 ±32	61 ±36	

AERP = atrial effective refractory perioid, AP = accessory pathway, APB = atrial premature beat, BCL = basic cycle length, CI = coupling interval, CL = cycle length, CMT = circus movement tachycardia, ES = extrastimulus, HRA = high right atrium, LS = left sided, RV = right ventricle, S_2A_T = first tachycardia interval, stim = stimulation, VPB = ventricular premature beat.

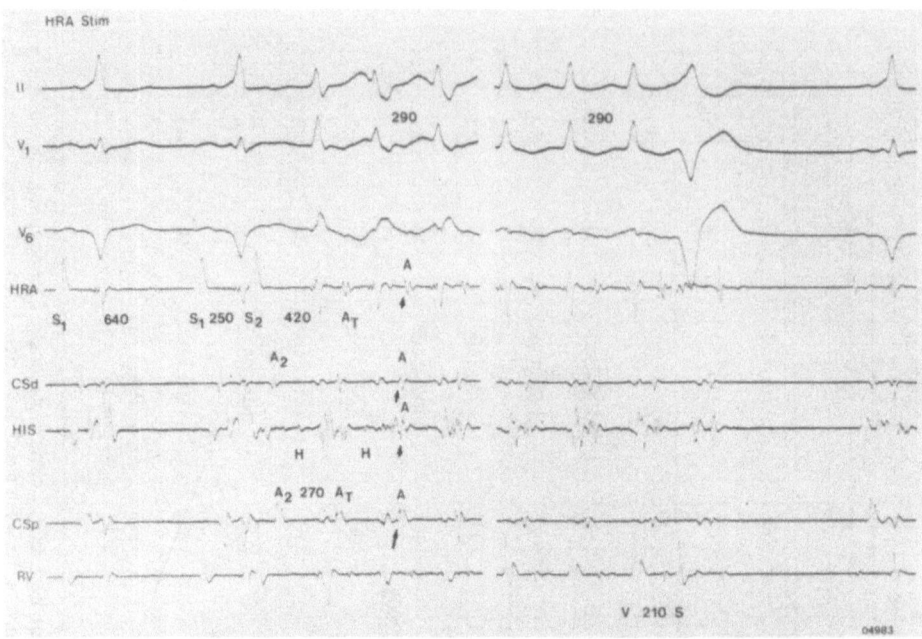

Fig. 2. Patient No. 3. Left panel: During basic pacing of high right atrium at a cycle length of 640 ms CMT is initiated by a single atrial extrastimulus delivered at an S_1S_2 interval of 250 ms. Initial tachycardia interval (S_2A_T) is 420 ms, preceding tachycardia cycle length of 290 ms. Arrows indicate retrograde atrial activation sequence during CMT, with earliest activity in proximal coronary sinus (CSp), followed by distal coronary sinus (CSd), His bundle (HIS), and high right atrium (HRA). Right panel: Tachycardia is terminated by single right ventricular premature beat (S), delivered at a coupling interval of 210 ms. Three surface electrocardiograms (II, V_1, V_6) are shown simultaneously with the endocardial recordings. Abbreviations as Fig. 1.

The mean length of the initial tachycardia interval S_2A_T was 432 ms for all 11 patients, with 425 ms for the 4 patients with a right-sided accessory pathway and 436 ms for those with a left-sided accessory pathway (difference statistically not significant). The mean tachycardia cycle length at 312 ms was significantly less ($p < 0.001$) than the initial tachycardia interval. There was no statistically significant difference in the mean tachycardia cycle lengths of patients with a right-sided accessory pathway (320 ms) and a left-sided accessory pathway (307 ms).

Linear regression of the width of the preventive zone on the initial tachycardia interval revealed a correlation coefficient of less than 0.5. Likewise, the width of the preventive zone was not found to correlate with tachycardia cycle length.

Figure 2 shows the initiation and termination of circus movement tachycardia in one of our patients (No. 3). Prevention of tachycardia in this patient by atrial extrastimuli delivered at the upper and lower limit of the preventive zone, respectively, is documented in the two panels of Fig. 3. Each atrial stimulus falling within the preventive zone leads to a single atrial depolarization (A_3) without re-initiating circus movement tachycardia. Reentrant tachycardia was prevented by each S_3 stimulus within this zone. Further shortening of S_2S_3 to 10 ms less than the lower limit of the preventive zone reaches refractoriness of S_2, and tachycardia is not prevented.

286

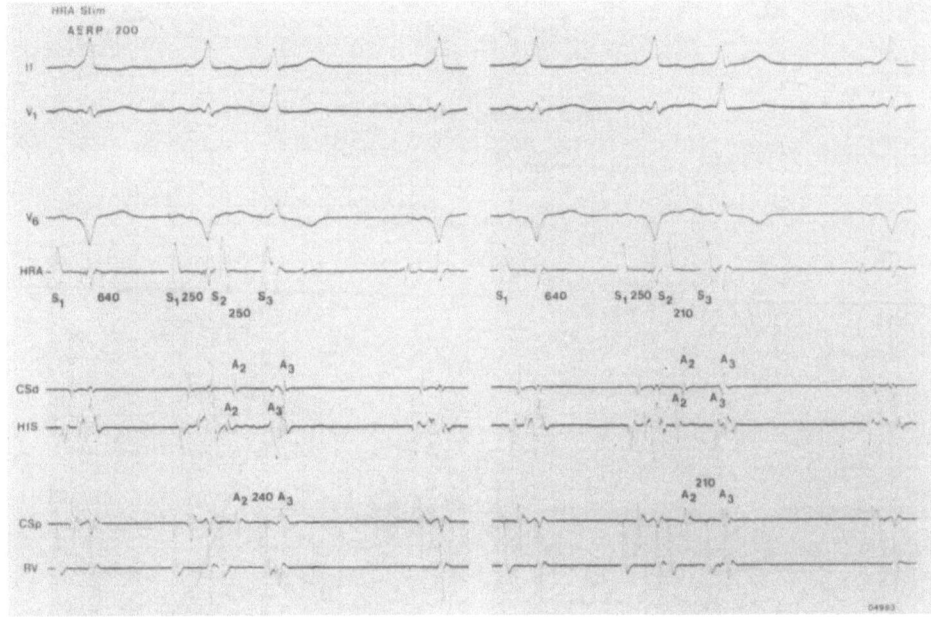

Fig. 3. Patient 3. Left panel: Introduction of second atrial extrastimulus (S_3) at a coupling interval of 250 ms prevents reentrant tachycardia. This coupling interval represents the upper limit of the preventive zone. Atrial effective refractory period of S_2 stimulus (AERP) is 200 ms. Right panel: Tachycardia is still prevented when S_2S_3 is decreased to 210 ms. This coupling interval represents the lower limit of the preventive zone. Note that it lies just 10 ms outside of AERP. Abbreviations as Fig. 1.

Figure 4 shows the effect of train stimulation in patient No. 1. On the left panel, a 100 Hz train of 100 ms duration is delivered 50 ms after the tachycardia-initiating stimulus S_2. Since the atrial effective refractory period of S_2 is 160 ms, this train fails to capture the atrium. Circus movement tachycardia is initiated. When delay of the train is increased to 100 ms (Fig. 4, right panel) single atrial capture occurs and circus movement tachycardia is prevented.

In none of the patients did a single extrastimulus S_3 or a train of stimuli completely within the refractory period of S_2 prevent tachycardia initiation. In none did single-beat or train stimulation initiate atrial flutter or fibrillation.

Discussion

This study shows that, in patients with an atrioventricular accessory pathway, initiation of reentrant tachycardia can be prevented by a single right atrial extrastimulus delivered during a critical interval after the tachycardia-initiating impulse. This interval is termed the "preventive zone". Prevention by single atrial capture can also be achieved by trains of stimuli, provided that any of the train stimuli falls within the preventive zone.

In animal experiments (6) protection against ventricular fibrillation has been demonstrated. In those studies, an extrastimulus delivered during a critical "protective zone" after a fibrillatory impulse and at a critical site was shown to prevent ventricular fibrillation. It

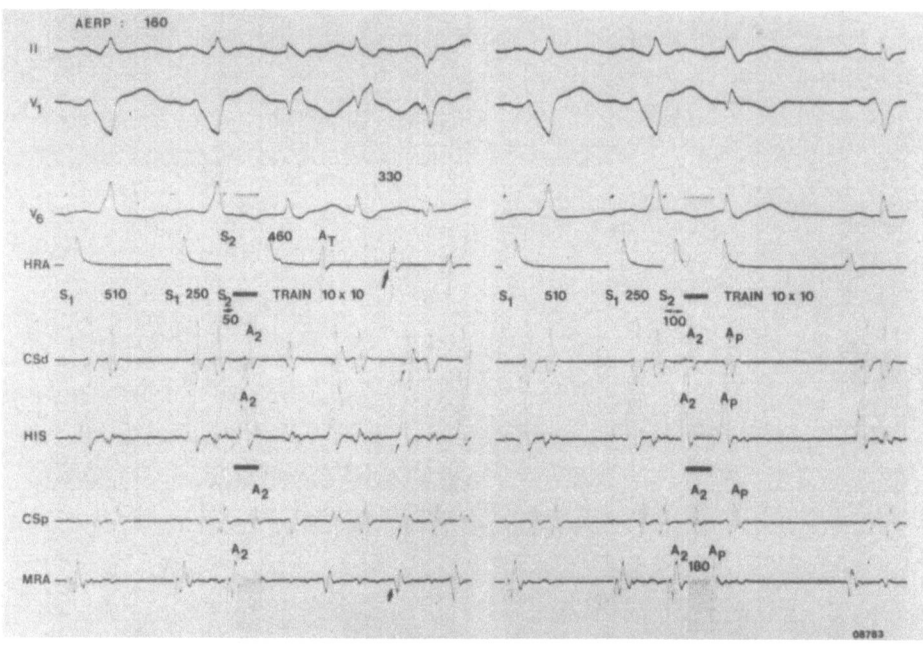

Fig. 4. Patient No. 1. Left panel: 100 Hz train (10 × 10 ms), delivered 50 ms after the tachycardia-initiating stimulus S_2 fails to capture the atrium, and CMT is initiated during HRA pacing at a cycle length of 510 ms, following an S_1S_2 interval of 250 ms. Initial tachycardia interval (S_2A_T) is 460 ms, tachycardia cycle length is 320 ms. Arrows indicate retrograde atrial activation sequence during CMT, with earliest activity in HRA and mid right atrium (MRA), followed by HIS, CSp and CSd. Atrial effective refractory period of S_2 is 160 ms. Right panel: Delay of train is increased to 100 ms. Single atrial capture (A_p) occurs and CMT is prevented. A_2A_p interval, measured in MRA, is approximately 180 ms, this outside ERP of A_2. Horizontal bar denotes train duration. Abbreviations as Fig. 1.

was postulated that the protective stimulus blocked the onset of ventricular fibrillation by a strictly localized phenomenon.

In patients with an accessory atrioventricular pathway atrial myocardium is part of the macro-reentrant circuit, and for tachycardia prevention to occur atrial myocardium must be rendered refractory in time to block the tachycardia wavefront. This can be achieved by a critically timed atrial extrastimulus.

In all patients, prevention of reentrant tachycardia was considerably easier than termination. This is due to the difference in cycle lengths between the initial tachycardia interval, allowing a relatively broad preventive zone of 61 ms, and the significantly shorter cycles of the ongoing tachycardia, which leave only short coupling intervals for terminating stimuli to become effective. Changes in heart rate and refractoriness due to alterations in autonomic tone following the initiation of tachycardia may also be responsible for the difficulties in tachycardia termination.

We have not yet studied the efficacy of preventive stimulation with variations of basic cycle length or tachycardia-initiating coupling interval within the tachycardia zone. Problems caused by variations in autonomic tone can probably be overcome by train stimula-

288

tion. Since the preventive zone begins just outside the effective refractory period of the tachycardia-initiating beat, trains beginning within the refractory period, with a duration calculated to result in single atrial capture, will consequently prevent tachycardia. Prevention should then be independent of day-to-day changes of the refractory period or changes due to various metabolic or antiarrhythmic drug conditions (7).

Furthermore, it is necessary to study the effect of different anatomical sites of origin of the initiating and preventing stimulus. Depending on the size of the reentrant circuit, timing *and* site of delivery of the preventive, with respect to the initiating, stimulus may be important.

Atrial flutter or fibrillation are potentially dangerous in WPW patients with a short antegrade refractory period of the accessory pathway because of the induction of high ventricular rates (8). These types of arrhythmia were not induced in any of our patients, either by single-beat or by train stimulation. However, because of this potential risk, preventive stimulation would be indicated only in patients with accessory pathways who have long antegrade refractory periods.

The external pacemaker system of Guize and Zacouto (9), which is based on automatic frequency adjustment, prevents tachycardia by pacing at higher rates, thereby either suppressing subsequent ectopic beats or leading to interference of the first paced beat with the tachycardia-initiating wavefront. However, suppression of ectopic beats is not necessarily rate dependent, and suppression of the first tachycardia beat will not succeed when an ectopic beat initiates tachycardia right away, so that frequency adjustment cannot occur.

In this study, we assessed preventive stimulation in circus movement tachycardia due to an atrioventricular accessory pathway. Further studies on other clinical types of reentrant tachycardia (e.g. AV nodal tachycardia) will be necessary to elucidate the general reliability of the preventive modes presented here. Prystowsky and Zipes (10) have recently shown that subthreshold stimuli can inhibit subsequent threshold stimuli if the inhibitory stimulis is applied close to the site of the threshold stimulus. Incorporation of this concept into preventive stimulation needs further investigation.

References

1. Wellens HJJ (1978) Value and limitations of programmed electrical stimulation of the heart in the study and treatment of tachycardias. Circulation 57: 845–53.
2. Fisher JD, Ostrow E, Kim SG, Matos JA (1983) Ultrarapid single-capture train stimulation for termination of ventricular tachycardia. Am J Cardiol 51: 1334–8.
3. Spurrell RAJ, Nathan AW, Bexton RS, Hellestrand KJ, Nappholz T, Camm AJ (1982) Implantable automatic scanning pacemaker for termination of supraventricular tachycardia. Am J Cardiol 49: 753–60
4. Den Dulk K, Bertholet M, Brugada P, et al. (1983) A versatile pacemaker system for termination of tachycardias. Am J Cardiol 52: 731–8.
5. Kuck KH, Brugada P, Wellens HJ (1983) Observations on the antidromic type of circus movement tachycardia in the Wolff-Parkinson-White syndrome. J Am Coll Cardiol 2: 1003–10.
6. Verrier RL, Brooks WW, Lown B (1979) Protective zone and the determination of vulnerability to ventricular fibrillation. Am J Physiol 234: H592–6.
7. Waxman MB, Sharma AD, Cameron DH, Huerta F, Wald R (1982) Reflex mechanisms responsible for early spontaneous termination of paroxysmal supraventricular tachycardia. Am J Cardiol 49: 259–72.

8. Dreifus LS, Haiat R, Watanabe Y, Arriaga J, Reitman N (1971) Ventricular fibrillation. A possible mechanism of sudden death in patients with Wolff-Parkinson-White syndrome. Circulation 43: 520–9.
9. Guize L, Zacouto F, Meilhac B, Le Pailleur C, Di Matteo J (1974) Stimulations endocardiaques orthorhythmiques. Interêt diagnostique et therapeutique. La Nouv Presse Med 3: 2083–2086.
10. Prystowsky EN, Zipes DP (1983) Inhibition in the humen heart. Circulation 68: 707–13.

Authors' address:
Karl-Heinz Kuck, M.D.
Department of Cardiology
University Hospital Eppendorf
Martinistr. 52
2000 Hamburg 20
West Germany

Hemodynamic and Antiectopic Effects of Long-term Dynamic Overdrive Pacing in Implanted VVI Pacemakers

U. J. Winter, D. W. Behrenbeck, Th. Brill, M. Höher, V. Hombach, H. Ebeling*, Hj. Hirche*, and H. H. Hilger

Summary: Overdrive pacing has been found to suppress repetitive arrhythmias or focal automaticity. Dynamic overdrive is a type of overdrive pacing in which the pacemaker continuously adjusts the overdrive stimulation rate to the underlying rhythm. Our own animal experiments revealed a significant reduction of direct current and ischemia-induced premature ventricular beats (VPB). Furthermore the threshold for the direct current induction of ventricular tachycardias was significantly increased during dynamic overdrive pacing.

The aim of the study was to investigate the clinical reliability of long-term dynamic overdrive pacing in patients with symptomatic bradyarrhythmias, premature ventricular beats (7/10 patients with VPB $\geqslant$ Lown II°) and antiarrhythmic drug treatment. Therefore, 10 patients (all male) were treated with a DPG 1 pacemaker and a Helifix lead (Vitatron). The antiectopic effect of the dynamic overdrive pacing mode was controlled by repeated, 24-hour Holter ECGs (Ela Medical: Anatec) and the premature beat counter in the DPG 1.

Five out of ten patients had a VPB reduction of more than 80% and 5/10 patients a reduction of the Lown grade to $\geqslant$ II°. During long-term application of the ventricular dynamic overdrive pacing mode, 3/10 patients revealed a manifest myocardial failure. After successful recompensation these 3 and an additional 2 patients were hemodynamically investigated by right heart catheter in the supine position (25 W; 3 minutes). The hemodynamic parameters of cardiac output and mean pulmonary artery pressure were compared during 70 ppm (VVI mode) and dynamic overdrive mode. The ventricular dynamic overdrive pacing mode led to a 10 to 15% reduction of the stroke volume, whereas the cardiac output remained equal due to the increased heart rate. Our data show that patients with reduced left ventricular performance (CO ↓, $\overline{PAP}$ ↑) at rest are particularly prone to develop myocardial failure during long-term ventricular dynamic overdrive pacing. *In conclusion:* Patients who might be candidates for ventricular dynamic overdrive require prior, careful investigation (Holter ECG; determination of the pump function). Atrial dynamic overdrive seems to have a better future, especially in dual chamber devices. Whether or not a significant reduction of premature beats also leads to prevention of tachycardia is still under discussion.

Introduction

Overdrive pacing is a commonly used method for terminating tachycardias. Furthermore, overdrive suppression of repetitive Purkinje fibre activity is a well known electrophysiological phenomenon. The working mechanisms of overdrive suppression on the cellular level are summarized in Table 1. Dynamic overdrive pacing, which means an overdrive stimulation with varying rate, was incorporated in the DPG 1 (Vitatron) for tachycardia prevention.

---

* Institute of Applied Physiology, University of Cologne, West Germany.

Table 1. Working mechanisms of overdrive pacing mode (see (1)).

Author	Year	Discussed mechanism
Han et al.	1966	Increase in heart rate leads to an increase of the fibrillation threshold and to better synchronization of repolarization.
Vassalle et al.	1967	Increase of heart rate leads to an increase of $[K^{\oplus}]$ in the coronary sinus.
Ten Eick et al.	1968	Increase in heart rate induces a higher threshold for the triggering of conducted potentials in the Purkinje fibres.
Krellenstein et al.	1969	Increase in heart rate influences the extracellular electrolytes.
Carpentier et al.	1971	A higher heart rate causes a $Na^{\oplus}$-efflux in the Purkinje fibres which leads to a higher RMP. This causes a delay in the diastolic depolarization.
Janse et al.	1971	Higher heart rate in local ischemia leads to lower fibrillation threshold and desynchronization of repolarization process.
Lüderitz	1983	High heart rate shortens the duration of diastole and reduces the probability of extrasystoles.
Camm et al.	1983	Increased heart rate leads to a reduction of coordinated impulse propagation of arrhythmias by increasing the depolarization between stimulation site and ectopic impulse generating tissue.

Objective

The aim of the study was to investigate the reliability of this new pacing mode, first in animal experimental set-ups with direct current and ischemia induced arrhythmias, and secondly in patients with CHD and premature beats.

Animal investigations

In 6 German domestic pigs (20 to 30 kg) we induced complex ventricular extrasystoles and sustained ventricular tachycardias by LAD occlusion and bipolar, epicardial, direct current (DC) application (up to 5000 μA). The method of this animal set-up has been previously described (2). During ventricular dynamic overdrive pacing (electrode positioned at the right ventricular apex), DC-induced complex arrhythmias disappeared in all the animals. Furthermore, we needed reproducibly significantly higher current strengths (before DO: about 2000 μA; during DO: more than 5000 μA) in all the pigs for the induction of sustained ventricular tachycardias. During DO pacing the atrial systolic blood pressure was reduced from 110 to 90 mm HG (Fig. 1). Very similar ventricular extrasys-

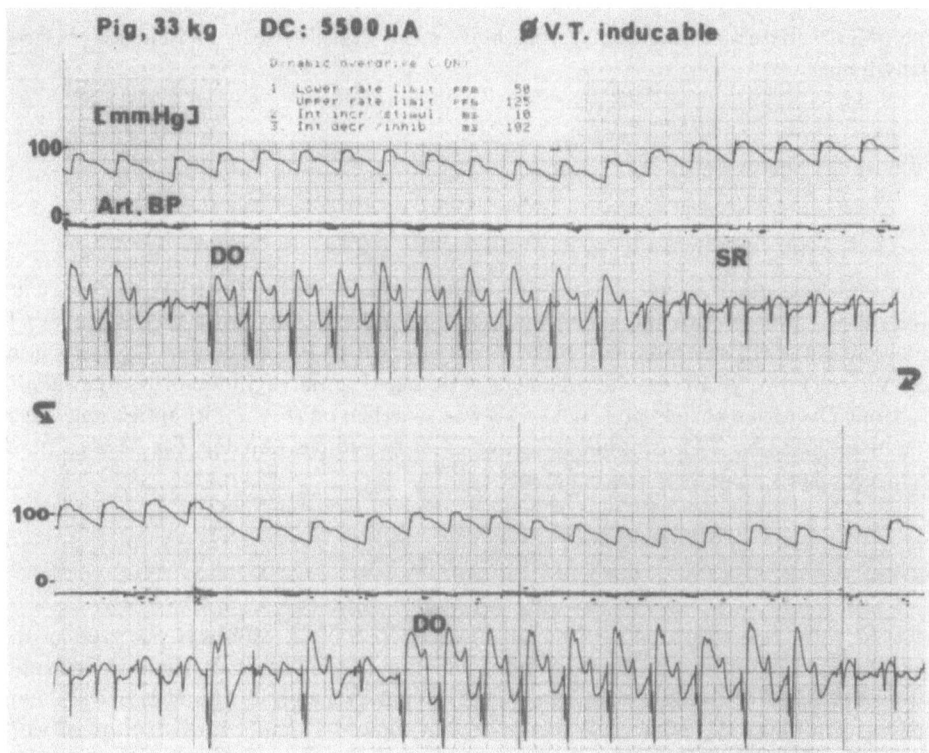

Fig. 1. In a pig heart, sustained ventricular tachycardias (V.T.), were inducible by epicardial DC application of 2100 μA. During ventricular dynamic overdrive pacing current strengths up to 5500 μA could not provoke sustained V.T. Furthermore DO pacing leads to a suppression of repetitive VES. (Vitatron DPG 1)

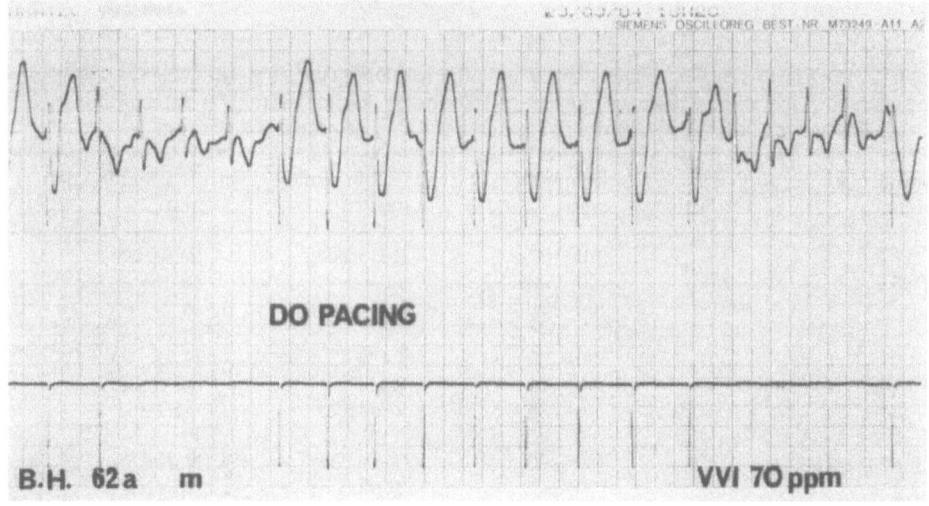

Fig. 2. Pacemaker Holter ECG recording (Ela Medical: Anatec) of a patient with ventricular dynamic overdrive pacing. In the second channel the pacemaker spikes are visualized, indicating the variable pacing interval during DO stimulation. (Vitatron DPG 1)

tole (VES) suppression and tachycardia prevention was also seen in ischemia-induced arrhythmias.

Clinical investigations

Methods

After these successful animal investigation findings, we decided to treat 10 (male) patients (age: 68 ± 11 years) with bradyarrhythmias and VES due to CHD with DPG 1-pm (VVI) and a Helifix lead (Vitatron). In 7 of the 10 patients with VES of Lown ≥ II°, 3 of whom had VES of Lown ≥ III° despite treatment with 1 to 3 antiarrhythmic drugs, the DPG's Dynamic Overdrive pacing mode (DO-PM) was switched on (Fig. 2). Its antiectopic effect was investigated by 24 h continuous Holter ECG recordings (Anatec, Ela Medical) and the pacemaker's premature beat counter.

Results

In 5/10 patients a reduction of the total number VES of ≥ 80% was observed in the pacemaker's premature beat counter and the Holter ECGs (Table 2). Only an insignificant reduction of VES could be achieved in 5/10 patients with low number of VES. One patient with Lown IV remained in this grade, but showed a significant reduction of VES. Another patient with VES of Lown Grade IV had a reduction of the total numbers, but remained at this Lown grade. Another 2 patients with Lown grade III b revealed only VES of Lown grade II during DO pacing. Two patients had VES of Lown grade III a, one of whom remained in this grade with significant reduction in VES incidence, but the

Table 2. Long-term ventricular DO stimulation (Vitatron DPG 1) with a significant VES reduction and a continuously high ventricular $\overline{\text{rate}}$ can lead to cardiac decompensation in patients with elevated mean pulmonary artery pressure ($\overline{\text{PAP}}$) and decreased cardiac output (CO) at rest.

Myocardial failure	VES reduction	DO [ppm] range	CO [l · min^{-1}] (rest)	$\overline{\text{PAP}}$ [cm H$_2$O] (rest)
Yes	81%	70–127	Reduced*	Increased*
N = 3	88%	90–100	3.01	25
	83%	100–120	4.08	28
No	0%	90–100	2.42	17
N = 7	9%	90–100	Reduced*	Increased*
	23%	70– 80	Reduced*	Increased*
	23%	80–100	3.18	10
	47%	80– 90	(Reduced)*	Normal*
	81%	70–100	(Reduced)*	Normal*
	98%	70–100	3.39	25

* No invasive studies possible, $\overline{\text{PAP}}$ and CO were concluded from the clinical examination.

other moved down to Lown grade I. Five patients with VES of Lown grade II demonstrated the following behavior: 3 remained at the same Lown grade without showing any change in total numbers, while 2/5 patients had VES of Lown grade I during DO pacing.

Clinical follow-up

Three of the ten patients showed a progression to myocardial failure during long-term DO pacing. This phenomenon was mainly seen when reduced cardiac output and elevated mean pulmonary artery pressure existed at rest (Table 2).
After recompensation the patients were examined by bicycle stress testing (20–25 W, supine position, right heart catheter) during repeated 4 minute periods. During exercise the DO pacing mode led to a 10 to 15% reduction of the stroke volume (as compared with spontaneous rhythm) which was balanced by the heart rate increase (Fig. 3). In comparison, atrial DO (n = 1) led to a higher cardiac output due to increased heart rate and atrio-ventricular synchrony.

Conclusions

Ventricular DO stimulation can reduce CHD-related extrasystoles significantly ($\geqslant 80\%$) in patients with VES $\geqslant$ Lown III° and a large quantity of ES, even during antiarrhythmic drug treatment. In 5/10 patients we saw a change to VES $\leqslant$ II° and a reduction $\geqslant 80\%$ of the total numbers of VES. In 5/10 patients with low Lown grade and few VES the reduction of premature beats was not significant. Cardiac output during ventricular DO pacing is not significantly influenced since the lower stroke volume (due to VVI pacing) is balanced by a higher ventricular rate. Pacemaker patients with elevated pulmonary artery

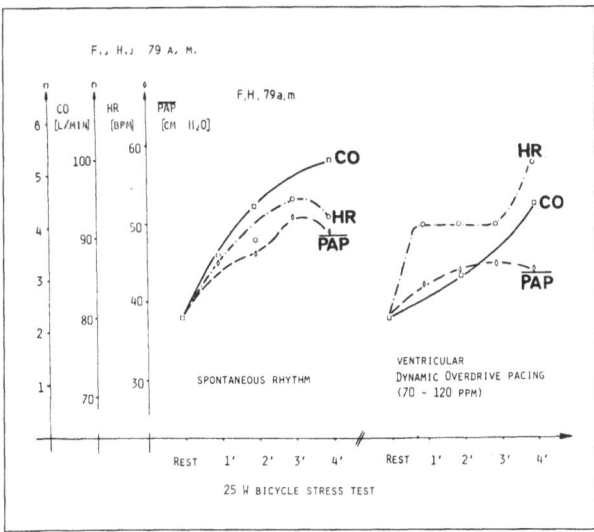

Fig. 3. The 10 to 15% reduction of the stroke volume is balanced by the heart rate increase during ventricular dynamic overdrive pacing, as compared with the values during spontaneous rhythm. (Vitatron DPG 1)

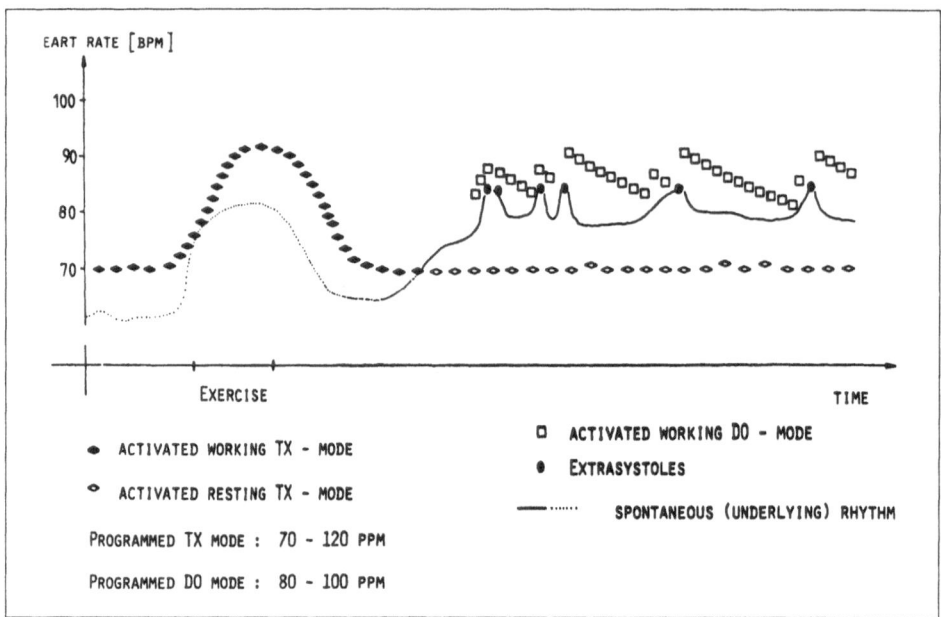

Fig. 4. Rate-variable pacing: dynamic overdrive and rate responsive pacing (TX). The DO mode is no real rate responsive pacing mode.

pressure at rest due to myocardial failure have to be excluded from long-term ventricular DO pacing. The continuously raised ventricular rate often leads to depressed cardiac pump function.

Patients who are to be treated with ventricular DO stimulation should be examined by continuous 24-h Holter ECG and a right ventricular catheter investigation before the implantation. For atrial DO pacing normal AV-conduction is a necessary prerequisite (3). In the pacemaker the lower rate limit and stand-by rate should be separately programmable to allow more physiological conduction. A sufficient, non-invasive control of rate-variable VVI pacemakers is only possible with special pacemaker Holter ECGs (4). Particularly in patients with sinus bradycardia and limited heart rate increase or reduced myocardial function a rate responsive VVI mode, such as TX mode, should be added to the DO mode in the pacemaker (see Fig. 4). Whether a significant VES reduction also leads to tachycardia prevention, has been under discussion for several years (5). Recently developed DDD pacemakers have the capability of atrial dynamic overdrive pacing (e.g. Quintech DDD, Vitatron).

References

1. Camm AJ, Ward D (1983) Pacing for tachycardia control. Telectronics Publications, p 45
2. Winter UJ, Ebeling H, Kebbel V, Arnold G, Schmahl M, Hirche Hj (1983) Induction of ventricular arrhythmias and ventricular late potentials by epicardial direct current application in pig heart in situ: importance of the stimulation position. Circulation 68 (Suppl II): 1151

3. Fontaine G, Frank R, Grosgogeat Y (1984) Value of a software pacemaker in the management of cardiac arrhythmias. In: Furlanello G (ed) Proceedings of the 6th International Congress on Cardiology, Marilleva, Italy, February 1984, pp 433–439
4. Höher M, Winter UJ, Behrenbeck DW, Vonderbank E, Verhoeven HW, Hombach V, Hilger HH (1985) Pacemaker Holter ECG: value and limitations in follow-up of pacemaker patients (this volume)
5. Josephson ME, Personal communication, Philadelphia

Authors' address:
U. J. Winter, M.D.
Medizinische Universitätsklinik III, Kardiologie
Josef-Stelzmann-Straße 9
5000 Köln 41
West Germany

Arrhythmias induced by antitachycardial pacing

G. Neumann and N. Bakels*

Summary: The chronic follow-up data of 52 patients with different types of antitachycardia pace-makers are discussed with special consideration of possible arrhythmogenic side effects. Follow-up ranges between a few weeks and eight years of observation after the implantation. From the available ECG, Holter and stress test recordings two categories of problems may be identified. One results from different types of abnormal pacemaker function. Sensing related problems which were particularly crucial during the early postimplantation period require specific postoperative care. Muscle potential detection, hyperpolarisation, postoperative signal amplitude alterations and a variety of different signal patterns during normal and irregular rhythms as well as rate overlap problems of sinus and arrhythmia rates are the basis of this rather difficult sensing problem. Some of the difficulties may probably be overcome by further tachycardia identification criteria such as hemodynamic tachycardia criteria. The second group of arrhythmogenic side effects represents an intrinsic rhythmological problem. Many of the tachycardias to be treated may in fact be enhanced, accelerated and may even degenerate into fibrillation under the influence of further pacemaker induced prematurity effects within and outside of a possible re-entrant circuit. This problem of course is specifically critical in ventricular applications, especially in the treatment of ventricular tachycardias on the basis of progressively diseased myocardium. There is no reliable method available to really predict future safety of interruptive pacing parameters in ventricullar application and in the treatment of ventricular tachycardias. Preoperative electrophysiological testing of interruptive atrial pacing parameters in the treatment of supraventricular tachycardias proved to be rather predictive in forecasting the possible inducibility of atrial fibrillation and also predicted the possible rhythmologic and hemodynamic tolerability of accelerated atrial rhythms and induced atrial fibrillation.

Antitachycardia pacing is now a well established therapeutic procedure in acute and chronic atrial and ventricular tachycardia control (1–3). The different antitachycardia pacing systems may however not only control but also induce arrhythmias in properly selected patients in the course of chronic stimulation treatment. Some of the typical arrhythmogenic side effects are discussed on the basis of chronic follow-up observations of a total group of 52 patients with different types of antitachycardia pacemakers and different intervention modes (see Table 1). The data base consists of 1,473 provoked antitachycardia interventions and 2,125 regular and irregular spontaneous interventions. Treatment time varied between 3 weeks and 8 years, with 35 of the patients already having been treated for more than 3 years.

Pacemaker controls and provoked interventions were repeatedly performed in all patients during the early postoperative period (3 weeks). Thereafter the procedure was performed in three monthly intervals during the year following the implantation, in half year intervals during the second year, and in yearly intervals thereafter unless specific problems required a different schedule. Continuous ECG recordings of 6 to 24 hours' duration were routinely performed from day 1 to day 4 after the implantation, once between days 5 and 15, once between days 16 and 30 and twice during the following 5 months after the implantation. The recordings were performed with 4 channel telemetry combined with a multichannel tape recorder with partial automatic tape evaluation (Siemens Meditape

---

* Medtronic BV, Kerkrade.

Table 1. Patients and antitachycardia systems.

Diagnoses	Systems	Leads	Modes
Overt WPW N = 17	IDP 64 SD N = 8	IE 65 N = 2	Burst 240 BPM (N = 41)
Concealed conduction N = 14	Medtronic 2402 N = 36	FY 61 (N = 24)	Adaptive burst
AV-nodal tachycardia N = 10	RF Medtronic N = 3	6990 (N = 39)	31% of cycle length (N = 7)
SVT with block N = 8	Cybertach N = 5	6960 (N = 2)	Permanent fixed high rate
Ventricular tachycardia N = 3	IDP 44 SD N = 1		(N = 1)
	SP 186 Medtronic N = 1		Scanning mode (N = 1)
	SP 500 Medtronic N = 7		Specific timing (N = 2)

AR 12). In all cases the analysis was performed by visual analysis of the tape recordings by very experienced investigators in combination with automatic event quantification by the Meditape device.

All patients with automatic antitachycardia intervention units were postoperatively observed during a specific pacemaker switch-off period in order to document the reoccurrence of persisting tachycardias without suitable pacemaker intervention.

Results

Two different types of arrhythmogenic stimulation were observed. Pacemaker malfunction of different degrees with consecutive abnormal stimulation was one of the main reasons for arrhythmogenicity. In this category of abnormalities parasystolic atrial stimulation due to detection problems of atrial spontaneous activity was the major problem. Respiration induced changes in signal amplitude, largely different signal amplitudes and slew rates of sinus and re-entrant atrial signals, abnormal signal parameters of ectopic atrial activity or variable P wave propagation in patients with sick sinus syndrome were the main reasons of poor or borderline atrial detection. In tachycardia pacing incidental parasystolic atrial stimuli, otherwise rather meaningless, may induce tachycardias if they are critically timed. If the tachycardia detection itself behaves normally these tachycardias are immediately terminated by a consecutive tachycardia intervention pacing pattern. The problem is related to the intracardial signal amplitudes and slew rates at the time of implantation. Signal amplitudes less than 3 mV measured under unlimited parallel ohmic resistance during sinus activity and or re-entrant activity predict a high probability of future sensing problems in the atrium. This is to a major degree a consequence of an average 50 percent decrease of signal amplitude in the atrium, in some cases even exceeding 75%, during the first two weeks after the implantation of different types of atrial leads. The definite signal amplitude level is normally established about two weeks after the implantation procedure. Therefore parasystolic pacing events with pacing induced tachyarrhythmias must be expected during the early postoperative period, specifically between days 1 and 5. This may cause considerable problems in a group of patients with easy inducible serious tachyarrhythmias. The wide spectrum of different sensitivity and output settings programmable in the new device generations as well as never elec-

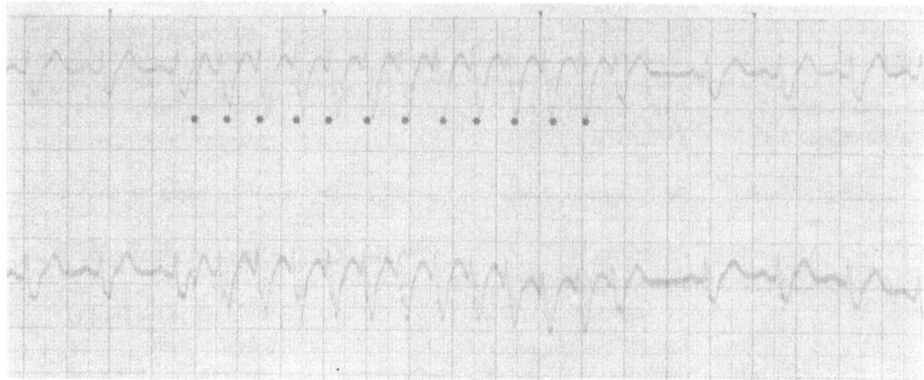

Fig. 1. Triggering of muscle activity by IDP 64 SD (unipolar unit). Abnormal activation of tachycardia mode.

trodes with better signal gain characteristics may minimize this problem. However, precaution must be taken to treat these patients suitably during this early postoperative period with rather limited reliability of pacemaker mediated tachycardia control.

Similar problems arise from different types of abnormal triggering of the tachycardia pacing modes. Myopotential detection and abnormal triggering of tachycardia pacing mode as a consequence was almost regularly observed with the first unipolar units (Fig. 1).

Another relevant reason of abnormal triggering of the tachycardia pacing mode was sinus and tachycardia rate overlap during physical exercise or in situations of postural hypotension.

The enormous problem with these types of abnormal tachycardia pacing mode is the fact that they persist throughout the entire treatment period. With the new devices available, specifically the bipolar units and the programmability of sensing and trigger parameters, many of these problems may be rather easily handled. The rate overlap problem may be overcome to a certain degree by supportive drug treatment (e.g. beta blocking agents, digitalis). It may be further optimized by more sophisticated tachycardia detection criteria than just a critical rate (e.g. rate increase patterns, signal analysis, analysis of depolarisation sequences of atria and ventricles, parallel detection of hemodynamic parameters like intracavitary impedance).

The myopotential detection problem cannot be overcome by pure electronic means, as it is fundamentally related to the necessarily extreme sensitivity of antitachycardia pacemakers, at least in atrial application. As a consequence only bipolar units should be implanted in atrial applications. In some rare cases false tachycardia mode activation also occurred in bipolar units. In these cases the possible cause was the detection of hyperpolarization induced phantom signals. This phenomenon was only observed with Cybertach units, when depleted 2404 devices were exchanged for the more programmable Cybertach units. The problem occurred in chronic leads showing excellent performance during the exchange procedure with highly reliable chronically stable lead characteristics. The problem was possibly a consequence of the different settings in the amplification circuitry of the two different devices, specifically enhanced by high stimulation rates and extremely high sensitivity settings. These problems could only be solved by the implantation of new leads allowing lower sensitivity settings of the pacemaker devices in the follow-up.

The second group of pacing induced arrhythmias occurs in spite of a completely normal pacemaker function. In these cases the induced arrhythmia results from the variations of the pacemaker induced interventional pacing rhythm response. One of the possible electrophysiological substrates of such induced arrhythmias as a consequence of interruptive pacing is the acceleration of a tachycardia which may then degenerate into fibrillation, flutter or normally unstable extremely high rate re-entry tachycardia. In atrial applications both types of acceleration are observed, although in the majority of such cases atrial fibrillation is the result of such an enhancement. Both reactions may also occur in ventricular application. This is the major limitation of the method in the treatment of ventricular tachycardias. Induction of atrial fibrillation may be a problem specifically in cases of overt Wolff-Parkinson-White (WPW) conduction and in patients with poor hemodynamic tolerance of atrial fibrillation. Careful patient selection should therefore include the consideration of these aspects and these points must be checked preoperatively by induction of atrial fibrillation and careful electrophysiological analysis of aberrant conduction behavior under this circumstance. In other cases induction of atrial fibrillation is the intended interruptive rhythm to convert atrial flutter or high rate supraventricular tachycardias with block into sinus rhythm or at least to reduce ventricular rates in these cases (Fig. 2).

Atrial flutter and fibrillation episodes have also been seen in burst pacing modes as well as in specifically timed premature single or double stimuli or in scanning modes during chronic follow-up. There was no difference in the incidence of these arrhythmogenic side effects between the different interruptive modes. With appropriate patient selection specifically in cases with overt WPW syndrome atrial fibrillation episodes did not provoke critical ventricular rates. Sometimes minor problems resulted from the time duration of atrial fibrillation attacks. Especially in patients with sick sinus syndrome these episodes sometimes lasted for some two or three hours. So far no event of pulmonary or arterial

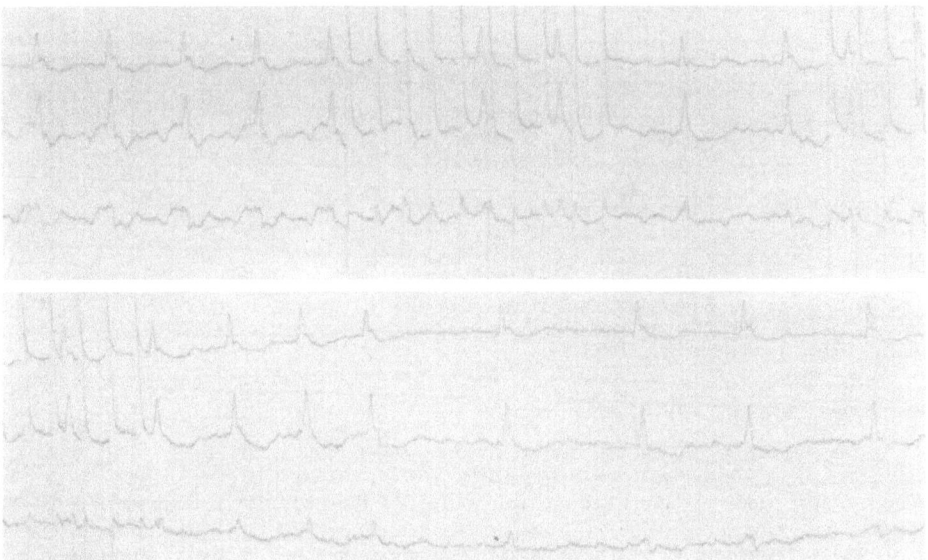

Fig. 2. Patient M. Pf. 2404. Induction of intentional atrial fibrillation for tachycardia conversion.

embolism has occurred in this group of patients. The rate increase effect of atrial fibrillation attacks led some patients to believe that the tachycardia pacemaker function was disturbed until they were examined in the pacemaker clinic. There was a good correlation between ventricular rate patterns during atrial fibrillation periods between preoperative and chronic follow-up fibrillation data.

Only one patient, who besides tachycardia pacing required a rather high chronic dosage of amiodarone (600 mg/day) for sufficient tachycardia control, developed critical ventricular rates during atrial fibrillation attacks after two years of sufficient upper rate control during atrial fibrillation. Amiodarone serum levels and the level of the metabolite were within the ranges of normality at this time***, at least proving the patient's compliance in drug consumption. The patient then needed Kent bundle dissection for further arrhythmia control.

In WPW cases in general, patients with cycle lengths shorter than 260 msec conducted via the abnormal pathway were excluded from chronic antitachycardia pacing therapy with atrial application of the device.

Acceleration of tachycardias by the interruptive pacing mode is of course a rather dangerous event in ventricular applications (Fig. 3). The upper panel of Fig. 3 shows a spontaneous and inducible ventricular tachycardia which could be easily interrupted with single stimuli between 280 and 320 msec of coupling interval in the right ventricular apex. After 12 weeks of successful treatment the ventricular tachycardia pattern changed. Spontaneous and inducible tachycardias were faster from this time on and could only be interrupted by paired stimulation in a scanning mode of coupling. This mode sometimes induced tachycardia acceleration as a transient rhythm before tachycardia conversion. This behavior coincided with the onset of pump failure. Another patient always showed tachycardia acceleration after 12 weeks of successful treatment without any change in drug therapy, pumping conditions and without any sign of a new ischemic event. He could no longer be treated by pacing, always required cardioversion from this time on

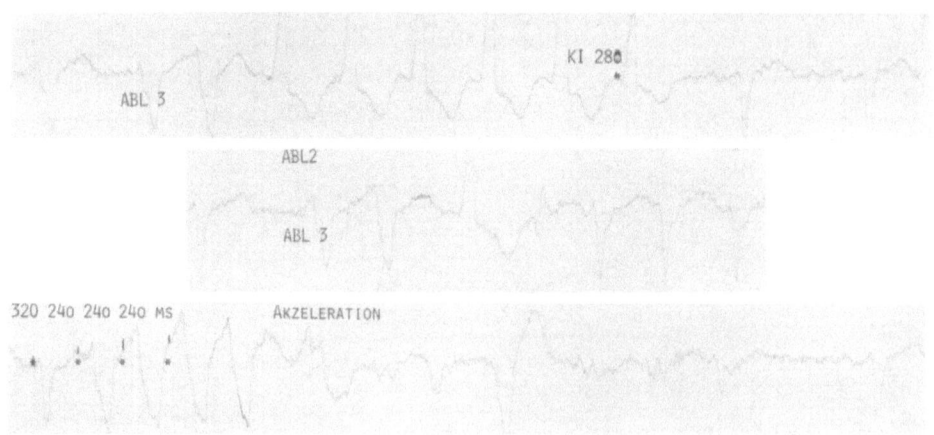

Fig. 3. Upper panel: uncomplicated interrruption of VT by single PVC*. Coupling interval 280 msec.
Mid and lower panels: accelerated tachycardia in the same patient after 12 weeks of stimulation therapy. Pacing interruption now required 4 PVC****. Coupling intervals 320, 240, 240, 240 msec. This program often initiated VT acceleration.

and definitely developed pump failure due to an incessant ventricular tachycardia. In both cases the change of the rhythmological conditions could not really be explained. Both patients had extremely poor ventricular function, each of them had a history of three severe myocardial infarctions, and both had inoperable aneurysms. A multiple antiarrhythmic drug therapy was concomitantly performed in both patients without any change in the dosage schedule at the time of abnormal electrophysiological response.

The incidence of undesired atrial tachyarrhythmias induced by interventional antitachycardia pacing during induced control tachycardias in the follow-up period was not significantly different from the incidence of these events during the preoperative acute testing in electrophysiological studies (Table 2).

The small number of 3 patients with pacemaker applications in ventricular tachycardias does not allow any reasonable quantitative comparison of pre and postimplant data.

Eighty percent of all analyzed spontaneous or induced control tachycardias during the follow-up period showed a totally normal pacemaker performance. During the first 4 days after the implantation this was only the case in 61% of the analyzed data. Abnormal P wave sensing occurred in 4% of all chronic data but in 23% of all recording during the first postoperative days. Abnormal tachycardia detection occurred in 4% of all chronic registrations but only in 2% of the early postoperative data. Tachycardia interruption failure was seen in 4% of all chronic and 3% of all acute potoperative registrations, undesired atrial fibrillation showed the same pattern of incidence, abnormal tachycardia triggering by muscle activity sensing or hyperpolarisation showed an overall chronic incidence of 3.7% of all registrations, and tachycardia acceleration was seen in 1.3% of all documented events. The data were calculated from the analysis of 2,127 tachycardia intervention recordings from 51 patients. All available ECG, Holter and induced tachycardia

Table 2. Comparison of induced arrhythmia incidence during acute studies and chronic follow-up. Data calculated from 1,473 induced control tachycardias in 51 patients.

Number of patients	51	51	48	47	42
Number of controls	255	255	233	231	499
Unintentional atrial fibrillation a) % of controls	3.14	2.75	6.01	4.76	5.41
b) Nr. of patients	4	3	6	6	7
Intentional atrial fibrillation a) % of controls	12.1	12.1	10.3	6.06	10.8
b) Nr. of patients	7	7	7	5	5
Acceleration a) Type of tachycardia	SVT		VT		SVT
b) Nr. of patients	2		2		3
	acute	3 weeks	3 months	12 months	13–36 months

registrations were taken as data base. While the majority of all abnormal sensing events occurred during the first three weeks of therapy, abnormal triggering of the tachycardia mode and induction of atrial fibrillation were randomly distributed over the follow-up period and real tachycardia acceleration was predominantly a late occurrence.

Conclusions

From these data the following conclusions seem reasonable.

1. Stimulation induced arrhythmias, depending upon some minor sensing and capture problems, must be expected during the early postoperative period. These arrhythmias may be rather difficult to treat because in general drug refractoriness or some degree of drug inefficacy is one of the indication criteria commonly selected for antitachycardia pacing. The occurrence of these sensing malfunction problems may be avoided if signal amplitudes of endocavitary atrial signals exceed 3 mV at the time of the implantation as well as in sinus rhythm and during re-entrant attacks. Sufficient atrial sensitivity should be programmed. 0.6 mV in general may be recommended, at least during the early post-operative period. Bipolar units are recommended in atrial application to avoid muscle activity sensing with abnormal activation of the antitachycardia pacing mode. In extremely critical cases it is useful to implant the electrodes in combination with lead extenders and to connect the implantable pacing device only during a second operative procedure. Tachycardia identification criteria besides a critical rate will presumably help to avoid tachycardia and sinus rate overlap problems.

2. Arrhythmias not induced by some degree of pacemaker malfunction are rather rare, at least in the treatment of properly selected patients with atrial tachycardias. Atrial fibrillation as a possible complication of interventive antitachycardia pacing may be quite reliably predicted by preoperative acute testing. In contrast to atrial applications in atrial tachycardias it is practically impossible to predict the risk of ventricular tachycardia enhancement, acceleration and degeneration into ventricular flutter and fibrillation. This was at least impossible in patients with extremely poor ventricular function. Thus in ventricular applications of antitachycardia pacing interventional pacing side effects may be hazardous and life threatening. Therefore indications should be considered very restrictively. Concerning this indication, we share the restrictive ideas of many other authors (4, 5). On the other hand, drug treatment as well as operative treatment or cardioversion and internal defibrillation are also not without serious side effects in these indications. So antitachycardia pacing is at least another therapeutic instrument if other approaches fail (6, 7). In combination with an implantable defibrillator this approach may even be one of the safest and most reliable instruments in the treatment of ventricular tachycardias.

There is little doubt that in atrial applications antitachycardia induced arrhythmias cannot be considered as a really relevant problem if critical cases of overt WPW syndrome are excluded from stimulation therapy.

References

1. Fisher JD, Mehra R, Furman S (1978) Termination of ventricular tachycardia with bursts of rapid ventricular pacing. Am J Cardiol 41 : 94

2. Barold SS, Falkoff MD, Ong LS, Heinle RA (1982) New pacing techniques for the treatment of tachycardias. In: Barold S, Mugcal J (eds), The Third Decade of Cardiac Pacing. Futura Publications, New York, pp 309–332
3. Neumann G, Funke H, Bakels N, Grube E, Schaede A (1982) Benefits and problems of chronic atrial tachycardia control pacing. In: Feruglio GA (ed) Cardiac Pacing. Piccin Medical Books, pp 269–272
4. Naccarelli GV, Zipes DP, Rahilly GT (1983) Influence of tachycardia cycle length and antiarrhythmic drugs on pacing termination and acceleration of ventricular tachycardia. Am Heart J 105:1–5
5. Fisher JD, Kim SG, Furman S (1982) Role of implantable pacemakers in control of recurrent ventricular tachycardia. Am J Cardiol 49: 194–206
6. Buxton AE, Josephson ME (1984) Ventricular tachycardia 1983. Pace 7,1: 96–108
7. Lüderitz B, Naumann d'Alnoncourt C, Steinbeck G, Beyer J (1981) Therapie von Tachyarrhythmien mit implantierbaren Schrittmachern. In: Lüderitz B (ed) Ventrikuläre Herzrhythmusstörungen. Springer-Verlag Berlin–Heidelberg–New York. pp 374–383

Authors' address:
Professor G. Neumann
Medizinische Klinik I
Städtisches Krankenhaus Solingen
5650 Solingen
West Germany

The Surgical Approach to Tachycardias

H. Klein, G. Frank, H. J. Trappe, P. C. Werner, E. Kühn, L. Jüppner,
P. R. Lichtlen, and H. G. Borst

Summary: In cases of unresponsiveness of supra- or ventricular tachycardia to antiarrhythmic drug treatment, antitachycardia pacemakers or map-guided surgical procedures may become alternative therapies. The Wolff-Parkinson-White(WPW) syndrome with episodes of atrial fibrillation and/or short refractory periods of the accessory pathway represent the main indication for surgical therapy of supraventricular tachycardias. We report on 19 patients undergoing surgical therapy for their atrial tachycardias. Sixteen patients had WPW syndrome and 3 had atrial flutter, junctional and left atrial ectopic tachycardia. A total of 20 accessory pathways were identified intraoperatively, 9 on the left and 11 on the right side. Eight patients were operated on using the closed heart technique without cardiopulmonary bypass. Fifteen of the 16 patients are free of tachycardias and PAT is not inducible. One patient had a delta wave without PAT and one had a spontaneous PAT relapse after surgery. Both patients had multiple accessory pathways identified intraoperatively. Endocardial resection or incision are the commonly used surgical procedures for medically refractory ventricular tachycardia. Sixty-eight patients, 62 with coronary disease, 5 with right and left ventricular dysplasia and one with sarcoidosis underwent map-guided surgery for their ventricular tachycardias. An encircling incision was performed in 14 patients, 48 of the patients had endocardial resection. In 18 patients, cryoablation was used either alone or in combination with other procedures. The early mortality rate was 12% (9 out of 68). The late mortality was 15% after a mean follow-up of 29 months. Five patients had a relapse of VT, one was reoperated successfully.
Electrophysiologically guided surgery for VT has an overall success rate of 75–80% and is preferable to blind aneurysmectomy. Patients with poor left ventricular function will have better therapeutic results with the automatic implantable defibrillator.

There is no doubt that antiarrhythmic drugs are the first treatment of choice in the management of atrial as well as ventricular tachycardias (1). However, the effectiveness of a drug is difficult to assess and long-term treatment is often disappointing (2, 3). Advances in pacemaker technology have led to promising results in the treatment of recurrent disabling episodes of tachycardia, particularly in cases in which prophylactic drug therapy failed to suppress the sudden onset of tachycardia. The group of patients who benefit from implantable antitachycardia devices is relatively small. There are more patients with supraventricular than with ventricular tachycardia in whom a device can be safely implanted.

We are still faced with a number of problems related to the antitachycardia devices. Despite enormous progress in the development of algorithms for better recognition of a tachycardia, shortcomings and potential hazards with antitachycardia pacing continue to exist. The rate and form of a tachycardia are often variable and therefore the mode of termination may be different, thus creating a need for different response mechanisms. An inappropriate sensing of the device can lead to spurious discharge and induction of the tachycardia. A major unsolved problem in antitachycardia pacing is the possible arrhythmia acceleration bearing the risk of deleterious ventricular fibrillation. Therefore, future pacing devices for ventricular tachycardia need a defibrillation back-up before pacemaker therapy can be generally recommended for ventricular tachycardia.

The surgical approach to tachyarrhythmias was initiated by Sealy in 1968 (4), when an accessory pathway in a patient with WPW syndrome was successfully divided. Due to more sophisticated electrophysiological mapping techniques for better localization of the accessory pathways, different surgical procedures were reported (5). The main difference between operative procedures for the WPW syndrome is either the epicardial or endocardial approach to the localized accessory pathway. Sealy and others (5) favour the endocardial approach, i.e. the endocardial incision directly above the mitral or tricuspid annulus, whereas Guiraudon (6) more recently propagated the epicardial approach for dissection of identified accessory pathways thus avoiding opening of the heart and preventing cardiopulmonary bypass. An important contribution was also made by Gallagher (7), introducing cryothermia and cryosurgical ablation for the treatment of atrial as well as ventricular tachycardia.

Indications for surgery of supraventricular tachycardia

The indication for surgical intervention in patients with recurrent episodes of supraventricular tachycardia continues to be a matter of debate. It is generally accepted that a life

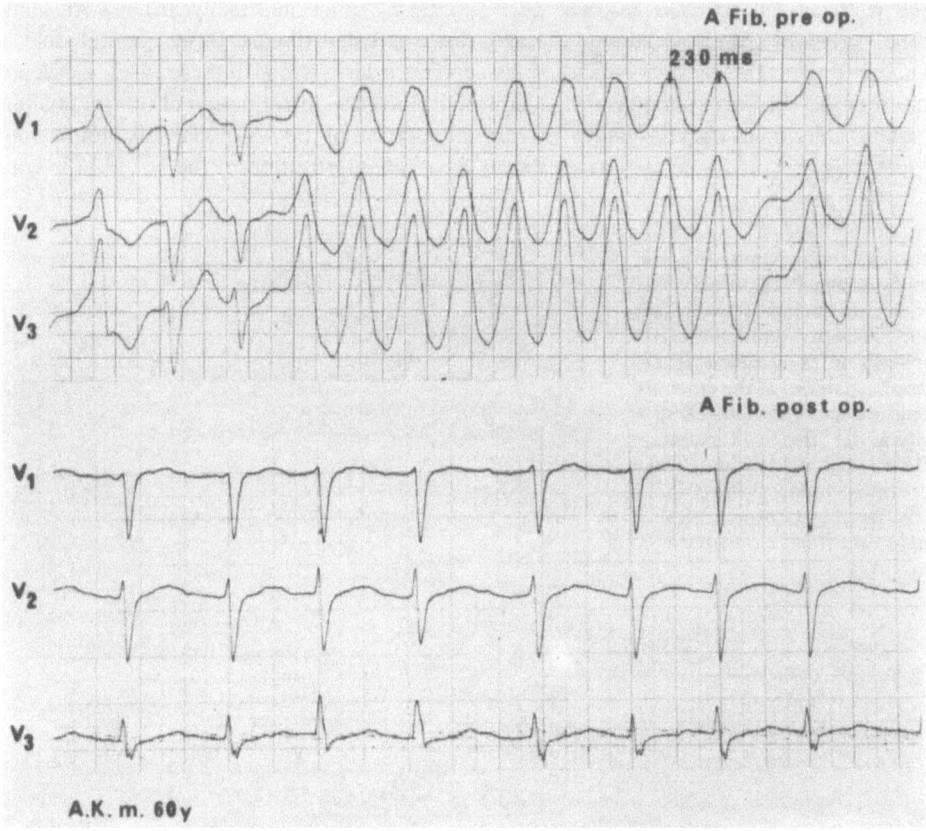

Fig. 1. ECG recording with unipolar leads V1–V3 of a patient with a left sided accessory pathway and recurrent atrial fibrillation. The upper tracing is recorded preoperatively. Note the very rapid antegrade conduction via the accessory pathway. The lower tracing represents the situation during atrial fibrillation after successful interruption of the abnormal pathway.

307

threatening tachycardia in the context of a preexcitation syndrome is represented by documented episodes of atrial fibrillation with rapid antegrade impulse conduction via an
accessory pathway (Fig. 1). These patients should have surgical ablation of their accessory pathways. There are patients who thus far did not develop atrial fibrillation, but
have had recurrent (more than once/month) episodes of paroxysmal atrial tachycardia
with heart rates greater than 200 bpm, symptoms of syncope, angina or had developed
cardiac failure with long lasting episodes of tachycardia. They often had very short accessory pathway refractory periods.

Surgical intervention is indicated when drug therapy fails to suppress these episodes. Although interruption of an accessory pathway should mainly be reserved for medically refractory patients, increasing experience and improved surgical technique will permit a
broader indication of surgical treatment. Why should a young patient take antiarrhythmic drugs lifelong with all the well known side effects when surgical treatment has a low
risk and high success rate?

There are patients who may need a surgical interruption of the normal atrioventricular
conduction, i.e. ablation of the AV-nodal or His bundle conduction. These patients have
fast and hemodynamically compromising AV-nodal tachycardias, atrial flutter or fibrillation with rapid ventricular response or reciprocating junctional tachycardias with additional problems, such as coronary artery disease, valve disease or congenital defects
which represent the primary indication for surgical intervention. In these cases, a cryoablation of the His bundle conduction is indicated. Since the introduction of transcutaneous
catheter ablation of the His bundle (8), surgical ablation of the AV-nodal-His bundle conduction has become a rare intervention (9). Surgical interruption of the His bundle con-

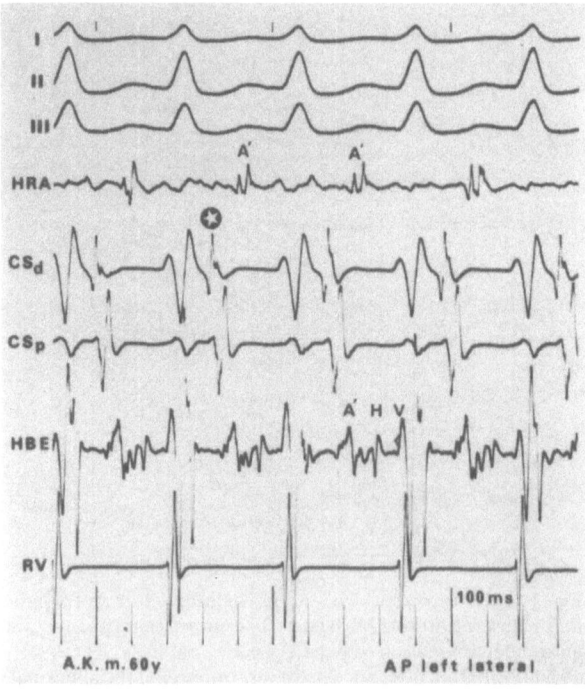

Fig. 2. Electrophysiological study during PAT of the same patient as in Fig. 1. Note that the shortest ventricular-atrial conduction is recorded at the distal electrodes of the coronary sinus catheter (CSd) indicating a lateral left free wall pathway. HRA = high right atrium, CSp = proximal coronary sinus, HBE = His bundle recording, RV = right ventricular electrogram.

duction may result, in some cases, as an unwanted result when accessory pathways run from the atrium to the ventricle contiguous with the His bundle (7).

Role of the preoperative electrophysiological study

In all patients in whom a surgical therapy for arrhythmias is considered, a thorough electrophysiological study prior to surgery is mandatory. Multiple catheters have to be introduced percutaneously to record electrical activity at different regions of the right atrium, the His bundle area, the coronary sinus and the right and/or left ventricle. It is necessary to localize the atrial and ventricular insertion of an accessory pathway during sinus rhythm and atrial and ventricular programmed stimulation as well as during induced tachycardia (Fig. 2) in order to determine the electrophysiological properties of various parts of a reentrant circuit. An electrophysiological study also serves as a useful tool to evaluate refractoriness, i.e. the influence of antiarrhythmic drugs on the mechanism of a tachycardia.

Supraventricular tachycardia: surgical experience

Nineteen patients underwent surgical procedures for their supraventricular tachyarrhythmias, 16 patients with WPW syndrome, one with recurrent atrial flutter, one with ectopic left atrial tachycardia and one with incessant junctional tachycardia.

The group of patients with WPW syndrome consisted of 13 males and 3 females, 3 of whom were children ages 3, 8 and 11 years. Nine patients had documented episodes of atrial fibrillation with rapid ventricular response due to fast antegrade conduction via the accessory pathway. Eight patients endured cardiac arrest or had syncopes. Seven patients had recurrent medically refractory paroxysmal atrial tachycardia and all patients had accessory pathway refractory periods of less than 250 msec.

Preoperative electrophysiological studies determined left sided accessory pathways in 7 patients. Intraoperative mapping revealed that 3 patients had additional pathways not clearly identified during the preoperative study. There were 20 localized areas of accessory pathways during intraoperative mapping. Nine pathways were situated on the left side (Fig. 2), 4 of which were located on the posterior septal side. Eleven pathways had a right atrial-ventricular conduction which consisted of 3 on the right anterior side, 3 septal, and 5 right free wall pathways. In 3 patients, 2 to 3 pathways could be localized.

A left lateral thoracotomy was performed without using cardiopulmonary bypass in 8 patients. In the other 8 patients, a median sternotomy was necessary; 4 of these were operated on without using cardiopulmonary bypass. In 2 patients, both with more than one accessory pathway, a reoperation was necessary within 2 days and 6 weeks due to recurrence of the delta wave and relapse of atrial tachycardia. Both reoperations were successfully performed and the additional bypass tracts dissected. There were no intraoperative deaths and the postoperative electrophysiological study revealed no delta wave and PAT was not inducible with the exception of one patient, who later showed no preexcitation after the second intervention. In the follow-up period of more than 15 months, 15 of the 16 patients were free of paroxysmal atrial tachycardia. In one patient, a relapse of PAT occurred, indicating that one accessory pathway was not interrupted successfully. None of the operated patients needs antiarrhythmic medication.

Of the three patients with cryoablation of the atrioventricular conduction, the patient with atrial flutter had an effective His bundle ablation in addition to a successful endocardial resection for his recurrent ventricular tachycardia. A two year old girl who suffered from congestive cardiomyopathy had incessant junctional tachycardia. Cryoablation of the His bundle region was performed intraoperatively creating a complete AV-block. The patient died 4 weeks later due to cardiac failure. The third patient with intraoperative His bundle ablation was a 20 year old woman with incessant ectopic left atrial tachycardia. Reliable mapping of the ectopic focus of the tachycardia was not possible and cryoablation of the AV-junction was considered suitable. An interruption of the His bundle conduction lasted for 6 days, rapid AV-conduction with atrial tachycardia then resumed. Percutaneous catheter ablation of the His bundle two weeks later was then successfully performed.

Taking into consideration the relatively small number of patients treated surgically for their supraventricular tachycardia in our institution, one can say that surgical treatment of WPW is a positive alternative to lifelong antiarrhythmic drug treatment. Also, in the view of other authors (10, 11), it is an intervention with low risk and a high success rate. Our approach to free wall right- and left-sided pathways without the need of cardiopulmonary bypass was recently confirmed by Guiraudon (12). None of our patients were candidates for antitachycardia pacemakers. One has to keep in mind that successful surgical intervention solves the tachycardia problem permanently, whereas pacemakers provide only a temporary solution.

The exact meaning of cryosurgical ablation still needs to be clarified, however, it will remain a diagnostic as well as a therapeutic approach.

The arrhythmogenic area, a basis for the surgical approach to ventricular tachycardia

The surgical procedure for ventricular tachycardia is directed to an arrhythmogenic area which has to be removed, ablated, isolated or electrophysiologically altered. This arrhythmogenic substrate is an area of delayed, heterogenous impulse propagation, some parts of it forming a undirectional block thus creating the condition for a reentrant circuit and onset of a ventricular tachycardia. Increasing heterogeneity of ventricular refractoriness and altered exitability in such an area may then lead to ventricular fibrillation. This arrhythmogenic area consists of subendocardial layers of islands of Purkinje fibers surviving a myocardial infarction, or straps of electrically conducting muscle cells within large areas of fibrous tissue in patients with cardiomyopathy or within fatty tissue in cases of ventricular dysplasia.

The important step to successful surgical therapy, therefore is the precise identification and localization of these areas. Bipolar electrogram recordings from arrhythmogenic areas demonstrate highly fractionated activity (Fig. 3) or delayed deflections indicating a slow desynchronized impulse conduction, that is, the electrophysiologic milieu where microreentry circuits originate (13). This area can be regarded as a necessary limb of the reentrant circuit of a ventricular tachycardia. Therefore, the earliest endocardial activation determined during a tachycardia is normally found in the close vicinity of an area of fractionated, delayed activity during sinus rhythm. Removal of such an arrhythmogenic area or alteration of the impulse conducting at this point by cryoablation or electrocautery should abolish a ventricular tachycardia. Although mapping during sinus rhythm

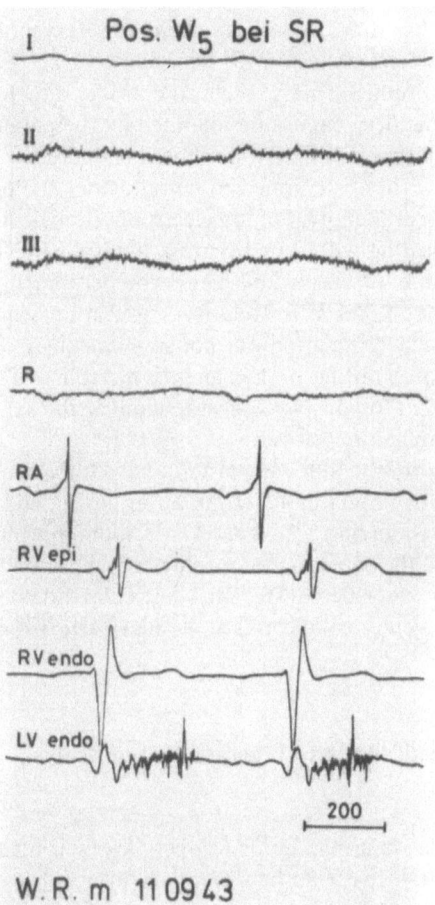

Fig. 3. Intraoperative endocardial mapping during sinus rhythm (SR) at the left ventricular posterior wall in a patient with ventricular tachycardia. Note the severely fractionated activity at the left ventricular endocardial recording (LV endo). R = aVR lead, RA = right atrial epicardial, RV epi = right ventricular epicardial, RV endo = right ventricular endocardial recording.

alone is certainly unreliable, it is a helpful guide for determining the earliest endocardial activation, that is the "onset" or "origin" of a ventricular tachycardia.

We believe that patients who are considered candidates for surgical therapy of their ventricular tachycardia should have endocardial catheter mapping during sinus rhythm, as well as during induced ventricular tachycardia, because it proves to be extremely helpful in cases in which the intraoperative mapping is incomplete or the tachycardia is not intraoperatively inducible (14).

Indication for surgical therapy of ventricular tachycardia

The most important question, who should have surgical therapy for ventricular tachycardia, has not yet been conclusively answered. This often makes it impossible to compare results of surgical therapy from different groups (15). The term "medical refractoriness" is generally accepted. This is defined as: 1. more than three episodes of a sustained ventricular tachycardia occurring within three months, 2. a spontaneous VT relapse under antiarrhythmic drug combination, and 3. a VT has to be inducible in spite of intravenous and oral drug administration. At least three electrophysiologic-pharmacological tests have to be performed in order to prove medical refractoriness. We also consider a tachycardia as drug refractory when an antiarrhythmic drug cannot be tolerated by the patient due to side effects, although the drug may be effective. Amiodarone should be included in the drug program of all patients before a tachycardia is claimed to be refractory. Under these conditions, an indication for a direct surgical therapy, i.e. the electrophysiologically guided intervention, is fulfilled when we are dealing with a tachycardia unresponsive to antiarrhythmic drugs and when the tachycardia is incessant and cannot be permanently terminated by stimulation or DC-shocks. We consider it a "relative" indication when there is a sustained VT inducible by programmed stimulation but not spontaneously occurring in a patient who needs coronary bypass grafting or LV aneurysmectomy. The same holds true for a spontaneously occurring VT reponsive to drugs, while at the same time an aneurysmectomy is indicated for hemodynamic reasons.

In order to have a positive benefit versus risk ratio, the following criteria have to be satisfied: The VT must be repeatedly inducible with programmed stimulation during endocardial catheter mapping; the spontanenously occurring VT should be a monomorphic sustained VT, and the induced VT should have the same monomorphic configuration as the inherent one. Two important factors to be considered are left ventricular function with an ejection fraction of at least 25% and severely compromised coronary artery anatomy.

Clinical experience with electrophysiologically guided surgical therapy for ventricular tachycardia

Sixty-eight patients, 62 men and 6 women, underwent map-guided surgery for their medically refractory ventricular tachycardia. Sixty-two patients had coronary artery disease and all endured myocardial infarctions. Six patients had no coronary disease, 5 of whom had right (4) and left ventricular dysplasia, and one patient suffered from sarcoidosis with a posterior aneurysm. Three patients with coronary disease had an incessant ventricular tachycardia. All patients had abnormally contracting left or right ventricles and preoperative hemodynamic measurements showing a mean left ventricular end-diastolic pressure of 22 mm Hg (range 6–40 mm Hg) and a mean LV-ejection fraction of 34% (range 19–58%).

In all patients an electrophysiological study was performed preoperatively, including endocardial catheter mapping in 50 of the patients. A sustained VT was inducible in all patients with the exception of 3 patients whith an incessant form of VT. In 14 cases (22%), more than one VT morphology was inducible. In all 65 patients at least one induced VT morphology was identical to the spontaneously occurring VT. In 47 of the 50 patients (94%) who underwent endocardial catheter mapping, we were able to localize the earliest endocardial activation of the tachycardia which we interpreted as an area next to the critical milieu or the "origin" of the tachycardia. The earliest endocardial activation was always found to be earlier than the onset of the QRS complex (mean of 35 msec).

Intraoperative mapping was performed in 66 patients. Two patients did not undergo intraoperative mapping due to a severely compromised left ventricle in one and a dangerous left main lesion in the other. In both cases, the surgical procedure was guided by preoperative endocardial catheter mapping. Epicardial mapping was done only in the first 16 patients. It was found (16) that epicardial breakthrough was often disparate from the endocardial origin of the tachycardia, thus misleading the surgical procedure.

We performed endocardial mapping during normothermic cardiopulmonary bypass during sinus rhythm (Fig. 4), as well as during induced ventricular tachycardia. A sustained tachycardia was inducible in 51 of the 63 patients (81%). In the other 12 patients, the induced VT was either unsustained or degenerated rapidly into ventricular fibrillation. The area of the earliest endocardial activation of the tachycardia could be determined in 50 of the 66 patients (75%) (Fig. 5). In 5 patients with 2 different VT morphologies, more than one area of earliest endocardial activation was identified. The surgical procedure in 16 of the patients was guided by the results of endocardial mapping during sinus rhythm, demonstrating an area of fractionated activity (Fig. 3) or delayed potentials (Fig. 4).

The surgical procedure was an encircling endocardial ventriculotomy (EEV) according to the Giraudon procedure (17) in the initial 14 patients, whereas a localized endocardial resection according to the Harken technique (18) was performed in 48 of the patients. An electrocautery knife was used for the endocardial "peel off". We believe that with this technique the deeper subendocardial layers will also be homogeneously ablated in order to reach a possible microreentrant circuit situated intramurally. In patients with right ventricular dysplasia, a rather large ventriculotomy was performed and extensive cryoablation was used (19). Cryosurgery alone or in addition to endocardial resection was used in 18 patients. We feel that cryoablation is extremely helpful in cases where the anatomical situation prohibits endocardial resection, in particular on the posterior wall and next

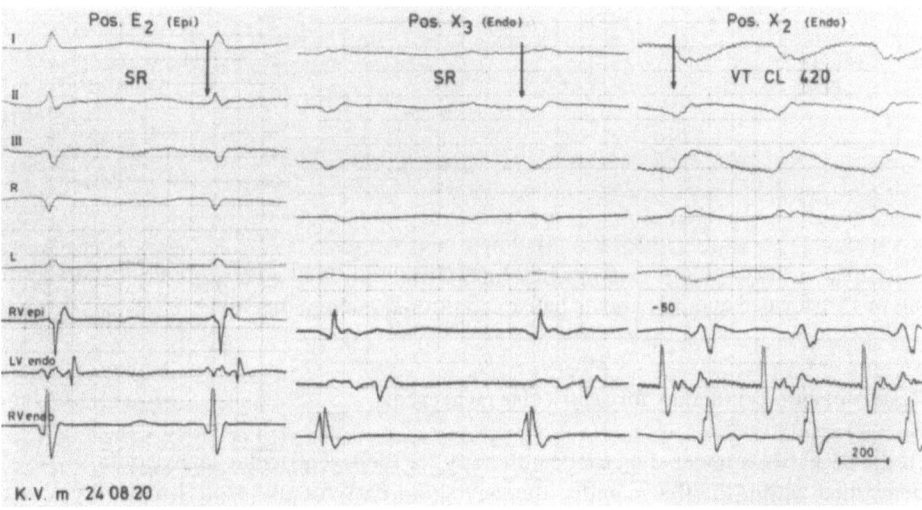

Fig. 4. Epicardial and endocardial mapping during sinus rhythm (SR) and ventricular tachycardia (VT). Tracings from top to bottom represent I–III, a Vr and a Vl standard leads, right ventricular epicardial, left ventricular endocardial and right ventricular endocardial recordings. Note the delayed potentials during SR on the left ventricular lateral wall (Position E2 and X3) and the earliest endocardial activation in close vicinity (Position X2) during ventricular tachycardia (VT), 50 msec prior to the onset of the QRS complex (vertical arrow).

Fig. 5. Endocardial activation times recorded intraoperatively during sinus rhythm (SR) and ventricular tachycardia (VT) in the same patient shown in Fig. 4. The endocardium of the left ventricle is depicted as the inside of a cyclinder as viewed from the wide-opened apex to the base of the heart. AO = aortic valve, MI = mitral valve. Note that the latest activation during SR is found in close vicinity to that of the earliest activation (50 msec prior to the onset of QRS, squared area) during VT.

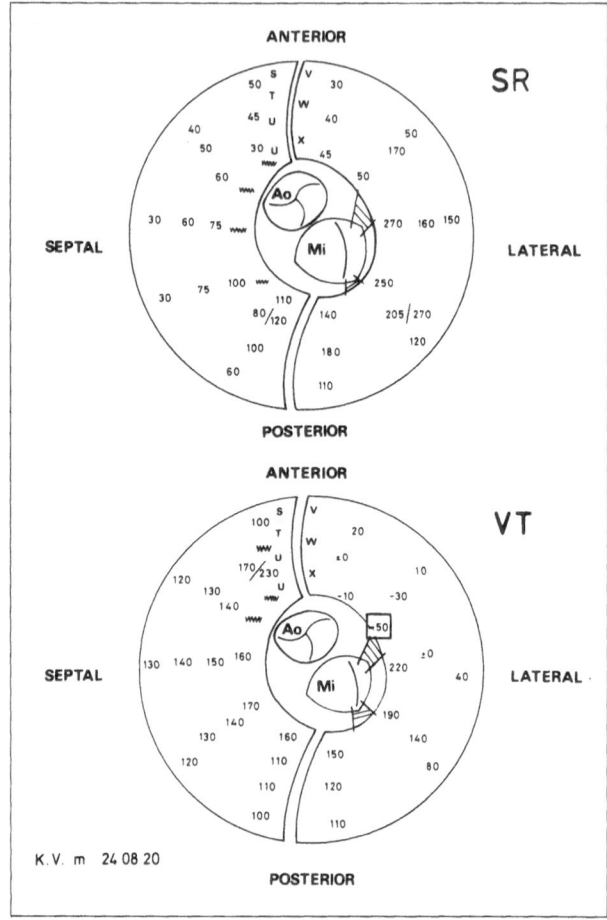

to or around the papillary muscles. In 22 patients, additional aortocoronary bypass grafting was performed and 38 patients had an additional aneurysmectomy.

Results of surgical therapy for ventricular tachycardia

Of the 68 patients undergoing surgical therapy for their ventricular tachycardia, eight patients died within the first months, thus giving an early or in-hospital mortality rate of 12%. The cause of death was low cardiac output and respiratory failure in 5, septic shock, ventricular fibrillation and cerebral embolus in the remaining patients. Sixty patients were discharged from the hospital. The mean follow-up was 29 months. Within this monitoring period, 9 patients died, giving a late mortality of 15%. The cause of death was pulmonary embolism and right heart failure in 3, cerebral embolism in one, reinfarction in 3 and sudden cardiac death in 2 patients.

314

Five patients had a relapse of their ventricular tachycardia (8%). One patient had a second intervention after 3 months and had no further VT episodes thereafter. Two patients received an antitachycardia pacemaker since the VT rate proved to be significantly slower after the surgical procedure. One device functions in automatic mode (Tachylog, Siemens) and the other is a patient-activated device (Orthocor, Cordis). In the other 2 patients, the VT was postoperatively controlled by antiarrhythmic drugs. All VT relapses occurred within the first 6 weeks after surgery.

Programmed ventricular stimulation was performed in 35 of the 60 surviving patients (58%) 3 to 6 months after surgery. In addition to the 5 patients with spontaneous VT relapse, 4 other patients had an inducible sustained VT which did not spontaneously reoccur. An unsustained VT or repetitive response phenomenon was inducible in 11 patients. Repeated ambulatory monitoring was performed in all surviving patients. Nineteen (31%) of the 60 patients are under antiarrhythmic drugs due to some form of complex ventricular arrhythmias.

Is the surgical approach to ventricular tachycardia recommendable?

Patients with recurrent episodes of sustained ventricular tachycardia have a poor prognosis, in particular when VT occurs in the context of coronary artery disease. They usually have abnormally contracting ventricles and therefore are prone to cardiac failure and sudden onset of ventricular fibrillation. This group of patients is extremely difficult to treat medically and are not ideal candidates for antitachycardia pacemakers. We know from earlier studies (20, 21, 22) that "blind" resection of ventricular aneurysms or scar tissue in patients with ventricular tachycardias yielded low success rates (less than 45%). Most centers involved in surgical therapy for arrhythmias turned to electrophysiologically guided procedures. After the initial enthusiasm of a new mode of tachycardia treatment, reports of larger groups of patients treated surgically under the guidance of electrophysiological mapping are now available. The risk of this type of surgery is expressed by a relatively high early mortality rate with a mean of 12% ranging from 6 to 16% (23, 24, 25). This, however, is not surprising due to the poor ventricular function, the history of repeated cardiac arrest and the treatment of antiarrhythmic drugs. The wide range of hospital mortality may be due to different surgical indications and procedures. It is still unknown which surgical technique – endocardial resection or endocardial incision – is most appropriate and therefore recommendable. Additionally, some groups have modified the originally described techniques. Some use semicircular incisions (15, 26) instead of complete encircling incisions. An electrocautery knife (27) for endocardial "peel off" was used, whereas others used a sharp knife (18). Some groups tried to resect the smallest endocardial area possible (28) defined through mapping, others resected all visible endocardial fibrosis (29) even without the assistance of mapping techniques. Surgical procedures without electrophysiological guidance are less effective as far as VT suppression is concerned (11). However, procedures with mapping guidance prolong cardiopulmonary bypass time and this, on the other hand, increases the risk of early hospital mortality (24, 25).

From the present available follow-up studies (15, 25), one can say that 75 to 85% of all patients undergoing VT surgery become free of ventricular tachycardia.

Some authors documented (30) that inducible VT early (10–14 days) after surgery was a reliable indicator for an unsuccessful intervention and spontaneous recurrence of the tachycardia. We are less rigid with early postoperative control stimulation but prefer a late (3 to 4 months) postoperative electrophysiological study. One must be aware that the early postoperative situation, particularly with epicardial wires, is completely different and difficult to compare with the preoperative electrophysiological situation.

It is generally agreed (23) that indicators for unsuccessful intervention are disparate sites of ventricular tachycardia origin, multiple morphologically distinct spontaneous VTs, absence of a discrete left ventricular aneurysm and a VT origin at the inferior wall. Some patients who had a tachycardia relapse exhibited a slower tachycardia rate and difficulty in inducing a tachycardia which now was responsive to antiarrhythmic drug therapy. This indicates that even in failures the surgical intervention has changed the condition or milieu of the arrhythmia genesis and one may also consider this as a therapeutic improvement.

The long-term survival or late mortality rate depends on the ventricular function and the grade of muscle damage produced by the procedure itself. Most of the late deaths, i.e. more than 6 months after the surgical intervention, occurred due to progressive left or right ventricular failure and rarely due to arrhythmia events.

We therefore believe that long-term survival, i.e. more than 2 years after the surgical intervention, is not a good parameter for or against surgical therapy for ventricular tachycardia.

With the increasing experience of all groups involved in arrhythmia surgery, a better selection of patients for different therapeutic modalities will achieve higher success rates. We believe that patients with a poor left ventricular function and high tachycardia rates are better treated with the automatic implantable defibrillator (31).

W. Sealy was certainly correct when he wrote 6 years ago (32): "The direct surgical treatment of arrhythmias could well be the last frontier in cardiology open to the surgeon." However, we can already say that with the automatic implantable defibrillator we have a promising new approach to the treatment of life-threatening ventricular arrhythmias.

References

1. Graboys TB, Lown B, Podrid PJ, De Silva R (1982) Long-term survival of patients with malignant ventricular arrhythmia treated with antiarrhythmic drugs. Am J Cardiol 50: 437
2. Spielman SR, Schwartz S, McCarthy DM, Horowitz LN, Greenspan AM, Sadowski LM, Josephson ME, Waxman HL (1983) Predictors of the success or failure of medical therapy in patients with chronic recurrent sustained ventricular tachycardia: a discriminant analysis. J Am Coll Card 1: 401–408
3. Swerdlow CD, Echt DS, Winkle RA, Griffin JC, Ross DL, Mason JW (1983) Clinical factors predicting successful electrophysiologic-pharmacologic study in patients with ventricular tachycardia. J Am Cardiol 1: 409–416
4. Cobb FR, Blumenschein SD, Sealy WC, Boineau JP, Wagner GS, Wallace AG (1968) Successful surgical interruption of the bundle of Kent in a patient with Wolff-Parkinson syndrome. Circulation 38: 1018
5. Sealy WC, Gallagher JJ, Pritchett ELC (1978) The surgical anatomy of Kent bundles based on electrophysiological mapping and surgical exploration. J Thorac Cardiovasc Surg 76: 804
6. Klein GJ, Guiraudon GM, Perkins DG, Jones DL, Yee R, Jarvis E (1984) Surgical correction of the Wolff-Parkinson-White syndrome in the closed heart using cryosurgery: a simplified approach. J Am Coll Cardiol 3: 405
7. Gallagher JJ, Sealy WC, Kasell J, Millar R, Campbell RWF, Harrison L, Pritchett ELC, Wallace AG (1977) Cryosurgical ablation of accessory atrioventricular connections: a new technique for correction of the preexcitation syndrome. Circulation 55: 471

8. Scheinmann MM, Morady F, Hess DS, Gonzales R (1982) Catheter induced ablation of the atrioventricular function to control refractory supraventricular arrhythmia. JAMA 248: 851

9. Harrison L, Gallagher JJ, Kasell J, Anderson RW, Mikat E, Hackel DB, Wallace AG (1977) Cryosurgical ablation of the AV-node-His bundle: a new method for producing AV-block. Circulation 55: 463

10. Gallagher JJ, Pritchett ELC, Sealy WC, Kasell J, Wallace AG (1978) The preexcitation syndromes. Prog Cardiovasc Dis 20: 285

11. Cox JL (1985) The status of surgery for cardiac arrhythmias. Circulation 71: 413

12. Guiraudon GM, Klein GJ, Sharma A, Jones D (1985) Surgical correction of the Wolff-Parkinson-White syndrome in the closed heart using cryosurgery: further observations and long-therm follow-up (Abstr). PACE 8: 304

13. Klein H, Karp RB, Kouchoukos NT, Zorn TN, James TN, Waldo AL (1982) Intraoperative electrophysiologic mapping of the ventricles during sinus rhythm in patients with a previous myocardial infarction. Circulation 66: 847–853

14. Josephson ME, Horowitz LN, Spielman SR, Waxman HL, Greenspan AM (1982) Role of catheter mapping in the preoperative evaluation of ventricular tachycardia. Am Cardiol 49: 207–220

15. Ostermeyer J, Breithardt G, Borggrefe M, Godehardt E, Seipel L, Bircks W (1984) Surgical treatment of ventricular tachycardias. Complete versus partial encircling endocardial ventriculotomy. J Thorac Cardiovasc Surg 87: 517

16. Horowitz LN, Josephson ME, Harken AH (1989) Epicardial and endocardial activation during sustained ventricular tachycardia. Circulation 61: 1227–1238

17. Guiraudon G, Fontaine G, Frank R, Escande G, Etievent P, Cabrol C (1978) Encircling endocardial ventriculotomy. A new surgical treatment for life threatening ventricular tachycardias resistent to medical treatment following myocardial infarction. Ann Thorac Surg 26: 438–444

18. Harken AH, Josephson ME, Horowitz LN (1979) Surgical endocardial resection for the treatment of malignant ventricular tachycardia. Ann Surg 190: 456–460

19. Gallagher JJ, Anderson RW, Kasell J, Rice JR, Pritchett ELC, Gault JM, Harrison L, Wallace AG (1978) Cryoablation of drug-resistant ventricular tachycardia in a patient with a variant of scleroderma. Circulation 57: 190

20. Mason JW, Stinson EB, Winkle RA, Griffin JC, Oyer PE, Ross DL, Derby G (1982) Surgery for ventricular tachycardia: efficacy of left ventricular aneurysm resection compared with operation guided by electrical activation mapping. Circulation 65: 1148–1155

21. Ostermeyer J, Breithardt G, Kolvenbach R, Borggrefe M, Seipel L, Schulte HD, Bircks W (1982) The surgical treatment of ventricular tachycardias. J Thorac Cardiovasc Surg 84: 704–715

22. Klein H, Bethge KP, Frank G, Borst HG, Lichtlen, PR (1979) Das Verhalten ventrikulärer Arrhythmien nach Aneurysmektomie. Z Kardiol 68: 10–16

23. Miller JM, Kienzle MG, Harken AH, Josephson ME (1984) Subendocardial resection for ventricular tachycardia: predictors for surgical success. Circulation 70: 624

24. Garan H, Ruskin JN, Marco JP, McGovern B, Levine FH, Buckley MJ (1982) Refractory ventricular tachycardia complicating recovery from acute myocardial infarction: treatment with map-guided infarctectomy. Am Heart J 107: 571

25. Swerdlow CD, Mason JW, Stinson EB, Oyer PE (1985) Results of map-guided surgery in 103 patients with ventricular tachycardia. J Am Coll Cardiol 5: 409

26. Waldo AL, Arciniegas JG, Klein H (1981) Surgical treatment of life-threatening ventricular arrhythmias: the role of intraoperative mapping and consideration of the presently available surgical techniques. Prog Cardiovasc Dis 23: 247–264

27. Frank G, Klein H, Lichtlen PR, Borst HG (1981) Direct surgical therapy of ventricular arrhythmias in coronary heart disease. Thorac Cardiovasc Surg 29: 315–319

28. Josephson ME, Harken AH, Harowitz LN (1982) Long-term results of endocardial resection for sustained ventricular tachycardia in coronary disease patients. Am Heart J 104: 51

29. Moran JM, Kehoe RF, Loeb JM, Lichtenthal PR, Sanders JH, Michaelis LL (1982) Extended endocardial resection for the treatment of ventricular fibrillation. Ann Thorac Surg 34: 538

30. Page PL, Arciniegas JG, Plumb VJ, Henthorn RW, Karp RB, Waldo AL (1983) Value of early postoperative epicardial programmed ventricular stimulation studies after surgery for ventricular tachyarrhythmias. J Am Coll Cardiol 2: 1046

31. Mirowski M, Mower MM, Reid PR, Watkins L, Langer A (1982) The automatic implantable defibrillator. PACE 5: 384
32. Sealy WC (1979) Direct surgical treatment of arrhythmias (Editorial), Chest 75: 536

Authors' address:
Helmut Klein M.D.
Abteilung für Kardiologie
Medizinische Hochschule Hannover
Konstanty-Gutschow-Str. 8
3000 Hannover 61
West Germany

Author Index

Subject Index

Ambulatory Blood Pressure Monitoring

M. A. WEBER and Jan I. J. DRAYER, Long Beach, Calif. (eds.)

1984. 248 pages. 108 figures. 29 tables.
Cloth DM 58, −; US $ 24.00 · ISBN 3-7985-0638-8

This book summarizes a broad experience utilizing differing technologies for measuring ambulatory blood pressure. It provides information about a new approach consisting of multiple blood measuring throughout the day in patients going about their routine activities. Emphasis has been placed on the differing techniques available; intra-arterial continuous blood pressure monitoring, intermittent but wholly automated non-invasive techniques, and patient-actuated techniques for repetetive measurements. The book also focuses on evaluating blood pressure in normal subjects, and in setting up standards against which patients with hypertension can be judged. Finally, it contains studies on the use of these automated techniques in evaluating the effectiveness of treatment. It illustrates the possibility of determining a blood pressure change with treatment, and considers the duration of the treatment effect.
It should be of interest to specialists in internal medicine, particularly cardiologists and nephrologists, but also general physicians.

Mild hypertension
Current controversies and new approaches

Proceedings of the International Titisee Workshop, October 13-15, 1983

M. A. WEBER, Long Beach, Calif. and C. J. MATHIAS, London (eds.)
With an introduction by W. S. PEART, London

1984. 176 pages. 45 figures. 13 tables.
Cloth DM 48, −; US $ 20.00 · ISBN 3-7985-0636-1

There has been a growing awareness that even mild hypertension can be a significant risk factor for premature heart disease, strokes, and other cardiovascular complications. This book addresses these problems in the patient with mild hypertension, presenting information not previously available. It should be of immediate and significant practical value to the physician.
Some of the basic mechanisms which might control blood pressure and explain hypertension are examined. The book looks at experiences with different approaches to treatment, and some contemporary ideas that might lead to more effective and better accepted modes of therapy. Innovative treatment methods, such as transdermal medications, are dealt with as possible new approaches for the management of hypertension.
The book is of interest to specialists in internal medicine, particularly cardiologists and nephrologists, and to general physicians.

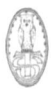 **Steinkopff** **Dr. Dietrich Steinkopff Verlag, Postfach 11 10 08**
Telefon 0 61 51/2 65 38, D-6100 Darmstadt